ELECTRONIC HEALTH RECORDS *for* Allied Health Careers

Susan M. Sanderson

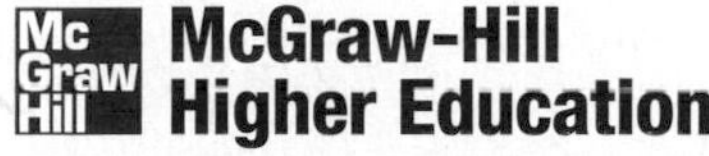

Boston Burr Ridge, IL Dubuque, IA New York San Francisco St. Louis
Bangkok Bogotá Caracas Kuala Lumpur Lisbon London Madrid Mexico City
Milan Montreal New Delhi Santiago Seoul Singapore Sydney Taipei Toronto

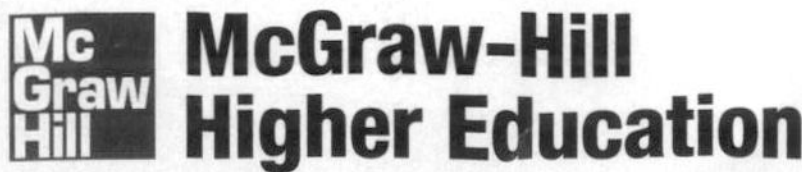

ELECTRONIC HEALTH RECORDS FOR ALLIED HEALTH CAREERS

Published by McGraw-Hill, a business unit of The McGraw-Hill Companies, Inc., 1221 Avenue of the Americas, New York, NY, 10020.

Some ancillaries, including electronic and print components, may not be available to customers outside the United States.

This book is printed on acid-free paper.

Printed in China
3 4 5 6 7 8 9 0 CTP/CTP 11 10

ISBN 978-0-07-340197-3
MHID 0-07-340197-8

Vice President/Editor in Chief: *Elizabeth Haefele*
Vice President/Director of Marketing: *John E. Biernat*
Senior sponsoring editor: *Debbie Fitzgerald*
Managing developmental editor: *Patricia Hesse*
Executive marketing manager: *Roxan Kinsey*
Lead media producer: *Damian Moshak*
Media producer: *Marc Mattson*
Director, Editing/Design/Production: *Jess Ann Kosic*
Project manager: *Marlena Pechan*
Senior production supervisor: *Janean A. Utley*
Designer: *Marianna Kinigakis*
Interior design: *Kay Lieberherr*
Cover design: *Kiera Cunningham Pohl*
Senior photo research coordinator: *Lori Hancock*
Media project manager: *Mark A. S. Dierker*
Outside development: *Wendy Langerud, S4Carlisle Publishing Services*
Typeface: *10.5/13 New Aster*
Compositor: *Aptara, Inc.*
Printer: *CTPS*

Credits: Figure 1.1: © Comstock/Picture Quest; 1.5: Courtesy of Healthcare Information and Management Systems Society www.himss.org/StateDashboard/; pp. 14–15: © American Health Information Management Association. Reprinted with permission; p. 30: Healthcare Information and Management Systems Society; photographer, David Collins; 2.2: © Royalty Free Corbis; p. 50: Intel Corporation; 2.4: Screen shot from CLUE Browser. CLUE and CliniClue® are available as freeware from The Clinical Information Consultancy Ltd, http://www.cliniclue.com; p. 62: Dept. of Defense Photo by Airman 1st Class Kurt Gibbons III, US Air Force; p. 99: © The McGraw-Hill Companies, Inc./Andrew Resek, photographer; pp. 118–119: © The Leapfrog Group; p. 130: InteleViewer Workstation, © Intelerad Medical Systems Incorporated; 5.1, 5.2, 5.3, 5.4, 5.5, 5.6, 5.7, 5.8, 5.9, 5.10, 5.11: Reprinted with permission. Copyright 2006 Medem, Inc.; pp. 152–153: Reprinted with permission. Copyright 2006 Medem, Inc.; 5.15: © Dossia; 5.16: © IndivoHealth; 5.17: Reprinted with permission. Copyright 2006 Medem, Inc.

Library of Congress Cataloging-in-Publication Data

Sanderson, Susan M.
Electronic health records for allied health careers / Susan M. Sanderson.
p. ; cm.
Includes index.
ISBN-13: 978-0-07-340197-3 (alk. paper)
ISBN-10: 0-07-340197-8 (alk. paper)
1. Medical records—Data processing. 2. Allied health personnel. I. Title. [DNLM: 1. Medical Record Administrators. 2. Confidentiality. 3. Forms and Records Control—methods. 4. Medical Records Systems, Computerized. 5. Practice Management, Medical. WX 173 S216e 2009]
R864.S263 2009
610.28′5—dc22

2007051786

The Internet addresses listed in the text were accurate at the time of publication. The inclusion of a Web site does not indicate an endorsement by the authors or McGraw-Hill, and McGraw-Hill does not guarantee the accuracy of the information presented at these sites.

All names, situations, and anecdotes are fictitious. They do not represent any person, event, or medical record.

www.mhhe.com

Brief Contents

Contents

Preface

Welcome to *Electronic Health Records for Allied Health Careers*. This text introduces you to the use of electronic health records in today's rapidly changing health care environment. Whether you plan to work as a medical assistant, a coding professional, a lab technician, or in any other area of allied health, this book is addressed to you.

YOUR CAREER IN ALLIED HEALTH

This is an exciting time to be entering the allied health field. In all work settings, from hospitals and physician group practices to laboratories, long-term care facilities, and pharmacies, allied health professionals are in demand. At the same time, major changes are taking place in health care. As costs continue to rise, there are greater demands for improved quality and safety in patient care. To tackle these problems, the U.S. health care system is turning to technology. This text focuses on one part of the technology initiative—the shift from paper-recordkeeping systems to electronic health records.

Why do allied health students need to know about electronic health records? The answer is simple—because you will use electronic health records to accomplish tasks once on-the-job. The transition from paper records to electronic records affects everyone working in health care today. Consider just a few examples of the changes electronic health records (EHRs) bring to these jobs:

- Medical assistants enter patient information, such as vital signs, into an EHR
- Coding professionals review electronic documentation in the EHR to determine the appropriate codes for an encounter
- Technicians working in blood and chemistry labs, radiology, nuclear medicine, cardiovascular medicine and other areas respond to electronic orders and send test results electronically using an EHR
- Billing professionals use information in the EHR to prepare insurance claims and patient statements
- Respiratory therapists, occupational therapists, physical therapists, and others review patient records, respond to orders sent from an EHR and enter treatment plans in an EHR
- Pharmacy technicans receive and process medication orders sent from an EHR

As you can see, many allied health careers require the use of computers, and because of this, there is great demand for graduates who have a background in health care as well as experience with computers. In addition, employers are seeking individuals who are capable of operating within a work environment that is always changing. To be successful, workers must be willing and able to learn new things throughout their career. In addition to education, certification from a nationally-recognized organization brings more employment options and advancement opportunities.

OVERVIEW OF THIS TEXTBOOK

Whatever your particular course of study in health care, this text provides you with a broad introduction to electronic health records. The intention of this book is not to make you an expert in one particular EHR program, although you will work with an EHR program in Chapter 7. The goal of the text is to explain the ways in which EHRs are used in different health care settings, and how they are changing the nature of the work performed by individuals throughout the health care field.

TO THE STUDENT

The chapters in this text follow a logical sequence. The first six chapters provide you with an understanding of electronic health records—what they are, who uses them, how they differ from paper records, and why have become so popular. The final chapter provides you with the opportunity to gain hands-on experience with an EHR program.

The chapter coverage is as follows:

- Chapter 1 introduces the topic of electronic health records. It explains what they are, why they are needed, and what they can do, as well as the impact of information technology on allied health careers.
- Chapter 2 explains how paper records are converted to an electronic format, and the computer hardware required to use an electronic heath record system. It also provides an overview of the common standards for clinical health information.
- Chapter 3 covers the use of electronic health records in outpatient settings, such as a physician's office.
- Chapter 4 explains how electronic health records are used in hospitals and how they interact with other hospital information systems.
- Chapter 5 explores personal health records (PHRs), including how they differ from electronic health records, and the different types of PHRs available.
- Chapter 6 covers the challenges to privacy and security that are created by the widespread use of electronic health record systems, including the HIPAA legislation.
- Chapter 7 introduces you to the features and functions of an outpatient electronic health record program, McKesson's Practice Partner. You will complete hands-on exercises working with the software.

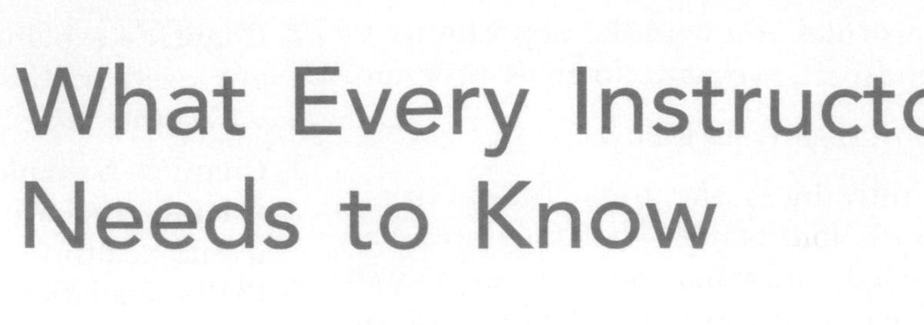

What Every Instructor Needs to Know

WELCOME TO ELECTRONIC HEALTH RECORDS FOR ALLIED HEALTH CAREERS!

As you know, the field of health care is in the midst of an enormous transition from paper-based recordkeeping systems to electronic health records. Your students are entering the allied health field at an exciting time, and you are teaching at an exciting time. While the demand for graduates with a background in allied health exceeds the supply, students entering the field today also need a basic understanding of health information technology, specifically, electronic health records. That is the purpose of this text, which was developed specifically for students in allied health programs.

TEACHING SUPPLEMENTS

For the Instructor

Instructor's Manual (0-07-3284297) includes:

- Course overview
- Chapter-by-chapter lesson plans
- Case Studies, Your Turn Exercises, and end-of-chapter solutions
- Correlation tables: SCANS, AAMA Role Delineation Study Areas of Competence (2003), and AMT Registered Medical Assistant Certification Exam Topics.

Instructor Productivity Center CD-ROM (packaged with the Instructor's Manual) includes:

- Instructor's PowerPoint® presentation of Chapters 1 through 7.
- Electronic testing program featuring McGraw-Hill's EZ Test. This flexible and easy-to-use program allows instructors to create tests from book specific items. It accommodates a wide range of question types and instructors may add their own questions. Multiple versions of the test can be created and any test can be exported for use with course management systems such as WebCT, Blackboard, or PageOut.
- Instructor's Manual.

Online Learning Center (OLC), www.mhhe.com/SandersonEHR, includes:

- Instructor's Manual in Word and PDF format
- PowerPoint® files for each chapter
- Links to professional associations
- PageOut link.

For the Student

Online Learning Center (OLC), www.mhhe.com/SandersonEHR, includes additional chapter quizzes and other review activities.

Acknowledgments

For insightful reviews and helpful suggestions, we would like to acknowledge the following:

Content Consultants

Coker Consulting, LLC
Alpharetta, GA

Beth Shanholtzer, BS, MA
Hagerstown Business College
Hagerstown, MD

Marsha Benedict, MSA, CMA-A, CPC
Indian River Community College
Brevard Community College
Jenson Beach, FL

Janet I. B. Seggern, M.Ed., MS, CCA
Lehigh Carbon Community College
Schnecksville, PA

Reviewers

Roxane M. Abbott, MBA
Sarasota County Technical Institute
Sarasota, FL

Dr. Judy Adams, PhD
Bowling Green State University
Bowling Green, OH

Catherine Marie Andersen, RHIA, CPHIMS
Eastern Kentucky University
Richmond, KY

Nina Beaman, MS, BA, AAS
Bryant and Stratton College
Richmond, VA

Norma Bird, M.Ed., BS, CMA
Medical Assisting Director
Idaho State University College of Technology
Pocatello, ID

Grethel Gomez, AS
Florida Career College
Miami, FL

Cheri Goretti, MA, BSMT (ASCP), CMA
Quinebaug Valley Community College
Danielson, CT

W. Howard Gunning, MS Ed, CMA
Southwestern Illinois College
Granite City, IL

Elizabeth A Hoffman, MA Ed., CMA, CPT (ASPT)
Baker College of Clinton Twp
Clinton Twp, MI

Carol Lee Jarrell, MLT, AHI
Department Chair-Medical
Brown Mackie College
Merrillville, IN

Donna D. Kyle-Brown, PhD, RMA, CPC
Virginia College
Biloxi, MS

Christine Malone, BS, MHA
Everett Community College
Everett, WA

Joy McPhail, RN
Fayetteville Technical Community College
Fayetteville, NC

Lisa Nagle, BSed, CMA
Augusta Technical College
Augusta, GA

Timothy J. Skaife, MA
National Park Community College
Hot Springs, AR

Lynn Slack, BS, CMA
Kaplan Career Institute-ICM Campus
Pittsburgh, PA

Barbara Tietsort, M.Ed.
University of Cincinnati
Cincinnati, OH

Cindy Thompson, RN, RMA, MA, BS
Davenport University
Bay City, MI

Marilyn M. Turner, RN, CMA
Ogeechee Technical College
Statesboro, GA

Marianne Van Deursen, BS, CMA
Warren County Community College
Washington, NJ

Denise Wallen, CPC
Idaho Career Institute
Boise, ID

Stacey Wilson, MHA, MT/PBT (ASCP), CMA
Cabarrus College of Health Sciences
Concord, NC

Introduction to Electronic Health Records

CHAPTER OUTLINE

A Mandate for Change
- *Frequency of Medical Errors*
- *Rising Health Care Costs*
- *Coordination of Care*

Trends in Technology, the Economy, and Government Policy
- *Advances in Technology*
- *Economic Pressures*
- *Government Health Information Technology Initiatives*

What Is a Medical Record?
- *Content of a Health Record*

The Purpose and Use of Health Records
- *Primary Purpose*
- *Secondary Uses*

Core Functions of an Electronic Health Record System
- *Health Information and Data*
- *Results Management*
- *Order Management*
- *Decision Support*
- *Electronic Communication and Connectivity*
- *Patient Support*
- *Administrative Processes*
- *Reporting and Population Management*

Advantages of Electronic Health Records
- *Safety*
- *Quality*
- *Efficiency*
- *Future Cost Reduction*

Implementation Issues
- *Cost*
- *Lack of Standards*
- *Learning Curve*
- *Workflow Changes*
- *Changes in the Software Market*
- *Privacy and Security Risks*

The Impact of Information Technology on Allied Health Careers
- *Certification and Lifelong Learning*
- *Outlook and Salaries*

LEARNING OUTCOMES

After completing this chapter, you will be able to define key terms and:

1. List three reasons why paper-based medical records are no longer adequate.
2. Discuss the economic pressures forcing changes in the health care system.
3. Describe the role of the government in bringing about changes in the health care system.
4. Explain the differences between electronic medical records, electronic health records, and personal health records.
5. Compare the content of a medical record in ambulatory and acute care settings.
6. List the eight core functions of an electronic health record.
7. Describe the advantages of electronic health records.
8. Explain the issues surrounding the implementation of electronic health records.
9. Explain how electronic health records will affect existing jobs in allied health as well as create new jobs.

KEY TERMS

acute care
adverse event
ambulatory care
continuity of care
electronic health record (EHR)
electronic medical record (EMR)
electronic prescribing
evidence-based medicine
health information exchange (HIE)
health information technology (HIT)
Health Insurance Portability and Accountability Act of 1996 (HIPAA)
medical error
medical record
Medicare Part D
Medicare Prescription Drug, Improvement, and Modernization Act of 2003 (MMA)
Nationwide Health Information Network (NHIN)
Office of the National Coordinator for Health Information Technology (ONC)
pay for performance
personal health record (PHR)
regional health information organization (RHIO)
standards

Why This Chapter Is Important to You

The information in this chapter will enable you to:

- Be aware of the problems with paper-based medical record systems.
- Understand how electronic medical records, electronic health records, and personal health records differ.
- Describe the core functions of an electronic health record.
- Understand how electronic health records reduce medical errors, increase the quality of care provided to patients, and bring down health care costs.
- Feel confident when discussing why electronic health records are so important to the reform of health care.

A man is injured in a car accident and is unconscious. Before he arrives at the hospital, the emergency department staff already knows that he has a potentially fatal allergy to penicillin.

A woman fainted while waiting for a commuter train. Paramedics who arrive on the scene know that she is a diabetic and is in her sixth week of pregnancy.

A man has been referred to an orthopedic specialist by his primary care provider. The specialist reviews copies of the X-rays from the primary care provider before the patient enters the exam room.

A few years ago, these scenarios would have sounded like something out of a futuristic movie. Today, however, information technology (IT) is changing the way doctors practice medicine, much as it has changed the way Americans buy airline tickets, pay bills, and listen to music.

One of the most important tasks in the practice of medicine is managing information, whether about a patient or about the latest developments in treating disease. To provide the highest quality of care, physicians need timely access to a patient's complete health record, including information from other doctors, laboratories, pharmacies, and hospitals that have treated the patient. The technology that integrates health information from these sources is known as an electronic health record. An **electronic health record (EHR)** is a computerized lifelong health care record for an individual that incorporates data from all sources that provide treatment for the individual.

electronic health record (EHR) computerized lifelong health care record with data from all sources.

A Mandate for Change

The health care field is undergoing enormous change as physicians and hospitals shift away from paper-based patient records and move toward electronic health record systems. This change affects more than the way doctors practice medicine; it changes the way almost everyone working in the field of medicine accomplishes daily tasks. Radiology technicians no longer develop film X-rays, MRIs, and CT scans but instead manage digital images. Medical assistants do not handwrite a patient's vital signs in a patient chart; they use a keyboard in the exam room to enter these data into a computer. Billing and coding staff members no longer code from paper encounter forms but review electronic documentation entered in the computer by the physician. No matter what the job, there is no doubt that this is an exciting, challenging time to be entering the field of health care.

Where did the call for change come from? During the 1990s and early years of the twenty-first century, there was a growing recognition that the current health care system, with its reliance on paper medical records, was no longer able to meet the needs of patients and their doctors. An increase in medical errors, rising health care costs, and the need for coordination of care all played a major role in the mandate for change.

FREQUENCY OF MEDICAL ERRORS

The Institute of Medicine defines an error as "the failure of a planned action to be completed as intended or the use of a wrong plan to achieve an aim" (*To Err is Human: Building a Safer Health System*, Institute of Medicine, 2000). In the field of medicine, patient harm that results from treatment by the health care system, rather than from the health condition of the patient, is known as an **adverse event.** All adverse events are not errors; they can also be side effects of medications. The term **medical error** refers to an adverse event that could have been prevented with the current state of medical knowledge and is also known as a preventable adverse event. Medication errors, including dispensing an incorrect dose of medication or prescribing a drug that is known to interact with another medication the patient is taking, are examples of preventable adverse events. Surgical errors, such as operating on the wrong site or performing the wrong procedure, are also preventable adverse events.

adverse event patient harm resulting from health care treatment.

medical error adverse event that could have been prevented.

Medical errors are the eighth leading cause of death in the United States. According to the same Institute of Medicine report, between 44,000 and 98,000 American deaths each year are a result of medical errors. This is more than the total deaths from automobile accidents, homicides, and AIDS combined.

Two-thirds of all errors in treatment and diagnosis occur because of communication problems, including:

- Misfiled or lost medical records
- Mishandling of patient requests and messages
- Inaccurate information in medical records
- Unreadable information due to poor handwriting
- Mislabeled laboratory specimens

Doctors' illegible handwriting results in more than seven thousand deaths a year, and preventable medication mistakes also injure more than 1.5 million Americans annually (see Figures 1-1 and 1-2). Medication errors are a major problem in the health care system, in

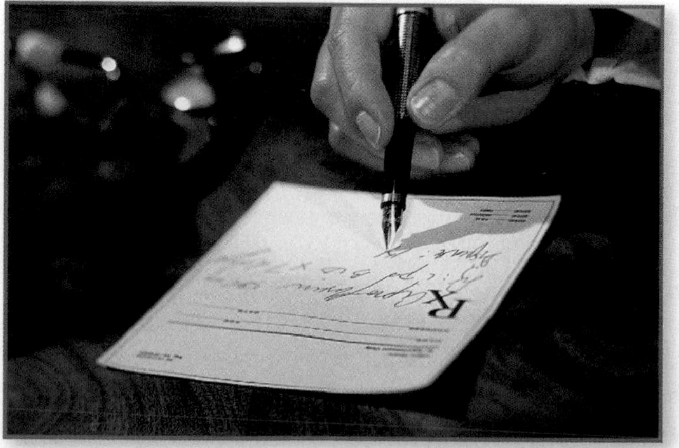

Figure 1-1
Handwritten prescriptions are not always easy to read.

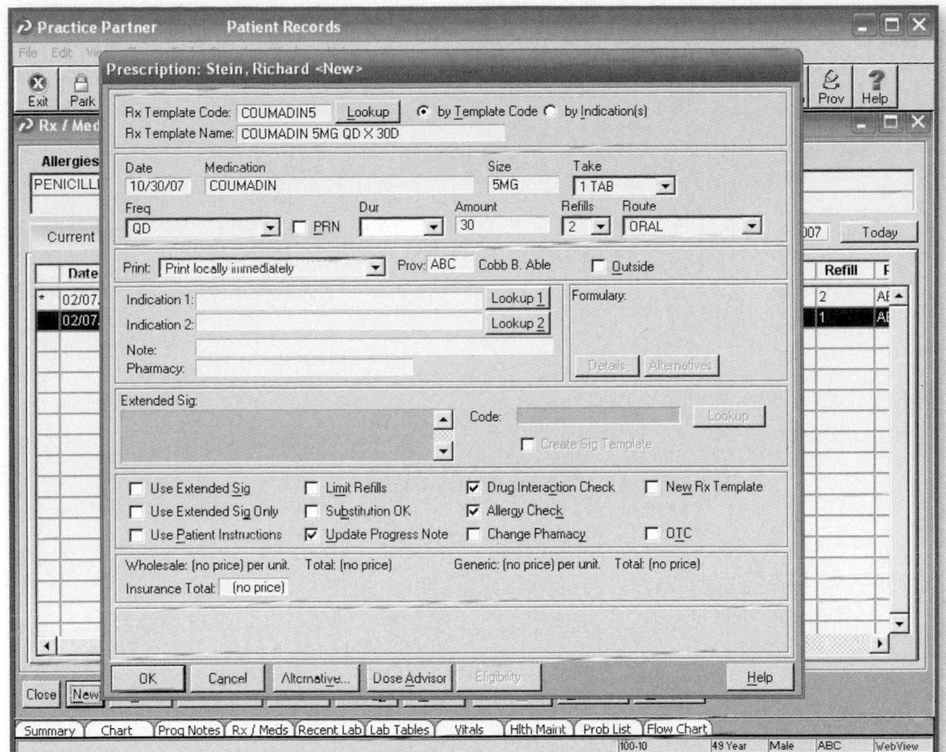

Figure 1-2

Prescription order in an electronic health record program.

part because the number of prescriptions continues to increase. In the United States, 3.6 billion prescriptions were filled between October 2004 and September 2005.

RISING HEALTH CARE COSTS

The United States spends 15 percent of its gross national product, or approximately $2 trillion a year, on health care. About 31 percent of all health care dollars are spent on administration instead of on the actual treatment of patients. Numerous studies identifying financial waste in the health care system have cited the use of outdated systems as a major factor. For example, $300 trillion is spent annually on treatments that are ineffective, duplicate another procedure, or are inappropriate. Despite the amount spent on health care in the United States each year, the American health care system ranks thirty-seventh in the world in quality and forty-eighth in life expectancy. On average, adults in the United States receive treatment from which they benefit only about half the time. See Figure 1-3 on page 6 for a comparison of the United States with other industrialized countries in safety, efficiency, and effectiveness.

COORDINATION OF CARE

Most patients today receive care from several medical professionals in a number of different settings. A teenager may have a primary care provider, a dermatologist for bouts of acne, a pulmonary specialist for asthma flare-ups, and an orthopedic doctor for a knee injured in a game of soccer. As the population ages, more and more Americans

Figure 1-3

Ranking of U.S. health care system in safety, efficiency, and effectiveness.

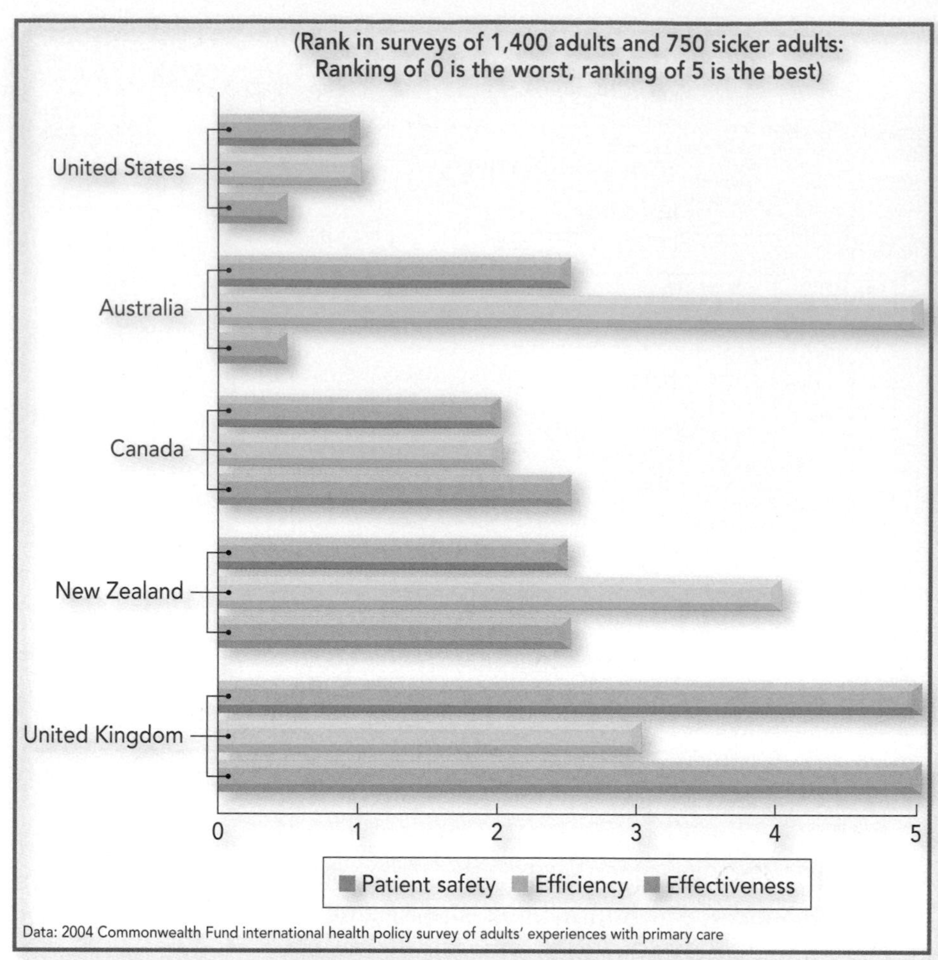

suffer from chronic health conditions such as cardiovascular disease, diabetes, and asthma. Like the teenager, the patient with a chronic condition receives treatment from multiple health care providers.

Most providers lack the information systems necessary to share and coordinate a patient's care with other providers. In these situations, it is likely that each physician maintains a paper-based medical record at his or her facility. The information that is in the patient's record at one provider's office is not part of the record at another. The physician currently seeing the patient does not have access to information about the treatments the patient received at another physician's office or in a facility such as a walk-in clinic.

Under this system of record-keeping, patients are often responsible for bringing copies of their relevant health records, such as lab reports or X-rays, to their other providers. If this does not happen, the doctors may end up treating them without a complete picture of their medical conditions. A patient may undergo a duplicate test because the physician does not know that another provider has already ordered the same test. Worse, a patient may experience a drug interaction if one doctor is not aware of the medication prescribed by another doctor. If these multiple providers cannot easily access a patient's complete health record, important treatment decisions will be made without all the necessary information.

Trends in Technology, the Economy, and Government Policy

It is widely believed that many of these problems could be overcome if information technology were applied to the business of health care in much the same way it was applied to the banking industry in the 1980s and 1990s. **Health information technology (HIT)** refers to the use of technology to manage information about the health care of patients. The widespread application of HIT has the potential to improve the quality of health care, prevent many medical errors, and reduce health care costs. Converging trends in technology, the economy, and government initiatives are all contributing to the demand for the increased use of HIT.

health information technology (HIT) use of technology to manage patient health care information.

ADVANCES IN TECHNOLOGY

The speed of computer processors, the vast amount of storage available, and the speed of data transmission make it efficient for physician practices to use computer technology. Wireless communications and high-speed Internet are now widely available. Software that can translate spoken words into word processing files, known as voice recognition software, makes it convenient and cost-effective for physicians to document patient care. Devices for storing files, such as CDs and flash drives, are smaller and require less physical space for storage. The cost of technology has also come down, making it more affordable than before.

ECONOMIC PRESSURES

A number of economic factors also contribute to the call for change in the health care system. Costs for patients, the government, physicians, and employers have been increasing at an alarming rate.

Administrative Costs

As discussed earlier, the burden of administrative costs in a paper-based system continues to put a strain on all parties in the health care system.

Medical Liability Premiums

Medical liability insurance covers doctors and other health care professionals in case of liability claims arising from their treatment of patients. Premiums for medical liability insurance are at an all-time high. In areas of the country with particularly high premiums, rising costs have driven some doctors to close practices or take early retirement.

Employer-Sponsored Insurance Premiums

Many people in the United States receive health insurance coverage through their employers. Premiums for employer-sponsored health coverage have increased dramatically (see Figure 1-4 on page 8). Since 2000, employer-sponsored premiums rose 87 percent. For some businesses, these costs are threatening not only profits but also the ability to

Figure 1-4
Employer cost of providing health insurance to employees.

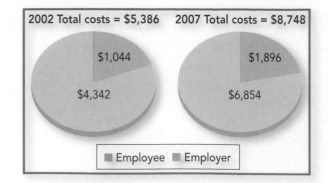

continue operating. At General Motors's annual meeting in 2005, it was revealed that providing health benefits for employees adds just over $1,500 to the sticker price of each new car. As financial pressure mounts on employers, workers are being asked to pay a larger share of the premiums. The annual cost of employer-sponsored health coverage for a family is about $11,500 annually. The amount of this cost paid by employees themselves has risen to almost $3,000 a year.

GOVERNMENT HEALTH INFORMATION TECHNOLOGY INITIATIVES

Health Insurance Portability and Accountability Act of 1996 (HIPAA) legislation to protect patients' private health information, ensure coverage, and uncover fraud and abuse.

standards set of commonly agreed-on specifications.

The federal government has taken a leadership role in pushing for the adoption of health information technology. Beginning in the 1990s, government officials began promoting the benefits of HIT. The **Health Insurance Portability and Accountability Act of 1996 (HIPAA)** was designed to protect patients' private health information, ensure health care coverage when workers change or lose jobs, and uncover fraud and abuse in the health care system. HIPAA also established standards for the electronic exchange of administrative and financial health information. **Standards** are commonly agreed-on specifications.

As one of its mandates, HIPAA requires the use of electronic rather than paper insurance claims, which has been made possible by the adoption of standards. This requirement put pressure on physician practices and hospitals to purchase and use computers for health care claims and patient billing if they were not doing so already. As a result, computer use by medical office staff members increased dramatically. HIPAA also set guidelines that protect the privacy of a patient's personal health information that is exchanged electronically (see Chapter 6).

Electronic Prescribing

Medicare Prescription Drug, Improvement, and Modernization Act of 2003 (MMA) legislation creating a prescription drug benefit that encourages electronic prescribing.

Medicare Part D voluntary prescription drug benefit under Medicare.

electronic prescribing computer-based communication system that transmits prescriptions electronically.

The **Medicare Prescription Drug, Improvement, and Modernization Act of 2003 (MMA)** created a voluntary prescription drug benefit, known as **Medicare Part D,** under Medicare. In an effort to encourage the widespread adoption of electronic prescribing, the MMA included a provision for an electronic prescription drug program. **Electronic prescribing,** also known as e-prescribing, enables a physician to transmit a prescription electronically to a patient's pharmacy. The system electronically checks for drug interactions and allergies and eliminates prescription errors caused by illegible handwriting. At the present time, e-prescribing is optional for physicians and pharmacies participating in the Medicare prescription benefit program, but drug plans that participate must support electronic prescribing.

Electronic Health Records

In his 2004 State of the Union address, President George W. Bush recommended greater use of information technology in health care and set the goal of establishing electronic health records for all Americans within ten years. In April 2004, the **Office of the National Coordinator for Health Information Technology (ONCHIT)** was established to work toward realizing President Bush's vision for health information technology. In 2005, ONCHIT funded research on several significant HIT initiatives, including:

Office of the National Coordinator for Health Information Technology (ONCHIT) government office established to oversee HIT initiatives.

- The development of industry-wide HIT standards
- The development of a certification process for HIT products
- The creation of a model of a widespread network to exchange health information

Advisory Role Formed in 2005, the American Health Information Community (AHIC) has the responsibility of making recommendations to the secretary of the Department of Health and Human Services on how to speed the development and adoption of health information technology. By the end of 2007, AHIC had made over 100 recommendations to HHS intended to speed the implementation of information technology in health care, such as:

1. *Consumer empowerment* Develop secure electronic health care registration information and medication history for patients that is responsive to consumer needs
2. *Chronic care* Ensure secure electronic communication between patients and their health care providers
3. *Electronic health records* Standardize laboratory test results in records that are available to authorized health professionals in a secure environment
4. *Biosurveillance* Enable public health agencies to communicate health information in a standardized, anonymous manner within twenty-four hours

Standards Development In 2006, the Health Information Technology Standards Panel (HITSP) announced standards in three of the four areas identified by AHIC, including consumer empowerment, electronic health records, and biosurveillance. HITSP is responsible for identifying the standards required for the electronic exchange of health information. In 2007, HITSP released a set of security and privacy standards designed to ensure the privacy of patient information that is transmitted electronically.

Software Certification The Certification Commission for Healthcare Information Technology (CCHIT) develops certification criteria for electronic health records software products. In 2006, CCHIT approved the first group of office-based EHRs. In 2007, more office-based products were certified, and criteria for certifying hospital-based EHRs were finalized. In 2008, CCHIT is working on certification in four additional areas, including health information exchanges, emergency departments, cardiology practices, and child healthcare requirements. In addition, CCHIT updates existing certification criteria on an annual basis.

Nationwide Health Information Network (NHIN) nationwide computer network facilitating the exchange of health care information.

Nationwide Network Trial The ONC has also led the efforts to develop a secure **Nationwide Health Information Network (NHIN)** to link health records across the country. The NHIN is expected to be a collection of networks rather than a single database of patient files. A nationwide health information network would make it possible for a doctor to access a patient's health record from any location at any time of the day or night.

health information exchange network that securely moves clinical information among a variety of health information systems.

regional health information organization (RHIO) group of health care organizations that share information.

Early in 2007, four corporations demonstrated NHIN models for the secure electronic exchange of health information. In late 2007, HHS awarded contracts to nine health information exchanges (HIEs) to begin trial implementations of a nationwide network. A **health information exchange** is a smaller, regional network that securely moves clinical information among a variety of health information systems while maintaining the meaning of the information being exchanged. HIEs are also known as **regional health information organizations.** HIEs are thought of as the building blocks of a future nationwide network, since it is hoped that by linking HIEs, a nationwide network can be formed. Figure 1-5 shows states that currently have one or more functioning HIEs.

Mandatory Compliance President Bush issued an executive order in August 2006 requiring federal departments and agencies that purchase and deliver health care to adopt HIT systems that use standards recognized by the secretary of HHS as their systems are updated. These groups include the Department of Veterans Affairs, the Office of Personnel Management, and the Defense Department, which provides

Figure 1-5
States with one or more HIEs.

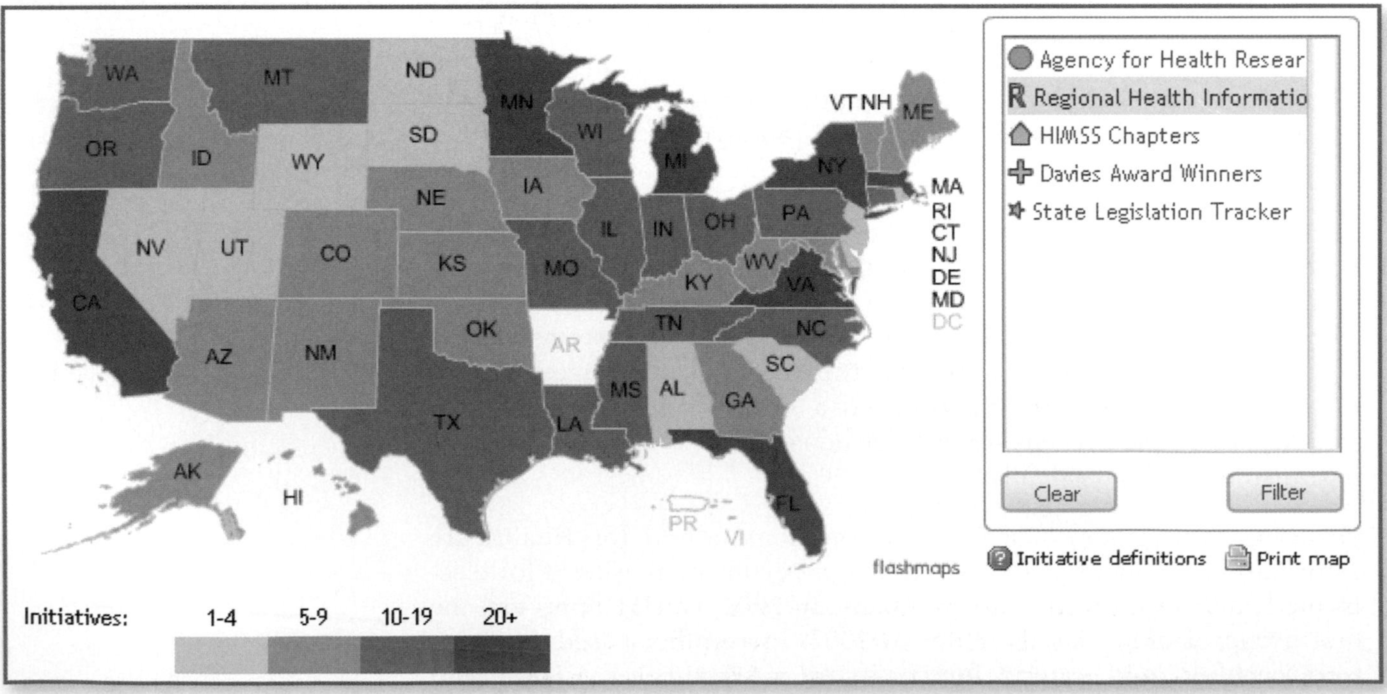

health care to active-duty members of the military as well as retirees and their families.

Regulatory Change The Stark Law prohibited physicians from referring Medicare patients to certain facilities, such as hospitals, with which the physicians have financial relationships. New regulations issued by HHS make it legal for hospitals and some other facilities to donate HIT systems and training to physicians, easing the financial burden physicians face when acquiring new HIT systems.

Financial Incentives In October 2007, the government announced that about 1,200 physicians participating in Medicare who switch from paper records to electronic records will receive extra pay for completing tasks online, such as ordering prescriptions or recording the results of lab tests. The physicians who most aggressively use the technology and who score the highest in an annual evaluation will receive the greatest increases.

What Is a Medical Record?

To fully understand the challenges of creating secure, interconnected electronic health records, it is important to review the content and purpose of a medical record, regardless of the form it takes. Every time a patient is treated by a health care provider, a record is made of the encounter. This record includes information that the patient provides, such as medical history, as well as the physician's assessment, diagnosis, and treatment plan. Medical records also contain laboratory test results, X-rays and other diagnostic images, a list of medications prescribed, and reports that indicate the results of operations and other medical procedures. This chronological **medical record** is an important business and legal document. It is used to support clinical treatment decisions, to document services provided to patients for billing purposes, and to document patient conditions and responses to treatment should a legal case arise.

medical record chronological record generated during a patient's treatment.

Since the idea of computer-based medical records came about, they have been referred to by a number of different names. In the 1990s, they were known as electronic patient records (EPRs), computerized patient records (CPRs), and computerized medical records (CMRs). These terms gave way to the current usage, which includes electronic health records (EHR), electronic medical records (EMR), and personal health records (PHR).

Although there is not universal agreement on definitions, the consensus is that **electronic medical records (EMR)** are computerized records of one physician's encounters with a patient over time. They serve as the physician's legal record of patient care. While EMRs may contain information from external sources including pharmacies and laboratories, the information in the EMR reflects treatment of a patient by a single physician.

electronic medical record (EMR) computerized record of one physician's encounters with a patient over time.

Electronic health records, on the other hand, are computerized lifelong health care records for an individual that incorporate data from all sources that treat the individual. As such, an electronic health record

Figure 1-6

A screen from an electronic health record program.

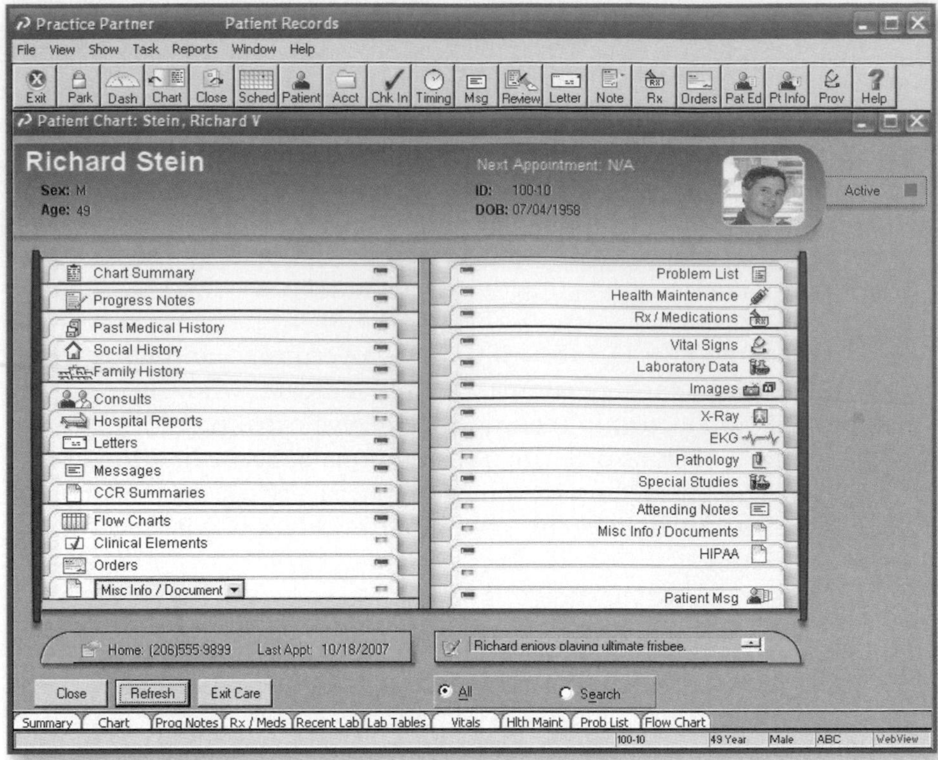

can include information from the EMRs of a number of different physicians as well as from pharmacies, laboratories, hospitals, insurance carriers, and so on. Information is added to the record by health care professionals working in a variety of settings, and the record can be accessed by professionals when needed. Figure 1-6 illustrates a screen from an office-based EHR program.

personal health records (PHR) individual's comprehensive record of health information.

Personal health records (PHR), on the other hand, are private, secure electronic files that are created, maintained, and owned by the patient. The patient decides whether to share the contents with doctors or other health professionals. PHRs typically include current medications and dosages, health insurance information, immunizations records, allergies, medical test results, past surgeries, family medical history, and more. Personal health records are created and stored on the Internet, but the files can easily be downloaded to a storage device such as a flash drive for portability. The topic of PHRs is covered in detail in Chapter 5.

CONTENTS OF A HEALTH RECORD

acute care inpatient treatment for urgent problems.

ambulatory care treatment provided without admission to a hospital.

The contents of health records vary depending on the setting where they are created and used. **Acute care** is most often used to refer to a hospital, which treats patients with urgent problems that cannot be handled in another setting. **Ambulatory care** refers to treatment that is provided without admission to a hospital. Ambulatory care settings include physician offices, hospital emergency rooms, and clinics. The records created and maintained in each type of facility vary. Hospital records, by nature, keep track of acute, time-limited episodes. Physician office charts, on the other hand, track less urgent ongoing health and wellness needs of individuals.

The ABCs of Electronic Records

EMR—Electronic Medical Record

Focus

- A computerized version of a paper chart with additional capabilities
- Document episodes of illness or injury

Origin of Information

- Created and maintained by a single provider or practice to keep track of that provider's treatment of a patient

Access

- Able to import data from external sources, including pharmacies and laboratory and radiology facilities
- Cannot be accessed by other providers or facilities

EHR—Electronic Health Record

Focus

- Broad focus on a patient's total health experience over the lifespan, rather than the documentation of episodes of illness or injury

Origin of Information

- Created and maintained by multiple providers and facilities

Access

- Can be viewed by multiple providers and facilities, including primary care physicians, specialists, hospitals, pharmacies, and laboratory and radiology facilities
- Information can be added to the record by any of these providers or facilities

PHR—Personal Health Record

Focus

- A computerized record about an individual patient's health and health care, including medications, health insurance information, immunizations, allergies, medical test results, and family medical history

Origin of Information

- Created and maintained by the individual patient

Access

- Able to import data from providers and facilities
- If permission granted, providers can access limited data

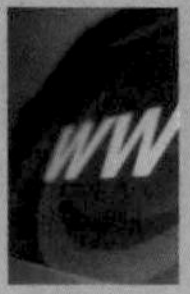

Chapter 1 Online Discovery

The American Health Information Management Association (AHIMA) hosts the website www.myphr.com. This site contains information about personal health—personal health records in particular. Open your Internet browser, and go to www.myphr.com.

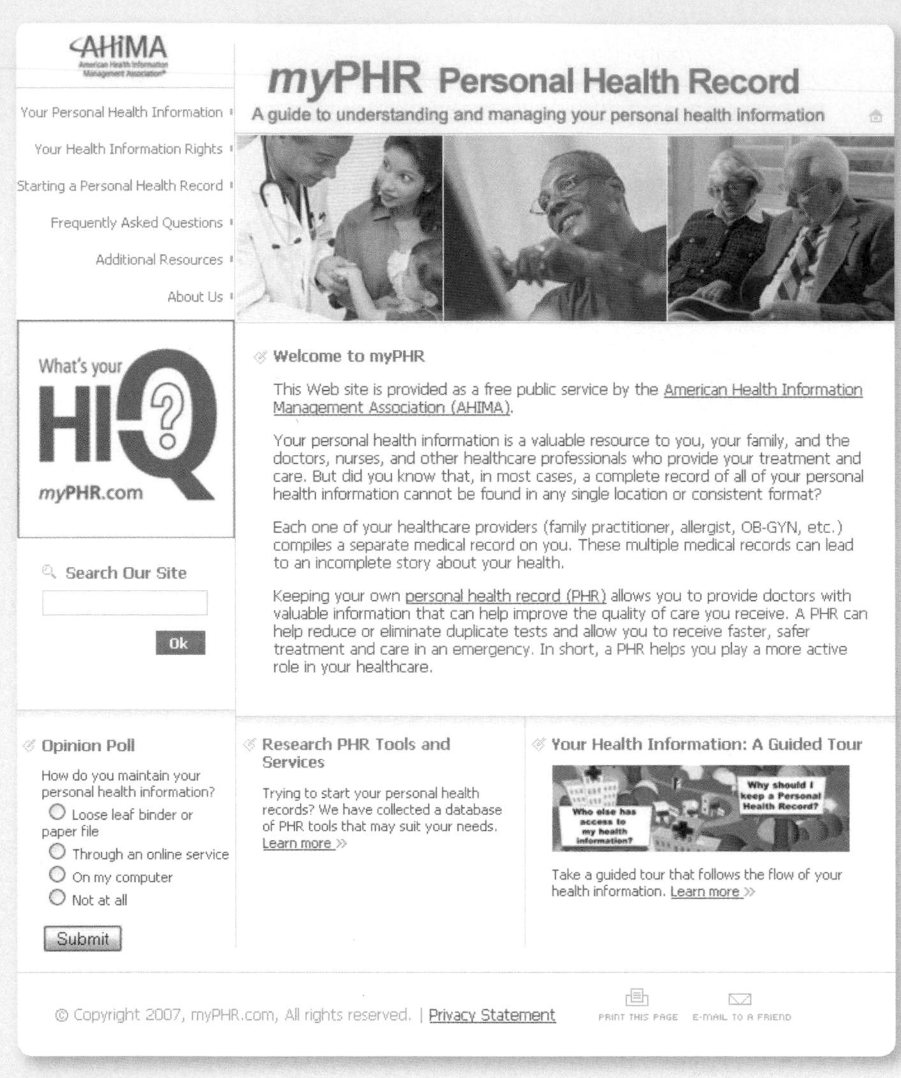

Thinking About It

1. How is your health information used?

____

2. Who owns your health information?

____

3. What does a health information management (HIM) department do?

____

Click the blue underlined words *Learn more* in the lower right corner of the window. A feature called "Your Health Information: A Guided Tour" will open. Read the instructions above the picture, and take the tour. Then answer the questions below.

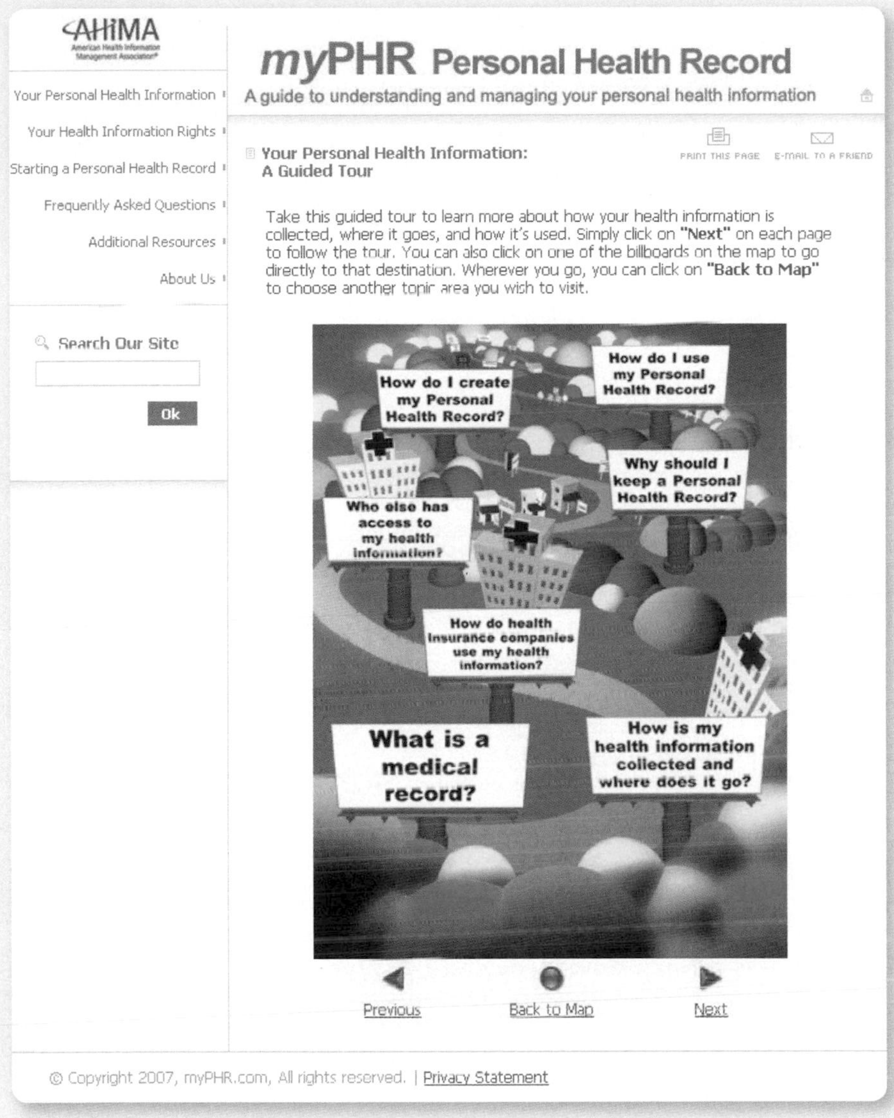

4. Who has access to your health record?

____

5. Why is it important to keep a personal health record (PHR)?

____

When you are finished viewing the tour and answering the questions, close your web browser.

Acute Care Records

In inpatient facilities such as hospitals, an individual's health record usually contains the following content:

Admission Record	The admission record contains identifying information such as the patient's name, address, and Social Security number. It also contains details about the patient's insurance coverage and information about whether the patient has an advanced directive or living will. The patient must acknowledge receipt of the hospital's notice of privacy practices.
Consents	Certain procedures and surgeries performed in a hospital require the signed consent of the patient. These forms are included in the health record.
Consultations	At the request of one physician, another physician may be asked to examine the patient and report the results. Information obtained in these consultations becomes part of the record.
Discharge Summary	The discharge summary includes a brief description of the patient's diagnosis and treatment, documentation of the outcome of treatment, the patient's condition when discharged from the facility, and follow-up care instructions.
Emergency Department	If the patient was admitted to the hospital after treatment in the emergency department (ED), the patient chart will include a report of the evaluation and treatment provided.
History and Physical	The history and physical portion of the patient chart includes the patient's medical history, chief complaints, a review of the important body systems, and the findings of a physical examination.
Laboratory Studies and Diagnostic Tests	The results of all laboratory tests, image studies, and other diagnostic procedures are part of the patient's health record.
Operative Notes	Physicians make notes before a patient undergoes surgery, including the purpose of the surgery, a preoperative diagnosis, and the procedure to be performed. After the surgery is completed, the physician adds a discussion of the actual surgery performed.
Pathology Reports	Pathology reports contain the pathologist's description of specimens from a patient and a diagnosis based on an examination of the specimen.
Physician Orders	Physician orders determine the treatment the patient receives while in the hospital, including tests, medications, and therapies.
Progress Notes	Progress notes document the clinical staff's observations of the patient, including regular updates of the patient's condition and responses to treatment.

Ambulatory Care Records

Patient records in an ambulatory care facility, such as a physician office, contain certain standard information, including:

Patient Identifying Information	This demographic and insurance information is obtained when the patient first comes to the practice and is updated regularly.
History and Physical	This section of the record contains information about the patient's past medical history, family medical problems, prior hospitalizations, current medications, and past surgeries. It also includes information from a physical examination.
Office Visit Notes	Office visit notes document the physician's findings during an examination, including observations of the patient's current medical problem, a diagnosis of the condition, and a plan for treatment. The notes also list physician orders. During each subsequent visit with the physician, notes about the patient's condition and response to treatment are added to the chart.
Lab Tests and Results	This portion of the patient record contains the results of all diagnostic procedures such as laboratory test results and pathology reports, including blood tests, X-rays, and biopsies.
Miscellaneous Consents and Releases	A number of miscellaneous forms are saved in the patient chart, such as release of information requests, acknowledgement of receipt of notice of privacy practices, and consents for certain procedures.
Prescriptions	The patient chart contains a record of all medications prescribed by the physician as well as patient requests for refills.
External Correspondence About Patients	Correspondence to and from the patient or a third party, such as a consulting physician, is part of a patient record. Physicians receive requests to sign forms for patients, such as applications for disability benefits and proof of immunizations.

The Purpose and Use of Health Records

In today's complex health care system, patient records are used by individuals and groups for a variety of purposes from communicating information about the patient's condition to researching the emergence of new diseases.

PRIMARY PURPOSE

The primary purpose of the heath record is to assist health care professionals in providing the most effective patient care. The record documents each encounter the individual has with a health care provider. It is used to communicate information about the patient from one provider to another, making continuity of care possible.

continuity of care delivery of appropriate and consistent care over time.

Continuity of care refers to delivering appropriate and consistent care to an individual over time. It is not limited to one provider or one illness during any one time period, but instead encompasses multiple illnesses over many years.

SECONDARY USES

Health records also provide information for other important purposes, which are known as secondary uses.

Billing and Reimbursement

The documentation in the health record is necessary to substantiate insurance claims and to collect reimbursement from government and private third-party payers. Reimbursement may be denied if documentation is incomplete or inaccurate.

Legal Issues

Information in the record may be used as evidence in a legal matter involving the patient, the physician, or the facility. For example, an individual may decide to sue an insurance company as a result of injuries sustained in an automobile accident. The insurance company would require access to the medical record to determine whether the individual was being treated for the condition before the accident.

Quality Review

pay for performance (P4P) use of financial incentives to improve health care quality and efficiency.

Individuals and institutions in the health care field must regularly evaluate the adequacy and appropriateness of the care they deliver. The health record is analyzed to obtain a measure of the quality of the services provided to the patient. Increasingly, data on quality are being linked to payment. **Pay for performance (P4P)** is the use of financial incentives to improve the quality and efficiency of health care services. For example, a hospital that is in the top 10 percent of statistics on postsurgery infections could receive additional compensation from a payer. In the physician office, a provider might be financially rewarded for significantly increasing the number of patients who receive annual mammograms.

Research

Health records provide information to medical researchers, who use the data to develop new methods of treatment and to compare the effectiveness of existing treatments. For example, researchers who are conducting clinical trials of a new treatment need access to medical records to validate that patients meet the criteria for the study.

Education

Health records provide case studies that are used to train a wide range of health professionals. For example, medical students are presented with cases developed from medical records during their training. In these cases, the patient's identity is removed *(redacted)* from the record. The identities of the individual patients are always deleted, so patient confidentiality is not at risk.

Public Health and Homeland Security

The records of physicians and hospitals are also important in determining the incidence of disease and in developing methods to improve the health of the population. The incidence and spread of disease can be followed closely using health records. For example, health records can help contain outbreaks of disease due to the contamination of food. In the event of an act of bioterrorism, such as the intentional spread of smallpox, health records would be critical in detecting the outbreak early and in containing its effects.

Credentialing

Health care professionals, such as physicians and medical assistants, must pass examinations before they begin practicing. After the initial credential is awarded, continuing education courses must be completed to maintain the license or certification. The Joint Commission (formerly JHACO) studies the quality and safety of health care organizations. Patient records are used by credentialing organizations to evaluate health care providers and facilities. The results of these evaluations determine whether the person or institution will be approved for licensing, certification, or accreditation.

Core Functions of an Electronic Health Record System

While paper and electronic health records serve many of the same purposes, the electronic record is much more than a computerized version of a paper record. The Institute of Medicine suggested that an EHR should include eight core functions:

1. Health information and data elements
2. Results management
3. Order management
4. Decision support
5. Electronic communication and connectivity
6. Patient support
7. Administrative processes
8. Reporting and population management

(*Key Capabilities of an Electronic Health Record System,* 2003)

HEALTH INFORMATION AND DATA ELEMENTS

An electronic health record must contain information about patients that enables health care providers to diagnose and treat injuries and illnesses. It has demographic information about the patient, such as address and phone number, as well as clinical information about the patient's past and present health concerns (see Figure 1-7 on page 20).

Figure 1-7

History and physical notes in an electronic health record.

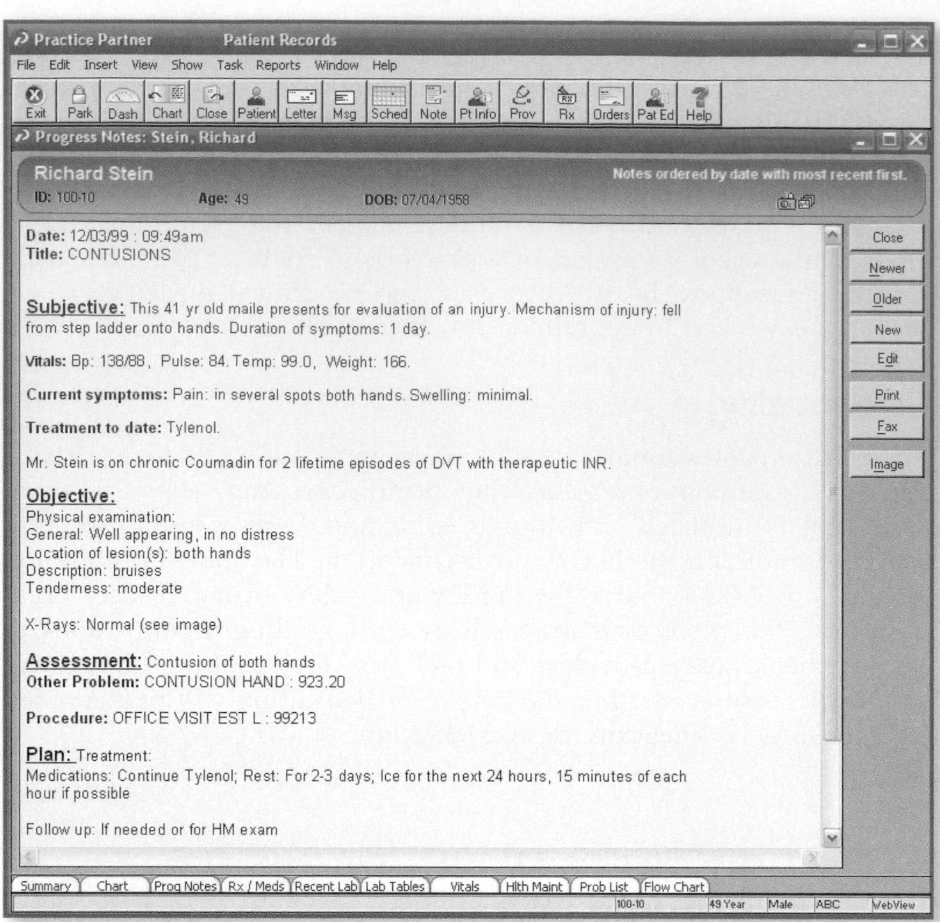
Practice Partner Patient Records
File Edit Insert View Show Task Reports Window Help
Exit Park Dash Chart Close Patient Letter Msg Sched Note Pt Info Prov Rx Orders Pat Ed Help
Progress Notes: Stein, Richard
Richard Stein
Notes ordered by date with most recent first.
ID: 100-10 Age: 49 DOB: 07/04/1958
Date: 12/03/99 : 09:49am
Title: CONTUSIONS
Subjective: This 41 yr old maile presents for evaluation of an injury. Mechanism of injury: fell from step ladder onto hands. Duration of symptoms: 1 day.
Vitals: Bp: 138/88 , Pulse: 84. Temp: 99.0, Weight: 166.
Current symptoms: Pain: in several spots both hands. Swelling: minimal.
Treatment to date: Tylenol.
Mr. Stein is on chronic Coumadin for 2 lifetime episodes of DVT with therapeutic INR.
Objective:
Physical examination:
General: Well appearing, in no distress
Location of lesion(s): both hands
Description: bruises
Tenderness: moderate
X-Rays: Normal (see image)
Assessment: Contusion of both hands
Other Problem: CONTUSION HAND : 923.20
Procedure: OFFICE VISIT EST L : 99213
Plan: Treatment:
Medications: Continue Tylenol; Rest: For 2-3 days; Ice for the next 24 hours, 15 minutes of each hour if possible
Follow up: If needed or for HM exam
Close
Newer
Older
New
Edit
Print
Fax
Image
Summary Chart Prog Notes Rx / Meds Recent Lab Lab Tables Vitals Hlth Maint Prob List Flow Chart
100-10 49 Year Male ABC WebView

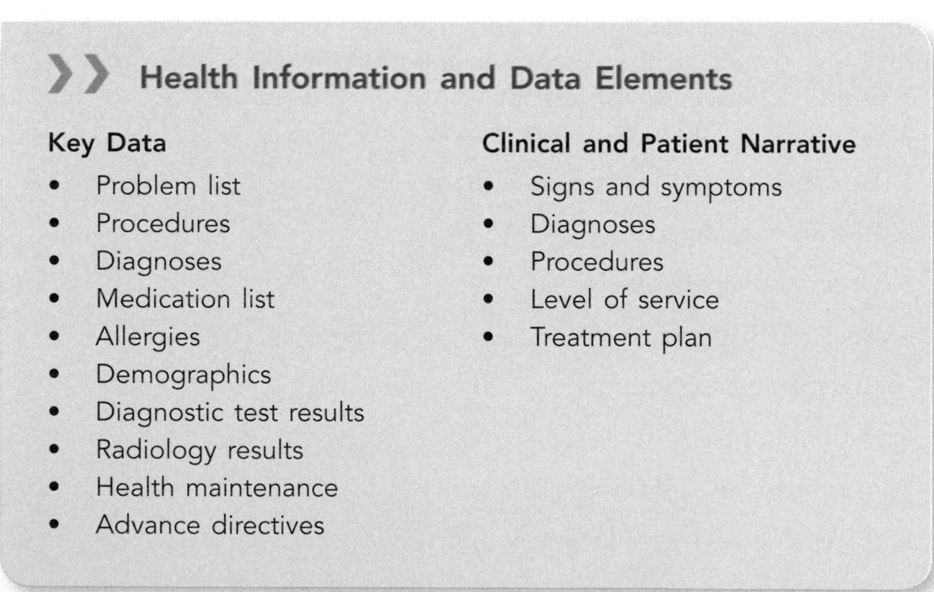

Health Information and Data Elements

Key Data

- Problem list
- Procedures
- Diagnoses
- Medication list
- Allergies
- Demographics
- Diagnostic test results
- Radiology results
- Health maintenance
- Advance directives

Clinical and Patient Narrative

- Signs and symptoms
- Diagnoses
- Procedures
- Level of service
- Treatment plan

RESULTS MANAGEMENT

Providers must have access to current and past laboratory, radiology, and other test results performed by anyone involved in the treatment of the patient. These computerized results can be accessed by multiple providers, when and where they are needed, which allows more prompt diagnosis and treatment decisions to be made.

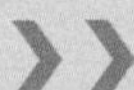

Results Management Elements

- Results reporting
- Results notification
- Multiple views of data/presentation
- Multimedia support (images, scanned documents)

ORDER MANAGEMENT

EHR programs must be able to send, receive, and store orders for medications, tests, and other services by any provider involved in treating the patient (see Figure 1-8). Staff members in different offices and facilities can access the orders, which eliminates unnecessary delays and duplicate testing.

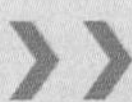

Order Management Elements

- Computerized provider order entry (CPOE)—electronic prescribing, laboratory, pathology, X ray, consultations

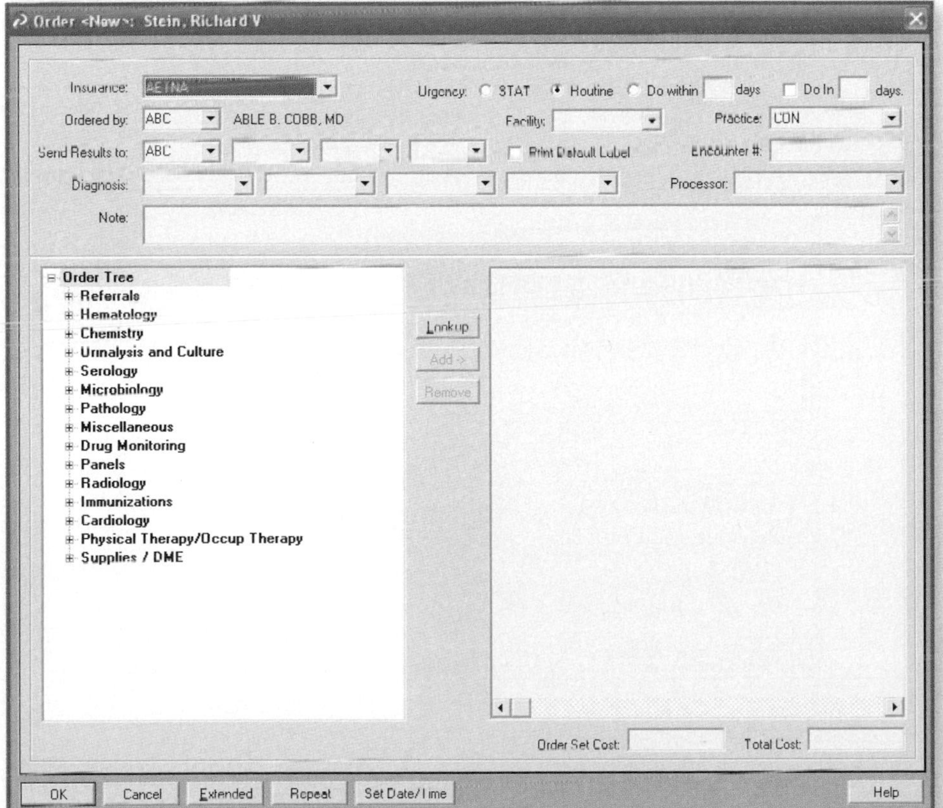

Figure 1-8

Order entry in an electronic health record.

DECISION SUPPORT

As the practice of medicine becomes more complex, the amount of information available to physicians continues to grow. Hundreds of new studies are published on a daily basis. It is not possible for a physician to remember all this information or to be aware of all the latest, most effective treatments. The latest medical evidence is incorporated into care only 50 percent of the time.

Electronic health records give physicians computer-based access to the latest clinical research for diagnosing and treating a patient while still in the examination room with the patient. The physician can also view the latest information on medications, including suggested doses, common side effects, and possible interactions.

In addition, electronic record systems provide a variety of alerts and reminders that physicians can use to improve a patient's health (see Figure 1-9 for an example of a medication alert). Physicians can, for example, see a list of all women over forty years of age who have not had mammograms in the past year. If the physician chooses, these women will all receive letters reminding them that they are due for this preventive screening.

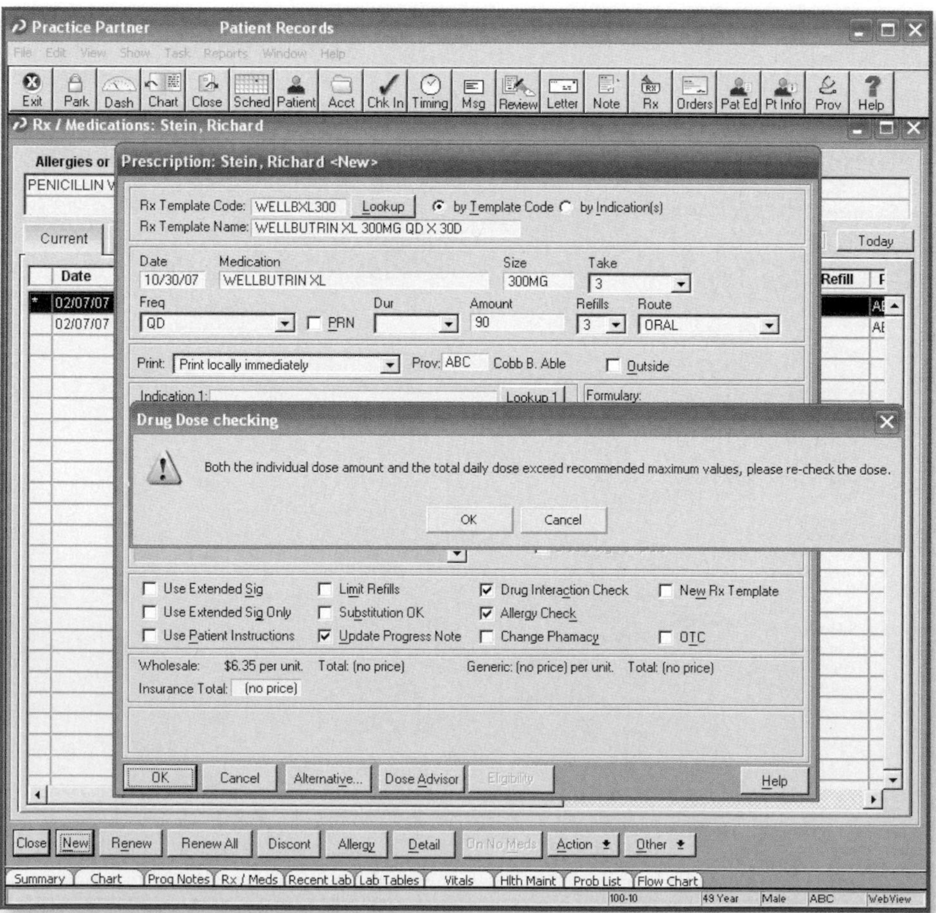

Figure 1-9

A drug alert in an electronic health record.

›› Decision Support Elements

- Access to knowledge sources
- Drug alerts
- Reminders
- Clinical guidelines and pathways
- Chronic disease management
- Clinician work list
- Diagnostic decision support
- Use of epidemiologic data
- Automated real-time surveillance

ELECTRONIC COMMUNICATION AND CONNECTIVITY

Patients are typically treated by more than one provider in more than one facility. Physicians, nurses, medical assistants, referring doctors, testing facilities, and hospitals all need to communicate with one another to provide the safest and most effective care to patients. Insurance plans also need information from the health record to process claims for reimbursement. Electronic health record systems offer a number of mechanisms to facilitate these communications, including e-mail and the Internet. Figure 1-10 illustrates an electronic message in an electronic health record.

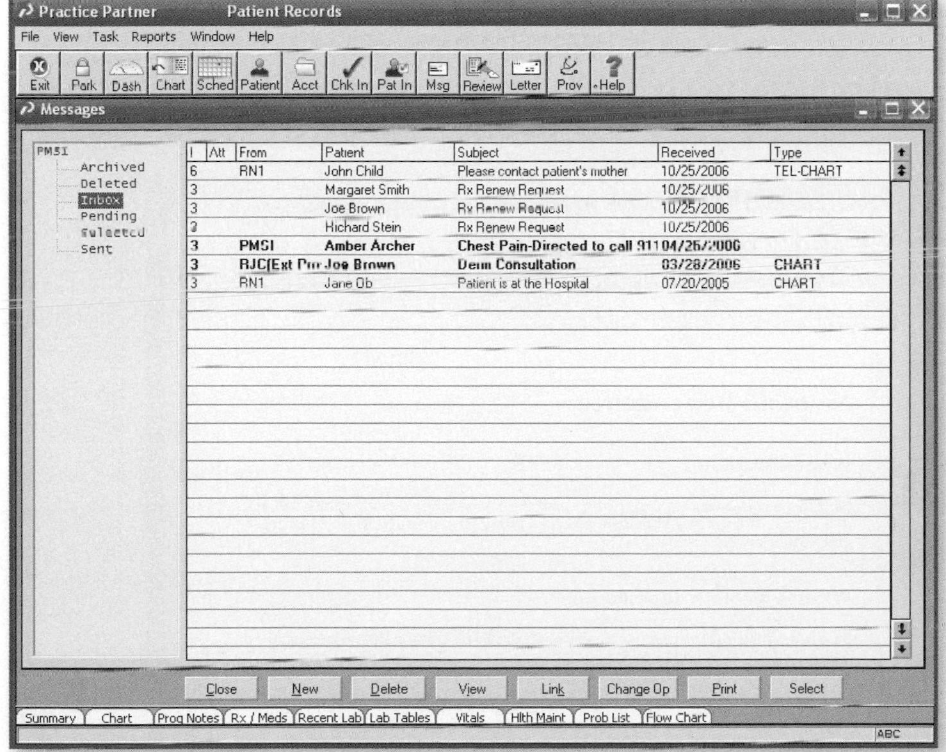

Figure 1-10
Electronic messaging in an electronic health record.

Electronic Communication and Connectivity Elements

- Provider-provider
- Team coordination
- Patient-provider
- Medical devices
- External partners (pharmacy, insurer, laboratory, radiology)
- Integrated medical record (within setting, across settings, inpatient-outpatient)

PATIENT SUPPORT

Electronic health records should offer patients access to appropriate educational materials on health topics, instructions for preparing for common medical tests, and the ability to report to their physician on home monitoring and testing. Figure 1-11 shows a sample patient education screen.

Patient Support Elements

- Patient education (access to patient education materials)
- Family and informal caregiver education
- Data entered by patient, family, and/or informal caregiver (home monitoring, questionnaires)

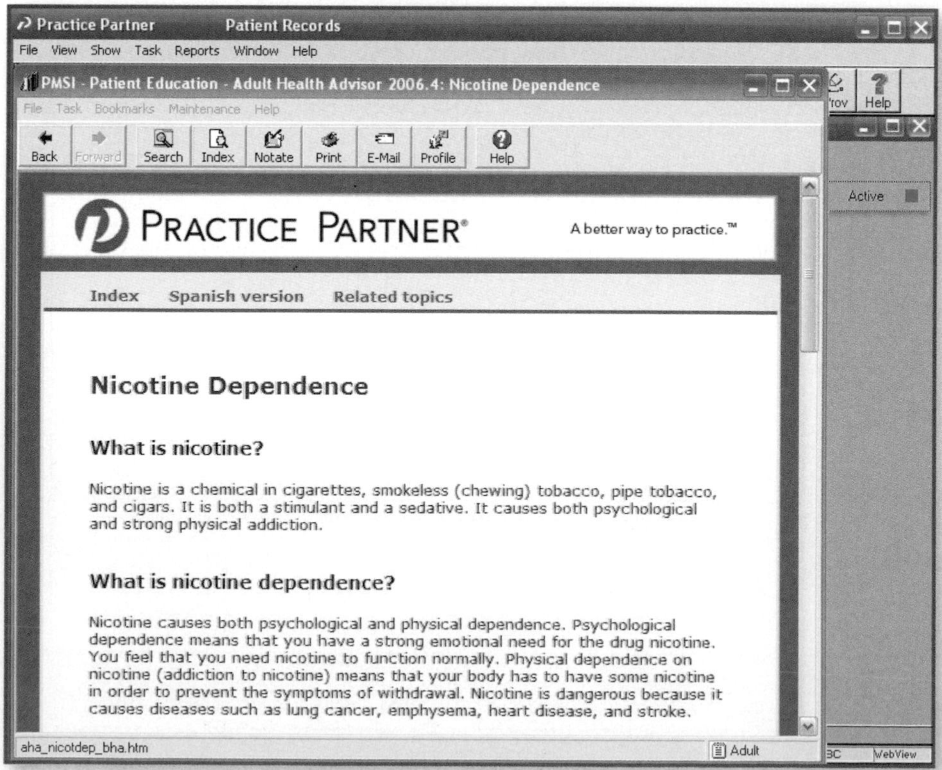

Figure 1-11
Patient education material available in an electronic health record.

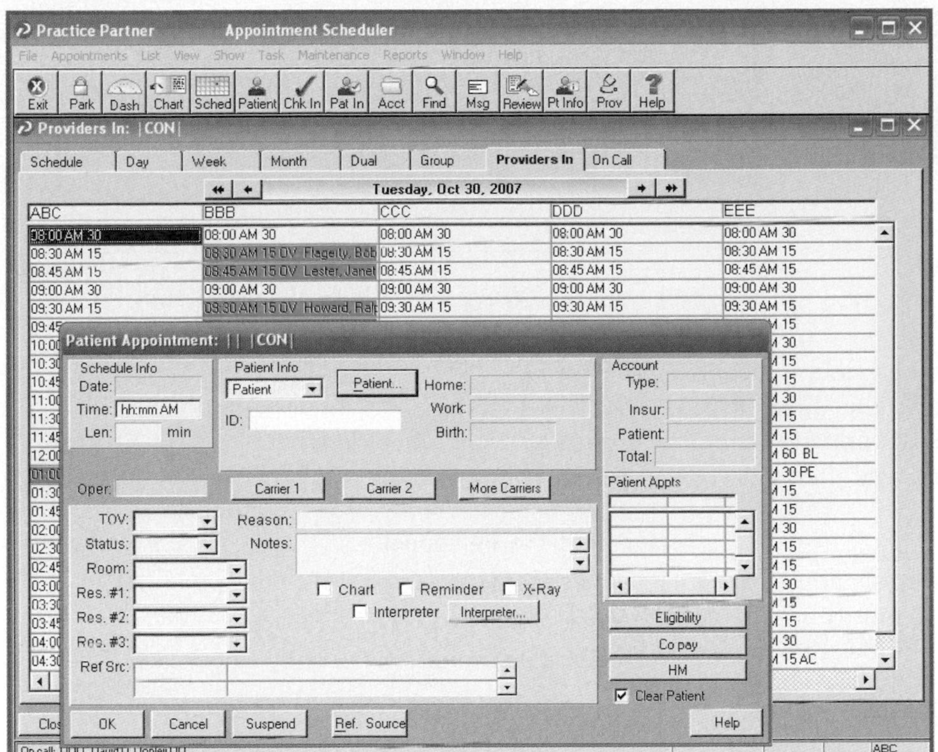

Figure 1-12

Scheduling window in an electronic health record.

ADMINISTRATIVE PROCESSES

The administrative area of health care also benefits from the use of EHRs. While most physician practices already use computers for billing and scheduling, an EHR streamlines the processes (see Figure 1-12). In addition to scheduling, the system electronically validates the patient's insurance eligibility before the patient is treated by the physician and checks whether prior authorizations are required.

Administrative Processes Elements

- Scheduling management (appointments, admissions, surgery and other procedures)
- Eligibility determination (insurance, clinical trials, drug recalls, chronic disease management)

REPORTING AND POPULATION MANAGEMENT

Electronic health record programs also enhance reporting capabilities both for internal use and for external reporting requirements. This makes it easier for physician offices and health care organizations to comply with federal, state, and private reporting requirements.

Electronic health records contain a wealth of information related to particular diseases and treatments. This information, as long as it does not include the patient's identity, can be used to advance medical knowledge through research. In addition, EHRs can assist in detecting

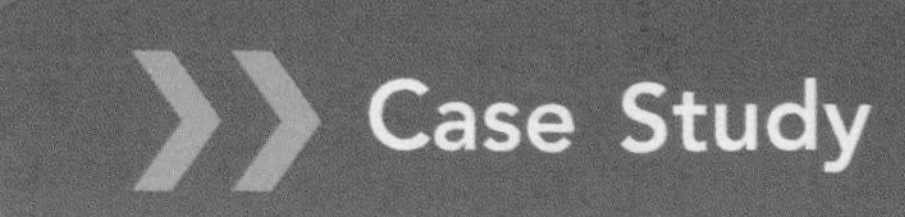

PATIENT CHECK-IN

Note to the student: Throughout the book, you will be reading case studies illustrating the differences between paper-based medical records and electronic health records. Read the entire case and then answer the questions that follow.

Amy Wilmot works as a medical assistant at West Side Medical Associates, a small family medicine practice located in Jacksonville, Florida, that serves approximately 4,500 patients annually. The staff consists of two physicians, a nurse-practitioner, a medical assistant, and a billing and coding person.

Amy's duties include registering patients, answering telephone calls, checking patients in, escorting patients to examination rooms, taking patients' vital signs, collecting information about patients' current condition, and going over the information in records to be sure it is up-to-date. She also performs simple procedures such as administering influenza vaccinations, processes referrals, fulfills doctor's orders for outside lab work and tests, monitors incoming test results, and manages the prescription renewal process.

Today, Amy is sitting at the front desk when an established patient, Denise Johnson, arrives for her appointment. Denise Johnson is a sixty-five-year-old female with a history of diabetes mellitus and clinical depression. She is currently taking Glucophage (metformin), 1500 mg daily, for her diabetes and 50 mg of Zoloft (sertraline hydrochloride) for depression.

West Side Medical Associates

About the Clinic

Clinic name: West Side Medical Associates
Specialty: Family Medicine
Location: Jacksonville, FL

About the Personnel

Physicians: David Chen, MD, Sheila Roth, MD
Nurse-practitioner: Sarina Perez
Medical assistant: Amy Wilmot, Roger LeGrande
Billing/coding department: Megan Riley, Teesha Johnson
Receptionist/front desk: Medical assistant and the billing/coding person share receptionist duty.

Johnson's address, telephone number, and insurance coverage must be verified before she is checked in for today's visit. She will see Dr. Chen, who is her primary care provider. Johnson has moved and changed jobs since her last visit, and her information must be updated. Her new insurance plan has a $30 copay per office visit. Johnson will use a credit card to pay. Once Johnson is checked in, she is taken to examination room 2, down the hall on the left.

The charts that follow lists the steps required to complete these tasks in a paper-based office, and in an office that uses electronic health records. Study the charts and answer the questions that follow.

Patient Check-in, Paper Office

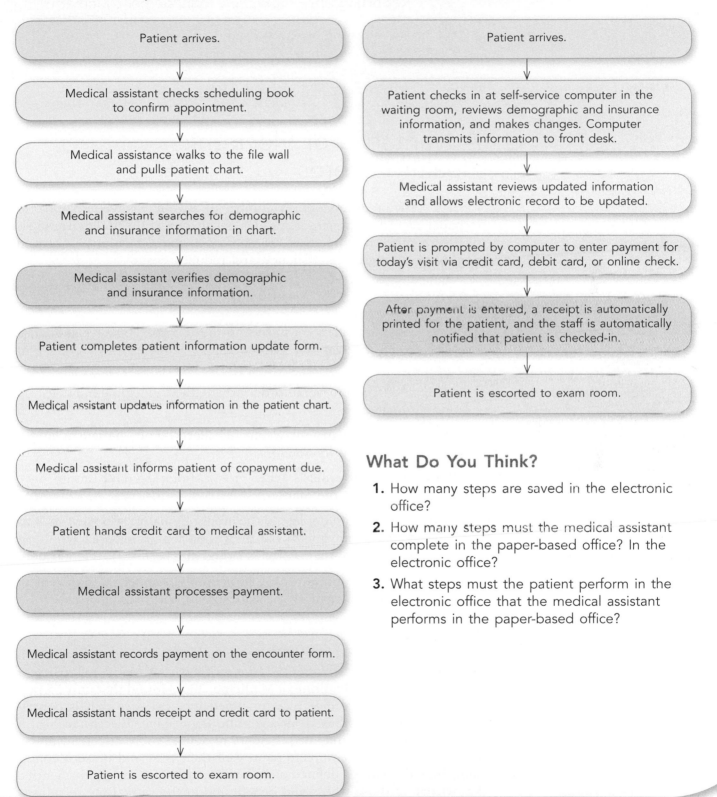

Patient arrives.

↓

Medical assistant checks scheduling book to confirm appointment.

↓

Medical assistance walks to the file wall and pulls patient chart.

↓

Medical assistant searches for demographic and insurance information in chart.

↓

Medical assistant verifies demographic and insurance information.

↓

Patient completes patient information update form.

↓

Medical assistant updates information in the patient chart.

↓

Medical assistant informs patient of copayment due.

↓

Patient hands credit card to medical assistant.

↓

Medical assistant processes payment.

↓

Medical assistant records payment on the encounter form.

↓

Medical assistant hands receipt and credit card to patient.

↓

Patient is escorted to exam room.

Patient Check-in, Electronic Office

Patient arrives.

↓

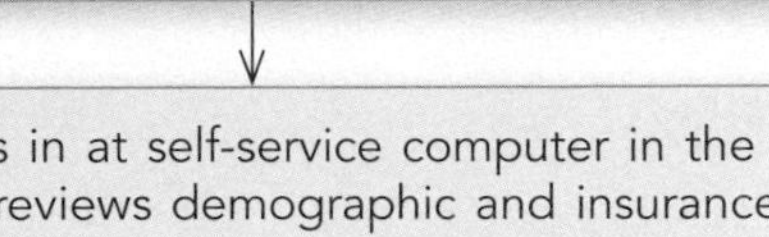

Patient checks in at self-service computer in the waiting room, reviews demographic and insurance information, and makes changes. Computer transmits information to front desk.

↓

Medical assistant reviews updated information and allows electronic record to be updated.

↓

Patient is prompted by computer to enter payment for today's visit via credit card, debit card, or online check.

↓

After payment is entered, a receipt is automatically printed for the patient, and the staff is automatically notified that patient is checked-in.

↓

Patient is escorted to exam room.

What Do You Think?

1. How many steps are saved in the electronic office?
2. How many steps must the medical assistant complete in the paper-based office? In the electronic office?
3. What steps must the patient perform in the electronic office that the medical assistant performs in the paper-based office?

threats to the health of the general population, such as bioterrorism or an outbreak of a new disease. For example, the immediate reporting of suspicious diseases to public health authorities may help identify a new influenza strain and prevent its spread.

›› Reporting and Population Management Elements

- Patient safety and quality reporting
- Public health reporting
- Disease registries

Advantages of Electronic Health Records

Clearly, EHR programs offer a number of advantages when compared to paper record-keeping systems. The most frequently cited advantages of electronic health records are increased patient safety, improved quality of care, greater efficiency, and reduced costs.

SAFETY

There is growing evidence that electronic record-keeping can reduce medical errors and improve patient safety. Some of the factors that contribute to greater safety include the following:

- Medication and physician order errors due to illegible handwriting are eliminated.
- Providers receive instant electronic alerts about patient allergies and possible drug interactions.
- Physicians receive alerts when medications deemed unsafe have been pulled from the market.
- Medical records are not lost in the event of a natural disaster, such as a hurricane, or an intentional attack such as a terrorist bombing, provided a copy of the records is stored at a secure, off-site location.
- Information is communicated in a timely manner in the event of an act of bioterrorism or the widespread outbreak of disease.

QUALITY

A 2001 report titled *Crossing the Quality Chasm: A New Health System for the 21st Century* (Institute of Medicine, 2001) found that only 55 percent of Americans receive recommended medical care that is consistent with guidelines based on scientific knowledge. Electronic health records make it possible for providers to deliver more effective care to patients based on a complete picture of their past and present condition. Effective care is defined as "providing services based on scientific knowledge to those who could benefit and at the same time refraining from providing services to those not likely to benefit" (*Crossing the Quality Chasm: A New Health System for the 21st Century,* 2001.)

With EHRs, physicians have access to evidence-based guidelines for diagnosing and treating conditions and to the latest clinical research and best practice guidelines. **Evidence-based medicine** refers to medical care that uses the latest and most accurate clinical research in making decisions about the care of patients.

evidence-based medicine medical care based on the latest and most accurate clinical research.

Electronic health records also enhance the quality of health care in the following ways:

- Patients are contacted with reminders for preventive care screenings.
- Patients suffering from chronic diseases, such as diabetes, are able to monitor their conditions at home and report results via the Internet, saving them numerous visits to the doctor.
- Health care consumers can review data about the quality and performance of providers and facilities and can choose facilities and providers accordingly.

EFFICIENCY

The retrieval of information from an EHR is immediate, which greatly improves efficiency and can be critical in emergency situations. Compared to sorting through papers in a folder, an electronic search saves critical time when vital patient information is needed.

Electronic health records also save valuable time for health care providers by reducing the time needed to enter information about patients. Currently, physicians spend almost 40 percent of their time writing up progress notes. With EHRs, physicians are finished entering notes when the patient leaves the examination room or shortly after. Nurses and medical assistants record information directly into the computer, so there is no need to copy information to a paper chart.

In regard to the efficiency of health care, electronic health records also:

- Improve the overall efficiency of the workflow in the physician practice or hospital
- Speed the delivery of diagnostic test results to the physician and the patient through electronic transmission
- Allow two or more people to work with a patient's record at the same time
- Eliminate the need to search for a misplaced or lost patient chart
- Permit physicians to review a summary of the patient's health information at a glance instead of flipping through pages
- Eliminate the need to manually enter diagnosis and procedure codes from a paper-based encounter form
- Reduce the time it takes to refill a prescription through electronic prescribing

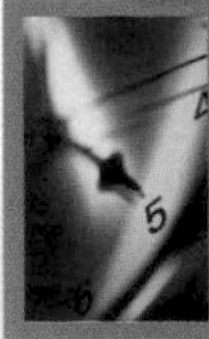

Making It Real

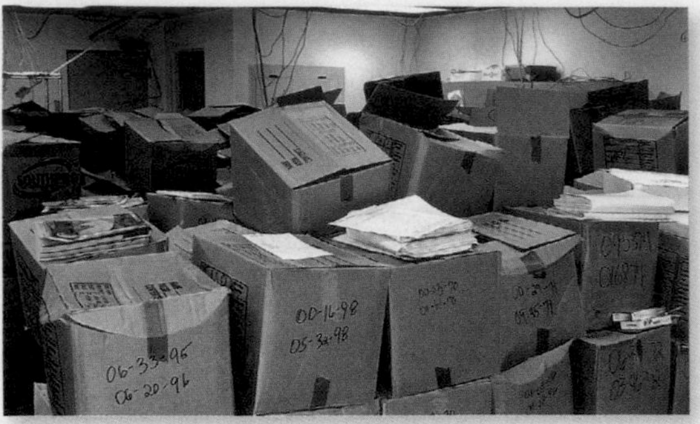
Boxes containing paper medical records salvaged during hurricane Katrina

Hurricane Katrina

Thousands of evacuees lost more than just their homes in hurricane Katrina—they lost their entire medical records, including medical histories, current conditions, test results, and lists of medications. Paper records were not the only records lost. Electronic records that were not backed up and saved at another location were lost as well when computers were hit by flood water. After the records were destroyed by the flooding, the only medical records available were those the evacuees took with them, and most did not keep copies of their health records. People with chronic diseases such as diabetes or asthma went without their medication for days. When they did receive care, health care providers lacked critical information needed to make accurate diagnosis and treatment decisions. In many cases, doctors had to start from scratch.

One bright spot amid the devastation was the Department of Veterans Affairs (VA). The VA has had some form of computerized medical records for over two decades. As the hurricane was approaching, employees at the VA made backup copies of electronic health records for their veterans in the Gulf Coast region. While the New Orleans VA Medical Center flooded, fifty thousand electronic medical records survived. Like other evacuees, veterans left the coastal areas and went to different states around the country. Many went to Florida and Texas. When they sought treatment at local VA facilities in these states, their complete medical records were available on the computer. No information had been lost.

The lessons of hurricane Katrina focused attention on the need for electronic medical records that can survive disasters, even when computers and medical offices do not.

- Organize all information in one place, including in-house messages, telephone call messages, requests for information, and referral letters
- Enable physicians to receive payment for services more quickly because patient encounter information is automatically transferred to the billing software

FUTURE COST REDUCTION

While the initial expense of an EHR system may be high, studies suggest that electronic health records contain or reduce health care costs over time. According to an estimate by the Center for Information Technology Leadership, an estimated $77.8 billion could be saved each year once nationwide interoperable electronic health care records are implemented (Walker, "The Value of Health Care Information Exchange And Interoperability," *Health Affairs*, January/February 2005).

Implementation Issues

Despite offering a number of significant advantages, electronic health records are not in widespread use in the United States today. According to an October 2006 report, approximately 17 to 24 percent of physicians in ambulatory settings use EHRs, while only 4 to 24 percent of hospitals have similar systems (*Health Information Technology in the United States: The Information Base for Progress,* Robert Wood Johnson Foundation, October, 2006). The migration from paper to electronic records has been slowed by a number of barriers.

COST

It is estimated that an electronic health record system costs approximately $33,000 per physician to install and roughly $8,400 per physician per year to maintain. These estimates include one-time costs associated with switching from paper records to electronic, such as the scanning of existing paper records into the new system. In addition, the hardware and software that are used to run the system need to be updated on a regular basis, which adds another expense.

LACK OF STANDARDS

The inability to share information due to the lack of standards is a major obstacle to EHR adoption. Standards make it possible for systems to effectively share information. Currently, few electronic systems can talk to one another, whether from one physician office to another or from a physician office to an inpatient facility such as a hospital. Major efforts are underway to create such standards (this topic is covered in detail in Chapter 2).

LEARNING CURVE

Providers are concerned that EHR systems are difficult to use and require time-consuming training. There is a significant learning curve for staff members to become proficient with new technology. Small practices especially may not have enough time to train staff members on a new system.

WORKFLOW CHANGES

Technology also alters the workflow in physicians' practices and hospital Health Information Management and billing departments, which can require staff members to make a difficult adjustment. For example, in a practice using an EHR, there is no need to pull charts of patients with upcoming appointments. Papers such as referral letters, lab reports, and copies of prescriptions are not filed in folders, and charts do not have to be filed at the end of the day. While these sound like benefits, the job responsibilities and tasks of staff members must be analyzed and altered as necessary. This is a time-consuming process, and individuals may be resistant to change.

CHANGES IN THE SOFTWARE MARKET

Another problem faced by physicians considering a move to electronic records in practices and hospitals is the possibility that the company providing the software will become obsolete within a year or two. According to some estimates, several hundred physician office EHR products are currently on the market. It is widely assumed that this number will drop below one hundred within the next few years.

PRIVACY AND SECURITY RISKS

One of the greatest challenges to EHR implementation is protecting private information about a patient's past and present health. By its nature, information contained in an electronic health record is stored on a computer and exchanged with other providers and facilities. There is always a risk that computers may be intentionally or unintentionally broken into, or "hacked." The frequent transfer of patient health information from one computer to another over a network, along with the number of people who have access to the record at any one time, increases the likelihood of the information's being obtained by an unauthorized party. In May 2006, over 25 million patient records were compromised when a laptop computer was stolen from a Department of Veterans Affairs employee. Stories like this may make providers and health care institutions hesitant to change their systems from paper to electronic.

Patients may also be wary of electronic health records. Patients share sensitive information with their health care providers and expect it to be kept confidential. There is concern among patients that the use of electronic health information jeopardizes the confidentiality of personal health information. Studies report that 70 percent of Americans believe that the nationwide implementation of an electronic health system would lead to inappropriate disclosure of personal health data as a result of inadequate security. Some individuals fear that their personal health information could be used to deny them employment or health

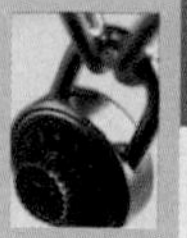

Privacy and Security Alert

Medical Identity Theft

Medical identity theft is a problem on the increase. While most people are familiar with identity theft involving Social Security numbers and credit card numbers, fewer are aware of the dangers of medical identity theft. Medical identity theft can take many forms, including seeking reimbursement for procedures that were never performed, impersonating the patient with the goal of receiving medication, and more. The real danger happens when false data are entered into a patient's health record. The next time the patient goes to the doctor's office, the false information can result in serious problems, such as prescribing the wrong medication or making an incorrect diagnosis.

insurance. If patients do not believe that their personal health information will be adequately protected, they may withhold important health information from their physician and endanger their treatment.

While the HIPAA legislation of 1996 addressed the issue of patient privacy and the security of electronic patient information, there are questions about whether these rules are sufficient to protect data stored in electronic health record systems. The privacy and security issues surrounding electronic health records are discussed in greater detail in Chapter 6.

The Impact of Information Technology on Allied Health Careers

As a profession, health care is an information-intensive field. Every encounter an individual has with the health care system—from seeing a physician, to having blood drawn at a lab, to picking up a prescription at a pharmacy—is documented. The accuracy and availability of this information plays a major role in determining the outcome of a patient's health care experience. Increasingly, health care providers and organizations are using technology to store and maintain patient data. On its own, technology does little to ensure a positive outcome for the patient. The usefulness and value of the information depends on a workforce of skilled professionals capable of creating, managing, and analyzing the data.

Health information technology (HIT) refers to the use of software and hardware to manage health information for clinical and administrative purposes. Students entering an allied health program may choose health information technology (HIT) as their area of concentration. Health information specialists can find employment in organizations that use and manage health information, including physician offices, hospitals, clinics, long-term care facilities, home health agencies, and others. In addition, opportunities exist in pharmaceutical companies, insurance carriers, and companies that provide products to the health care industry.

Whether he or she chooses to specialize in HIT, every graduate of an allied health program will be required to use health information technology once on the job. As the United States moves toward the adoption of electronic health records, the demand for allied health graduates with skills in information technology and familiarity with computers exceeds the supply.

The application of information technology to health care will also result in new careers that have not existed in the past. Some of these new positions include:

- *Clinical analyst:* Designs clinical content for software applications
- *Clinical applications coordinator:* Implements and supports clinical software programs and provides training to new users
- *Enterprise applications specialist:* Facilitates the creation, implementation, and maintenance of organization policies and procedures related to EHR

- *Health information technician:* Provides technical and administrative support for health information services
- *Information privacy coordinator:* Assesses risks to health information security and privacy; monitors privacy compliance issues; and establishes policies and procedures to address privacy and security risks
- *Records and information coordinator:* Provides reference services on electronic systems to departments and individuals, and approves materials for integration into current systems

CERTIFICATION AND LIFELONG LEARNING

The field of health care is always changing. This makes it an exciting area for employment, but it also presents challenges. To keep pace with rapid change, professionals must keep their knowledge and skills current. Education does not end with the awarding of a certificate or a degree; in the health care field, it is a lifelong commitment.

As in other medical fields, individuals with certification generally have an easier time finding employment. Certification acknowledges that an individual has mastered a standard body of knowledge and meets certain competencies. Employers look for certification when filling open positions, and certified individuals usually earn higher salaries than those who are not certified. Certification is offered in most allied health specialties. The field of health information technology offers a number of certifications, including:

- The *Registered Health Information Technician (RHIT)* certification is offered by the American Health Information Management Association (AHIMA; www.ahima.org). RHITs work with patient medical records on a daily basis, performing a range of tasks depending on the setting. Those wishing to take the certification examination must have an associate's degree.
- The *Registered Health Information Administrator (RHIA)* certification, also offered by AHIMA, is intended for individuals who want to work in managerial positions related to HIT. In addition to skills in collecting, interpreting, and analyzing health information, RHIAs are also capable of assuming management positions in which they work with people at all levels of an organization. Individuals must possess a baccalaureate degree to be eligible to take the certification examination.
- The *Certified Professional in Healthcare Information and Management Systems (CPHIMS)* designation is offered by the Healthcare Information and Management Systems Society (HIMSS; www.himss.org). It is intended for healthcare information and management systems professionals who possess a combination of educational and work experience.
- A *Certification in Healthcare Privacy and Security (CHPS)* is offered by AHIMA and signifies competence in designing, implementing, and administering privacy and security measures. A minimum of a baccalaureate degree is required to be considered for the certification.

- Health IT Certification, LLC (www.healthitcertification.com), offers a *Certified Professional in Electronic Health Records (CPEHR)* credential. Individuals who pass the certification examination demonstrate competency in the planning and implementation of electronic health record systems.
- *Medical coding:* A number of certifications in coding are available from AHIMA (www.ahima.org) and from the American Academy of Professional Coders (www.aapc.com). A coder who completes an education program may become an apprentice coder, but full certification is reserved for individuals with on-the-job experience.
- *Tumor registrar:* The *Certified Tumor Registrar (CRT)* certification in tumor registry is available from the National Cancer Registrars Association (NCRA) (www.ncra-usa.org).

OUTLOOK AND SALARIES

The health care field remains one of the fastest growing segments of the economy. From 2004 to 2014, the number of people in older age groups will grow faster than the total population. These individuals generally have higher-than-average health care needs, so more jobs will be created. In addition, people are living longer. As a result of advances in medical technology, patients with serious illnesses will survive longer than they had in the past, and they will require care. Employment growth is predicted to account for approximately 3.6 million new jobs in the 2004 to 2014 time period.

The 2006 AHIMA Salary Study ("The Results Are In: 2006 Salary Study." *AHIMA Advantage* 10, no. 7, 2006) reports the following median annual incomes for HIT professionals:

Medical records analyst	$40,419
Tumor/cancer registrar	$41,072
Coding professional	$43,995
Data quality analyst	$50,190
Information security officer	$55,655

While these are reported as median salaries, it is important to note that salaries vary according to a number of factors, such as the location of the job (urban or rural), the size of the organization, the education and experience of the individual, and other factors.

CHAPTER REVIEW

CHAPTER SUMMARY

1. Paper-based medical records are no longer adequate. Individuals are more likely to be treated by multiple providers in multiple facilities. To receive safe and effective care, all providers need access to information in the patient's health record. This is not possible with paper records. Many medical errors are a result of misplaced or lost medical records and handwriting errors, particularly in prescriptions for medication. The cost of health care is rising, and a significant amount of money is spent on administrative processes still based on paper record-keeping.

2. Medical liability premiums for health care providers have become more costly, causing some doctors to leave the field. Corporations that provide health insurance coverage to their employees are finding it more difficult to pay for these benefits, and workers are being asked to pay more of the cost.

3. The federal government has played a significant role in bringing about changes in the health care system. HIPAA legislation passed in 1996 established standards that made it possible for insurance claims to be submitted electronically in a common format. HIPAA also set standards for ensuring the privacy and security of personal health information. The Medicare Prescription Drug, Improvement, and Modernization Act of 2003 encourages the use of electronic prescribing technology. In 2004, President George W. Bush set a goal of establishing electronic health records for all Americans by the year 2014.

4. Electronic medical records are computerized versions of paper charts. They are created and maintained by a single provider. Electronic health records are a computerized lifelong health care record that includes information from multiple providers and facilities. The information in the record is shared among providers treating the patient. Electronic health records are used by health care professionals. Personal health records are online files created and maintained by individuals. They contain information such as current medications, allergies, health insurance details, medical history, and test results.

5. Medical records in acute care settings focus on short-term events, while records in ambulatory care settings track a person's symptoms, diagnoses, and treatment over time. Acute care records include admission and discharge notes, which are not part of an ambulatory care record. A major part of an ambulatory care record is the physician's notes created during a patient encounter.

6. The eight core functions of an electronic health record are:
   1. Health information and data elements
   2. Results management
   3. Order management
   4. Decision support
   5. Electronic communication and connectivity
   6. Patient support
   7. Administrative support
   8. Population reporting and management
7. Electronic health records offer a number of advantages when compared with paper records. These advantages include a reduction in the number of medical errors, a higher quality of care for patients, and time and cost savings due to increased efficiency and productivity.
8. Electronic health records are not in widespread use today for a number of reasons: the cost of implementation, the lack of standards, a significant learning curve for staff members, workflow changes, and privacy and security risks to personal health information.
9. Students entering the field of health information technology may choose from a number of specialties, including medical record coder/abstractor, discharge analyst (acute care), tumor registrar, and quality analyst.

CHECK YOUR UNDERSTANDING

Part 1. Write *T* or **F** in the blank to indicate whether you think the statement is true or false.

_____ **1.** The use of outdated systems has been cited as a cause of financial waste in the American health care system.

_____ **2.** Patients purchase medical liability insurance to protect themselves from being victims of medical errors.

_____ **3.** The Medicare Prescription Drug, Improvement, and Modernization Act of 2003 (MMA) requires individuals covered by Medicare to participate in a prescription drug program.

_____ **4.** The users of electronic health records are health care professionals.

_____ **5.** A personal health record (PHR) contains admission and discharge summaries.

_____ **6.** A physician office and an outpatient clinic are examples of ambulatory care facilities.

_____ **7.** Health information exchanges (HIE) are nationwide health-care networks.

_____ **8.** Electronic health record systems are inexpensive and easy to learn.

_____ **9.** Electronic health records are less prone to privacy and security issues than are paper-based records.

_____ **10.** Certification in a field of study represents mastery of a body of knowledge.

Part 2. Match each term below with its correct definition.

_____ **11.** continuity of care

_____ **12.** electronic prescribing

_____ **13.** standards

_____ **14.** electronic health record (EHR)

_____ **15.** pay for performance

_____ **16.** evidence-based medicine

_____ **17.** Nationwide Health Information Network (NHIN)

_____ **18.** electronic medical record (EMR)

_____ **19.** personal health record (PHR)

_____ **20.** acute care

a. A computerized, record of one physician's encounters with a patient over time, including medical history, diagnosis, treatment, and prognosis.

b. The delivery of appropriate and consistent care to an individual over the course of time.

c. The use of financial incentives to improve the quality and efficiency of health care services.

d. Treatment provided in an inpatient setting, such as a hospital, for urgent problems that cannot be handled in another setting.

e. A comprehensive record of health information that is created and maintained by an individual over time.

f. A computer-based communication system that allows prescriptions to be transmitted electronically from physician to pharmacist.

g. A set of commonly agreed-on specifications.

h. A computerized lifelong health care record for an individual that incorporates data from all sources.

i. Medical care that is based on the latest and most accurate clinical research in making decisions about the care of patients.

j. A nationwide interconnected computer network that facilitates the secure exchange of health care information.

THINKING ABOUT THE ISSUES

Part 3. In the space provided, write a brief paragraph describing your thoughts on the following issues.

21. Why is there a need to change from paper records to electronic records?

___

___

22. Why have physicians been slow to change to electronic records?

___

___

23. Can you think of any instances in which paper medical records would be preferred over electronic records?

___

___

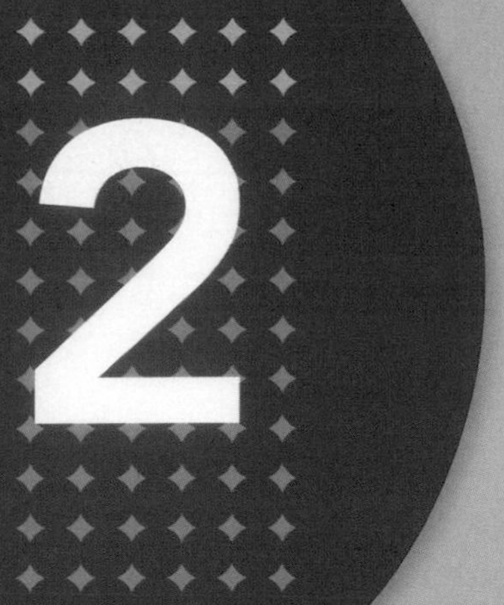

2 Transitioning to an Electronic Health Record and the Need for Clinical Information Standards

CHAPTER OUTLINE

Converting Existing Charts to an Electronic Health Record
- *Total Conversion*
- *Incremental Conversion*
- *Hybrid Conversion*

Entering Live Data in an Electronic Health Record
- *Dictation and Transcription*
- *Clinical Templates*
- *Voice Recognition*
- *Scanning*

Computer Requirements for Electronic Health Records
- *Input Devices*
- *Networks*

EHR Hosting Choices: Local Versus Application Service Provider
- *Locally Hosted Model*
- *Application Service Provider (ASP) Model*
- *Blended or Hybrid Systems*

The Importance of Clinical Standards

Types of Clinical Information Standards
- *Clinical Vocabularies*
- *Classification Systems*
- *Messaging Standards*
- *Electronic Health Record Content Standards*

Voluntary Versus Mandatory Standards

LEARNING OUTCOMES

After completing this chapter, you will be able to define key terms and:

1. Describe the major strategies for converting paper-based charts to EHR.
2. List the four ways of entering live patient data into EHR.
3. Explain how desktop, laptop, and tablet computers differ.
4. Discuss the advantages of wireless networks in health care.
5. Explain the major difference between locally hosted and ASP hosting models.
6. Discuss why the adoption of clinical standards is critical to the successful implementation of electronic health records.
7. Describe the difference between clinical vocabularies and classification systems.
8. List four messaging standards used with electronic health records.
9. Describe the significance of the Medicare Prescription Drug and Modernization Act of 2003 in the adoption of clinical standards.

KEY TERMS

application service provider (ASP)
classification systems
clients
clinical templates
clinical vocabularies
Current Procedural Terminology (CPT)
content standards
desktop computer
Digital Imaging and Communications in Medicine (DICOM)
Healthcare Common Procedure Coding System (HCPCS), Level II
Health Level Seven (HL7)
hybrid conversions
incremental conversion
Institute of Electrical and Electronics Engineers 1073 (IEEE1073)
International Classification of Diseases, Ninth Revision
interoperable
laptop computer
locally hosted
Logical Observation Identifiers Names and Codes (LOINC)
messaging standards
National Council for Prescription Drug Program (NCPDP)
network
outsourcing
personal digital assistant (PDA)
picture archiving and communication system (PACS)
scanning
server
smart phones
Systematized Nomenclature of Medicine Clinical Terms (SNOMED-CT)
tablet computer
total conversion
Unified Medical Language System (UMLS)
voice recognition
wired network
wireless networks
workstations

Why This Chapter Is Important to You

The information in this chapter will enable you to:

- Understand the ways to convert existing paper-based patient charts to electronic health records.
- Understand how information is entered in electronic health records.
- Understand how computers share information.
- Understand the advantages of application service providers (ASP).
- Understand why clinical standards are so important.
- Understand the types of standards necessary for electronic health records.

The greatest value of an electronic health record (EHR) is its ability to provide complete, accurate, and timely access to patient information. Medical providers use information in the EHR to diagnose a patient's condition and make decisions about the best treatment. For this reason, the accuracy and completeness of the data are critical not only to a successful EHR, but also to the health and well-being of patients.

The information in an EHR comes from many different sources—physicians, nursing staff, medical assistants, technicians, and other allied health professionals working in laboratories, hospitals, insurance companies, and government agencies, among other settings. The words to describe a patient's condition may differ depending on who is capturing the information, the method used to record the information, and how the information will be used. The use of different terms to indicate the same condition or treatment makes it difficult to share patient data. For clinical information to be useful, it must use common terminology so that words have the same meaning to all individuals and organizations in the health care system. This requires the use of a set of clinical standards that can be incorporated into such information systems as electronic health records.

At the same time, most clinical information about medical practices' patients is still contained in paper charts. These charts contain descriptions of problems, diagnoses, assessments, interventions, test results, procedures, and outcomes, as well as telephone messages, copies of insurance cards, referral letters, and more. Moving from paper charts to electronic health records is a major undertaking. Each piece of data in the patient chart has a value and a cost associated with conversion to an electronic format. Before beginning any conversion of paper records, it is important to determine which patient records will be included in the transfer and what information within each record should be converted.

Converting Existing Charts to an Electronic Health Record

There are a number of conversion strategies to choose from, and the decision about which strategy to choose depends on the unique needs of the health care facility. When considering the transition of paper records to an EHR, it is important to determine how much historical information in the patient record should be converted. For example, routine cholesterol tests taken once a year may not be important after they are three or four years old.

TOTAL CONVERSION

total conversion paper to electronic document conversion method by an external company.

In the **total conversion** approach, a practice outsources the conversion process to an external company. Some companies specialize in converting paper charts to digital images, with prices ranging from $0.25 per page to as much as $1.00 a page. If a practice has two thousand patient charts and each chart averages thirty pages, total data conversion will cost between $15,000 and $60,000.

The advantages of total conversion include the following:

- All patient data are converted at once and are available in the EHR.
- Office staff members do not need to take time away from regular tasks to manually enter data.

The disadvantages of total conversion include:

- Cost
- The conversion of unnecessary data, such as data for patients who will not visit the practice again
- A higher error rate because of lack of in-house oversight of conversion

INCREMENTAL CONVERSION

An alternate approach to the total conversion strategy is to convert the data incrementally, based on the assumption that electronic access to the record is required only for those patients for whom appointments are scheduled. This is known as **incremental conversion.**

incremental conversion gradual paper to electronic document conversion process.

Practices commonly classify patients as active or inactive. While the exact definitions vary, a patient who has not visited the practice for certain period of time is considered inactive. Records for inactive patients can be archived in storage and not converted to the EHR system. If the charts are needed in the future, they can be retrieved and converted at that time. This saves the practice the expense of converting records that may not be needed. For patients classified as active, paper records can be converted to the EHR in advance of their next scheduled office visits. Once the desired information from paper charts has been entered into the EHR system, the paper record can be archived.

The advantages of an incremental approach are:

- Cost savings because the conversion is done by the office staff
- A smoother transition with less impact on day-to-day practice operation because the data are converted gradually

The disadvantages of an incremental approach are the following:

- Occasional use of archived paper charts may be necessary.
- Not all patient data are available in the EHR at once.

HYBRID CONVERSION

Many practices use a combination of strategies, which are called **hybrid conversions.** In a hybrid approach, some records may be outsourced, and others are converted in-house. **Outsourcing** is the process of an organization contracting with an outside company for completion of all or part of a job. For example, a practice may outsource the conversion of charts of active patients who do not have

hybrid conversions paper to electronic document conversion process that combines approaches.

outsourcing is the process of an organization contracting with an outside company for completion of all or part of a job.

appointments within ninety days, while preferring to convert patients with near-term appointments internally. In another hybrid scenario, a practice begins the conversion process in-house, in part to help identify the specific data that are required for the practice's needs. Once the key information has been identified, the entry of the remaining patient charts may be outsourced.

Entering Live Data in an Electronic Health Record

Once existing paper charts have been converted to the electronic health record system, "live" data must be recorded when patients visit the practice. There are a number of ways for patient information to be entered in an EHR, including dictation, clinical templates, voice recognition, and document scanning. Physicians do not have to choose one of these methods; most EHR systems accommodate more than one. Each approach has advantages and disadvantages.

DICTATION AND TRANSCRIPTION

Even after a successful transition to an EHR, many physicians prefer to continue using dictation as a means of entering progress notes. Dictation and transcription have been the traditional method of documenting patient encounters. The flow of dictation is illustrated in Figure 2-1. A medical provider dictates the medical note into a telephone or a recording device. A medical transcriptionist receives the dictation and transcribes it on a computer. After review, the final computerized word processing file is then e-mailed to the health care provider, or the file is transferred to a website and is later downloaded by the provider. It is then added to the patient's electronic record.

Dictation corresponds intuitively to the physician's usual way of working. It allows the physician to describe a patient's condition in his or her own words, reflecting both content and context. Physicians can dictate anytime, anywhere, using a telephone, a computer, or another recording device. By using this traditional method of documenting

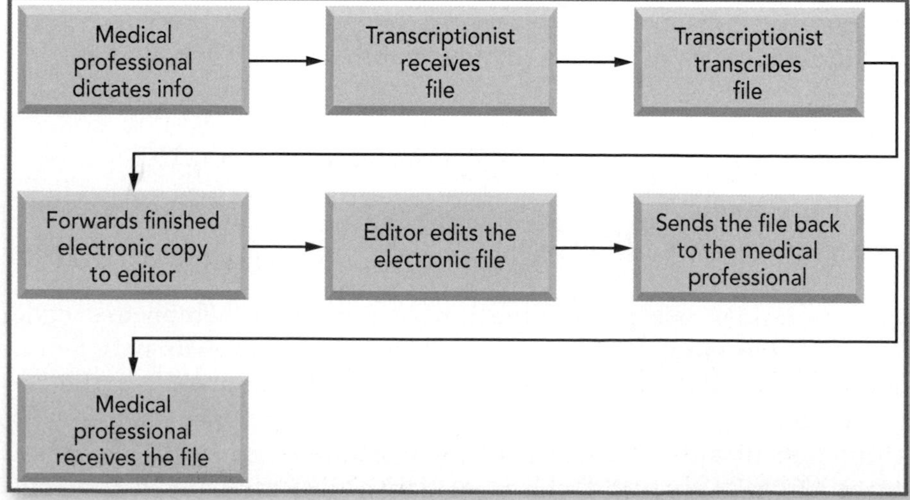

Figure 2-1
Flow of dictation and transcription.

patient care, providers need not change the way they practice to accommodate an EHR system.

The benefits of dictation and transcription are as follows:

- Physicians who are uncomfortable with computers in the examination room can still use an EHR.
- Dictation retains the narrative form of documentation that promotes detail, context, and comprehensiveness.
- The method does not require additional training for physicians.

The drawbacks of dictation include these:

- Transcribed reports are not immediately accessible.
- Dictation incurs transcription costs.
- The physician or an assistant must review and edit files.
- Detail is more likely to be omitted or forgotten if data are not captured at the point-of-care.

CLINICAL TEMPLATES

Most EHR systems allow providers to generate clinical documentation by making selections from clinical templates. **Clinical templates** are structured progress notes that physicians use to document patient encounters in an EHR. In response to options on the computer screen, providers point and click to select conditions observed in a given patient. The end result is a file that closely resembles a traditional progress note.

clinical templates structured progress notes that document patient encounters in an EHR.

The advantages of clinical templates include the following:

- Repetitive information, such as review of systems, problem lists, and patient history, is quickly documented.
- Data appear in the patient's record as soon as the information is captured.
- Templates can be customized to meet the needs of the practice.
- Transcription costs are reduced.
- Data are standardized and consistent.

The disadvantages of clinical templates include these:

- The physician must change his or her standard way of documenting the patient encounter.
- The physician may not be comfortable using the computer while in the examination room with the patient.

VOICE RECOGNITION

Voice recognition offers the promise of reducing the need for keyboard entry while providing a cost-effective alternative to traditional

voice recognition method of entering information via a microphone connected to a computer.

transcription. With **voice recognition,** providers dictate using a microphone connected to a desktop or laptop computer equipped with special voice recognition software. The software converts the recording into an electronic file, which is then reviewed and entered into an EHR. With recent technological advances, voice recognition is becoming a viable means of data entry.

The advantages of voice recognition are these:

- Transcription costs are reduced.
- Information is available in medical record in less time than with standard dictation and transcription methods.
- Physicians are comfortable with the approach because it is similar to traditional dictation.

The disadvantages of voice recognition include:

- The possibility of an unacceptable accuracy rate if interference such as background noise is present
- The need for the physician or an assistant to review and edit the files
- The costs associated with purchasing voice recognition equipment and software

SCANNING

scanning method for electronically capturing text and images from paper documents.

Scanning is a method of capturing electronic text or images from paper documents. A sheet of paper is fed through a scanning device, and whatever is on the paper appears on a computer screen. If the paper contains an image, it can be saved in a graphics file format such as JPG and stored in an EHR system. If the paper contains text, an optical character recognition (OCR) software program translates the text into a word processing document that can be stored in the EHR.

The benefit of scanning is the efficient entry of text and images into an EHR.

The drawbacks of scanning include these:

- Additional hardware is required if scanning is done in-house.
- Text files captured by OCR software must be reviewed for accuracy.

Computer Requirements for Electronic Health Records

Implementing an EHR system often requires the medical practice or hospital to upgrade its computer system. Two of the most important types of hardware for EHR systems are input devices and communications networks. Input devices are used to enter information into the EHR; networks allow different devices to exchange information electronically.

INPUT DEVICES

Workstations are the hardware devices used to access the electronic health record software as well as the word processing, practice management, and other software. There are three common types of workstations: the desktop computer, the laptop computer, and the tablet PC. The personal digital assistant, or PDA, while not considered a workstation, can also be used to enter information in an EHR.

workstations hardware devices used to access the electronic health record and other software.

Desktop Computers

The **desktop computer** is a fixed, hardwired computer that stays in one location and cannot easily be moved from room to room. It usually has a standard configuration consisting of a central processing unit (CPU), a monitor, a keyboard, and a mouse. The desktop computer can function independently or can share data with other devices in a network.

desktop computer fixed, hardwired computer.

Desktop computers have the following advantages:

- They do not cost a lot.
- They are relatively inexpensive to repair and replace.
- They are capable of running almost all software programs.
- Additional devices such as microphones, speakers, and headsets can be added at a low cost.

Their disadvantages are that they:

- Must be purchased for each location in the office that requires access to the EHR
- Take up more physical space than other workstations

Laptop Computers

A **laptop computer** is a fully functioning computer that is small enough to be portable. Like desktop computers, laptops can function as a stand-alone computer or can connect to a network. A laptop can also serve as a desktop machine if it is connected to a larger monitor and a standard keyboard through a hardware device known as a docking station.

laptop computer fully functioning portable computer.

A laptop computer:

- Is portable—can be carried from room to room
- Requires less space than a desktop computer
- Can easily be turned to allow patients to view information on the screen
- Accepts standard computer inputs such as a keyboard and a mouse

However, a laptop computer has a relatively high initial cost, and repairs and maintenance are usually more expensive than for desktop computers. It is also more likely than a desktop computer to be lost or stolen, putting information at risk.

Tablet Computers

tablet computer portable computer with built-in handwriting and voice recognition software.

The **tablet computer,** or tablet PC, is a third type of workstation that contains voice recognition software and that also has built-in handwriting software. Using the handwriting recognition feature, a user can write on the screen using a stylus, much as he or she would write on a piece of paper. The handwritten words are then saved as a word processing file. The voice recognition feature allows physicians to record their notes directly into the tablet PC, which saves the recording as a text file.

Tablet PCs offer physicians a workflow that is similar to the traditional dictation methodology—handwriting notes or dictating them into a recording device. This ability to capture patient information at the point-of-care reduces the possibility of errors in clinical documentation.

A tablet PC:

- Is portable and lightweight, usually weighing less than a laptop
- Does not require a keyboard
- Can translate poor handwriting into legible text

There are disadvantage to tablet PCs:

- Writing with a stylus takes practice.
- Handwriting recognition dictionaries have not yet fully integrated medical terminology and acronyms, so editing is required.
- There is limited availability of software designed to take advantage of tablet capabilities.
- More likely than a desktop computer to be lost or stolen.

Personal Digital Assistants (PDAs) and Smart Phones

personal digital assistants (PDA) handheld devices used to search for information, write prescriptions, and handle e-mail.

smart phones handheld devices similar to personal digital assistants (PDAs) that are also cell phones.

Personal digital assistants (PDAs), also known as handheld PCs, are used for tasks such as searching for medical reference information, writing prescriptions, sending and receiving e-mail, and accessing the Internet (see Figure 2-2). **Smart phones** are are similar to PDAs, but can also function as cell phones. PDAs and smart phones are most useful for activities that do not require a large screen for viewing data. Because of their small size and portability, physicians are likely to be carrying them when information is needed. The ability to access tools such as clinical guidelines and drug interaction databases at the point-of-care represents one of the most valuable features these portable devices.

PDAs and smart phones are small and easy to carry, so they are more likely than workstations to be available when needed.

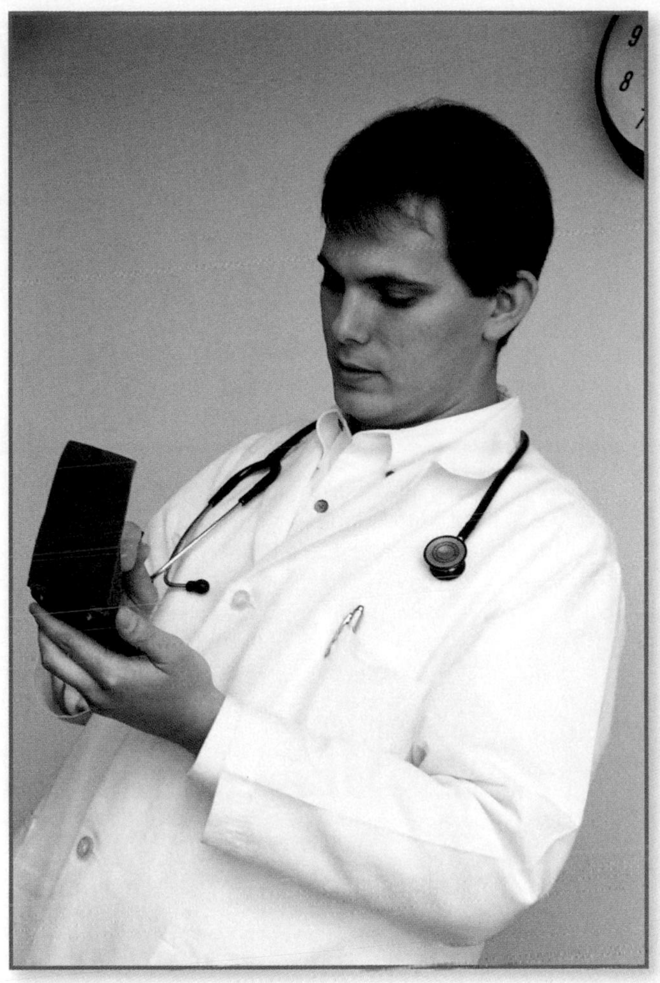

Figure 2-2

A healthcare professional using a portable digital assistant (PDA).

The downside is that these devices have:

- Limited screen size
- Limited functionality (not all programs run on a PDA)
- Restricted battery life

NETWORKS

Once patient information has been entered in the EHR program using a workstation, it needs to be shared among appropriate health care professionals. This requires a network. The term **network** refers to all the equipment required to enable computers and other types of hardware to exchange information electronically.

network equipment that enables computers to exchange information electronically.

Key hardware components in the network are the server and the clients. A **server** is a powerful computer that houses software applications and data. It is connected to other computers through the network. The computers that access the server through the network are called **clients.** The client computer makes a request to the server, and the server transmits the information to the client. The server provides the clients with access to EHR programs, practice management programs, word processing software, e-mail programs, and so on, as well as to such practice data as patient records and scheduling information. A

server powerful computer that houses software applications and data.

clients computers that access a server through a network.

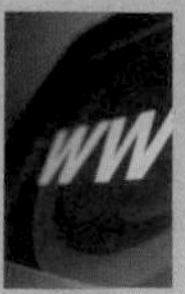

Chapter 2 Online Discovery

To address the unique needs of providers, some manufacturers are developing tablet PCs that are designed specifically for the health care field. One example is the Motion C5. Open your Internet browser, and go to www.motioncomputing.com/flash/intel/index.html to view a video about the device.

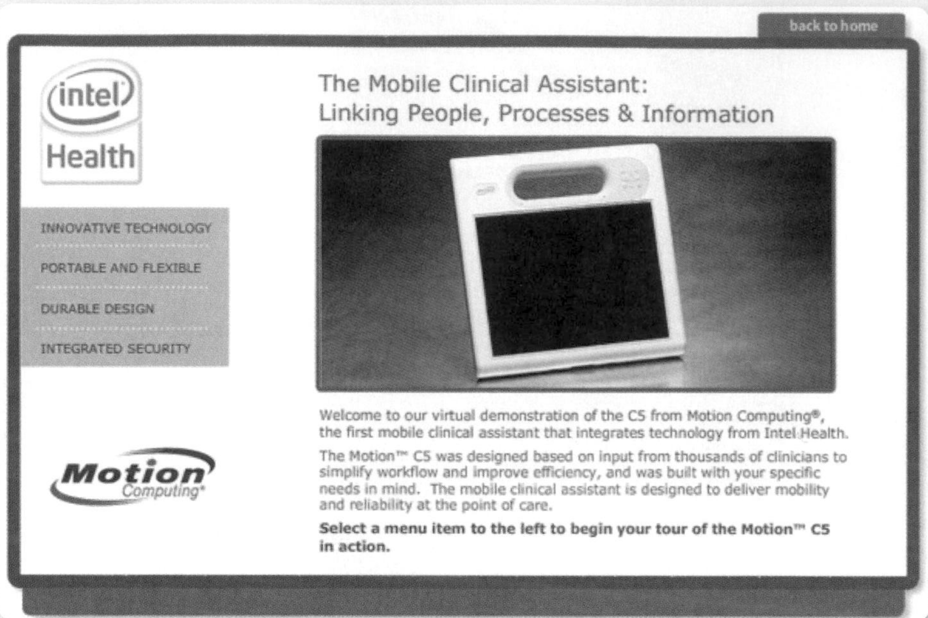

After the first video finishes, click the phrase "Innovative technology" in the blue area on the left side of the screen to start another brief video. When it is finished, click the other topics listed in the blue area, one at a time. Then answer the questions below.

Thinking About It

1. What are the advantages of a tablet PC over other workstations?

____

2. How can the use of a tablet PC reduce the chance of errors?

____

3. What are the security features of this tablet PC?

____

When you are finished viewing the videos and answering the questions, close your web browser.

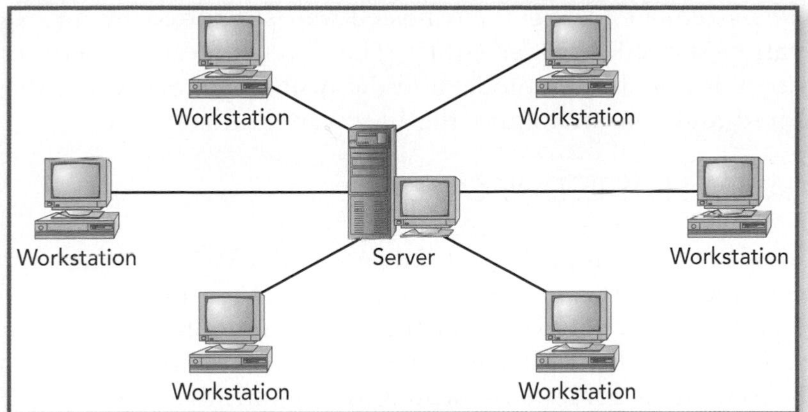

Figure 2-3

A client-server network.

server allows simultaneous access from more than one computer. When someone with a computer accesses the Internet to perform a search using Google, client-server technology is involved (see Figure 2-3). The search is not performed on the person's desktop computer. It is conducted on one of Google's servers, and the results are returned to the desktop computer, which in this case is the client.

Wired and Wireless Networks

The network that connects the server to the clients can be wired or wireless. On a **wired network,** all the client computers are connected with physical wiring called Ethernet cable that transports data to and from the server.

wired network network in which computers are connected via Ethernet cable.

Wireless networks, also known as "Wi-Fi," allow multiple computers to access a server or the Internet without using cables. Computers have wireless adapters that send information via radio signals and an antenna. The signals are received by an antenna and a wireless adapter in another computer, decoded, and then translated back into radio signals and sent back to the original computer.

wireless network network in which computers access servers without cables.

With a wireless network, portable computers, such as laptops and tablet PCs, can be transported from room to room and still maintain a network connection. This offers major advantages in the health care environment. A wireless network makes it possible for physicians to access medical reference tools in the examination room or at a patient's bedside. Other tasks, such as basic charge capture, prescription writing, clinical documentation, and messaging, are more convenient with a wireless network.

Wireless networks are susceptible to security breaches. A number of security features are available that can make breaking into wireless networks almost impossible. This topic is covered in Chapter 6.

EHR Hosting Choices: Local Versus Application Service Provider

In recent years, the emergence of reliable broadband technology has allowed medical professionals to choose between having their computer hardware and software applications housed and maintained on-site (locally hosted) or having them hosted and supported by an external application service provider (ASP). The core differences between the traditional locally hosted model and the ASP model are where the data are stored and who maintains the hardware and software.

LOCALLY HOSTED MODEL

locally hosted hosting model in which hardware and software are housed on-site.

In a **locally hosted** model, the hardware and software required to run an electronic health record program are located on-site at the provider's location. The EHR software and the data are stored on a centralized server. The medical staff accesses the programs and information on the server from client computers located throughout the office or facility.

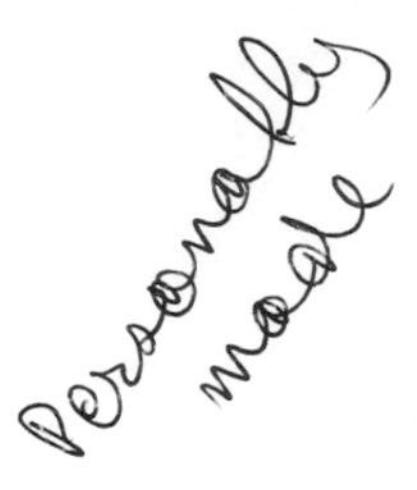

Advantages of locally hosted systems include these:

- The practice maintains direct control of systems.
- Ongoing maintenance fees are lower.
- There is reduced reliance on external sources.

Disadvantages of locally hosted systems include:

- Higher start-up costs
- Need to purchase computer hardware (servers, backup devices, uninterruptible power supplies)
- Greater IT support costs for system administration and maintenance
- Need for office space to house hardware

APPLICATION SERVICE PROVIDER (ASP) MODEL

application service provider (ASP) model in which software and data are housed on an external company's servers.

An alternative to the traditional approach of purchasing, installing, and maintaining computer hardware and software is the **application service provider (ASP)** model. In an ASP, an external company houses the software and data on servers at its site. Medical providers usually access the application via the Internet using a web-based browser such as Internet Explorer. The software can also be installed and run on computers in the health care facility. In either case, data are stored and maintained at the vendor's site rather than on a file server at the medical facility.

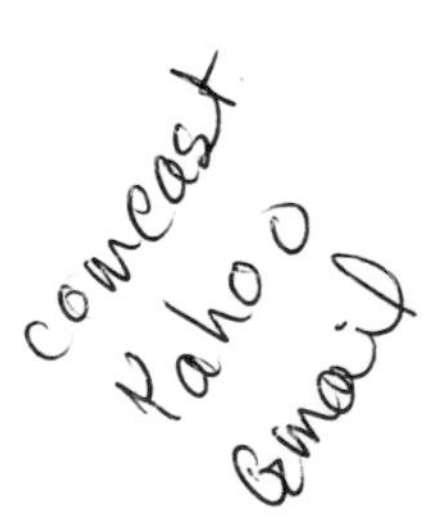

In an ASP environment, the user pays a monthly fee for use of the ASP. In return, the hosting company assumes responsibility for supporting both the hardware and the software, including software maintenance and upgrades, server maintenance, data backup, and technical support. This reduces the information technology burden on the medical office.

Because of the advantages offered by this approach, ASPs are becoming more popular in health care organizations. Their advantages include the following:

- Users do not have to purchase expensive computer hardware or hire information technology personnel.
- Spending can take place in increments (monthly payments) rather than all at once.

- Data are backed up by the vendor on a regular basis.
- The EHR can start running more quickly than with locally hosted models.
- Energy costs are lower since there is less in-house equipment to run.

There are several drawbacks to ASPs, including:

- The need for a broadband Internet connection to access data, with the risk of outages.
- Possible slowdown of the system when transferring large files, such as scanned images.
- Greater privacy and security concerns, since patient data are stored off-site.

BLENDED OR HYBRID SYSTEMS

Some users choose a blended or hybrid approach; they select an ASP model but have a server located in their offices that receives a backup of data from the ASP provider every night. This eliminates the risk of losing access to data should an Internet connection go down.

The Importance of Clinical Standards

Once paper charts have been converted to electronic files and current encounters are recorded electronically, the information in the patient's record can be accessed wherever and whenever it is needed. However, for the information to be useful to different providers in different settings, different computer systems must be **interoperable;** that is, they must be able to exchange information and use the information in a meaningful way. For computer systems to be considered interoperable, they must share the same clinical data standards.

interoperable systems that can exchange information and use the information in a meaningful way.

Clinical information encompasses the details of a patient's health information, including:

- The patient's health problems
- The physician's observation of the patient
- The results of tests performed to determine the patient's illness
- The patient's diagnoses
- The procedures performed or treatment given
- The outcome of the interventions

Standards exist in all aspects of life. During a typical day, we wake to an alarm clock that follows universal time, obey traffic signals while driving to work, and use seven- and ten-digit telephone numbers when making phone calls. Standards ensure consistency, reliability, and safety. Developing a standard for traffic signals was relatively simple—green for go, yellow for caution, and red for stop. Medical information, in contrast, is detailed and complex.

Case Study

CONVERTING PAPER RECORDS TO AN ELECTRONIC HEALTH RECORD

West Side Medical Associates

About the Clinic

Clinic name: West Side Medical Associates

Specialty: Family Medicine

Location: Jacksonville, FL

About the Personnel

Physicians: David Chen, MD, Sheila Roth, MD

Nurse-practitioner: Sarina Perez

Medical assistant: Amy Wilmot

Billing/coding department: Megan Riley

Receptionist/front desk: The (medical assistant and the billing/coding person share receptionist duty).

Note to the student: This is one of a number of case studies illustrating the differences between a paper-based medical office and an electronic medical office. These case studies will take you through many of the everyday events in a medical office. This particular case revolves around issues with an incremental approach to converting paper charts to electronic records.

Dr. David Chen, the senior physician at West Side Medical Associates, is excited about the new technology. He has been using a tablet PC to record patient encounters for the last six months. Amy Wilmot, his medical assistant, transcribes and prints his notes and files the paper record in the patient's chart.

After much persuading, Dr. Chen has convinced the rest of the staff that it is time to convert to an EHR. During the past month, the small staff of the West Side Medical Associates has received training in EHR from a local medical software vendor. Last week Megan Riley, who generally does billing and coding, and Amy Wilmot successfully converted the paper files for all the patients scheduled to see Dr. Chen and Dr. Roth today and tomorrow.

Consider a patient's visit to a physician's office. A physician may indicate that a patient has low blood sugar by referring to the condition as hypoglycemia, while the report from the lab would read "Glucose 60 mg/dl." The terms used can also vary from one doctor to another. One physician might use the abbreviation *MI* in the patient record to indicate a myocardial infarction, while another physician might record the same incident as 410.00, which is a diagnosis code for myocardial infarction. In both instances, health care professionals would understand that the two concepts refer to the same condition. A computer, however, would not know that *hypoglycemia* and *Glucose 60 mg/dl* refer to low blood sugar, or that *MI* and *410.00* indicate myocardial infarction. To solve this problem, a set of common clinical standards must be used by all providers and institutions that contribute information to a patient's record. While use of standard code sets for administrative functions such as billing became a requirement with the passage of HIPAA legislation in 1996, no such mandatory standards have been adopted for clinical information.

Today was the big day when the practice would test the EHR system. Dr. Chen took his tablet PC into the examination room to meet with Joshua Hart. Joshua is a fifty-five-year old elementary school principal diagnosed with hypertension. He has recently been put on medication. The purpose of his visit today is a three-month review of the effectiveness of the medication.

Upon her arrival at the medical practice, Amy checked Joshua's vital signs and entered the information directly onto her laptop. As Dr. Chen entered the examining room, he pulled up Joshua's electronic chart on his tablet PC and immediately saw that his blood pressure was within the normal range. After a brief conversation with Joshua, in which he asked him a series of questions (prompted by a template in the EHR) and recorded his responses on the tablet PC with a stylus, Dr. Chen feels comfortable renewing the medication for another three months. Using the e-prescribe feature of the EHR, he enters the prescription information and clicks the send button. The order to refill the medication goes directly to Joshua's local pharmacy, and the medication will be available for him to pick up when he arrives.

A flashing button on the toolbar of his PC monitor alerts Dr. Chen that his next patient is waiting, and he says good-bye to Joshua and leaves the examining room. Dr. Chen is glad he persuaded the staff to go through the costly and time-consuming process of converting some of the paper charts to an electronic system. This first encounter worked like a charm.

Dr. Roth, another physician at West Side, is examining Angelo LoSapio, who was in a minor car accident over the weekend. Mr. LoSapio called the office early this morning complaining of shoulder pain. Since this was an unscheduled visit, Mr. LoSapio's chart had not been converted to the EHR. Dr. Roth must wait while Amy retrieves the paper chart from the filing room.

What Do You Think?

1. What information did Dr. Chen have available to him when he pulled up Joshua's EMR?
2. What paper-based steps were eliminated in the patient encounter with Joshua Hart?
3. How does EHR also benefit the patient?

Types of Clinical Information Standards

For electronic health record systems to share clinical information, clinical information standards are needed for vocabularies, classifications, messaging, and content. Vocabularies provide the common medical language necessary, and classification systems group these terms into categories. Messaging standards enable computer systems to exchange information with one another. Content standards specify the type of information that is included in an information system.

CLINICAL VOCABULARIES

Clinical vocabularies, also known as *nomenclatures*, are sets of common definitions for medical terms that facilitate communication by minimizing ambiguity. A shared vocabulary leads to consistent descriptions of a patient's medical condition regardless of where the data were

clinical vocabularies common definitions of medical terms that minimize ambiguity.

created. Much like a dictionary does for language, vocabulary standards define the terms and codes used for clinical information.

The use of a shared vocabulary helps in the clinical care delivery process by facilitating the understanding of information. Without a common vocabulary, information can be transmitted from one system to another, but the data may have different meanings in each system. Clinical vocabularies that are particularly relevant to electronic health records include SNOMED-CT, LOINC, and UMLS.

SNOMED-CT

Systematized Nomenclature of Medicine Clinical Terms (SNOMED-CT) comprehensive clinical vocabulary of all terms used in medicine.

Systematized Nomenclature of Medicine Clinical Terms (SNOMED-CT) is a comprehensive clinical vocabulary designed to encompass all the terms used in medicine, including procedures and diagnoses. SNOMED-CT provides a mechanism to capture the detail needed to support classification systems and much more. It was developed by the College of American Pathologists (CAP).

Vocabularies such as SNOMED CT provide the complete clinical detail of a health care encounter. SNOMED CT is used for many health care applications, including electronic medical records, clinical decision making, medical research, and clinical trials.

Using SNOMED-CT, all information in a patient medical record can be coded, including signs and symptoms, diagnoses and procedures, and occupational history, as well as the origins of illness including infectious conditions, genetic conditions, and physical causes of injury. Figure 2-4 shows a sample SNOMED-CT screen.

LOINC

Logical Observation Identifiers Names and Codes (LOINC) universal terms and codes for electronic exchange of laboratory results and clinical observations.

Logical Observation Identifiers Names and Codes (LOINC) is a set of universal terms and codes used for the electronic exchange of

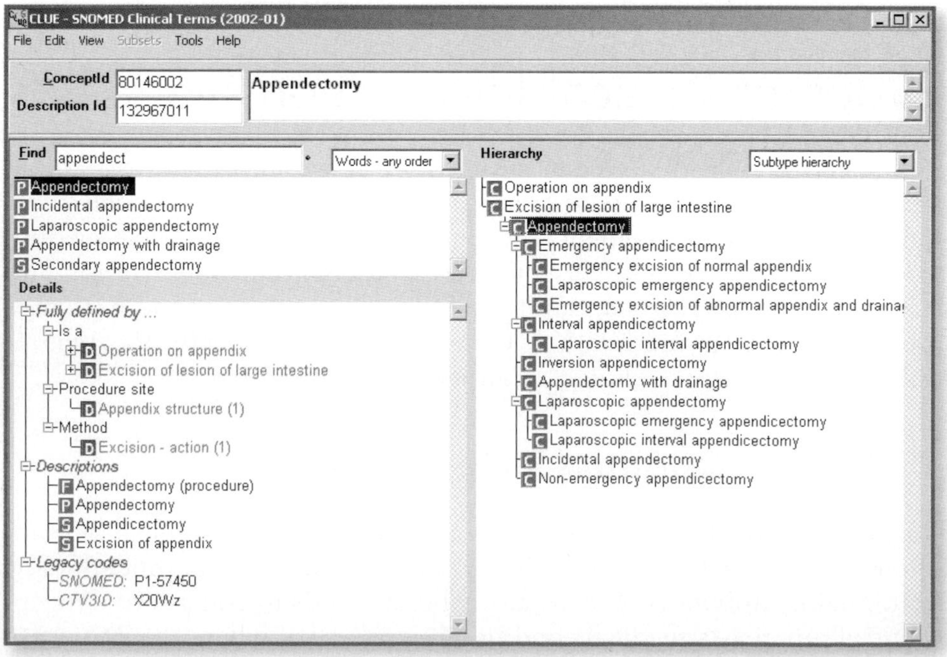

Figure 2-4
SNOMED-CT screen for appendectomy.

laboratory results and clinical observations. The LOINC standards allow results from different laboratories to be recognized and understood regardless of their origin. For example, one laboratory uses the code C1231 for serum sodium, while a different lab uses the code SNA. Before LOINC was developed, every laboratory had its own unique code for every test observation. This made it difficult for office practices, hospitals, public health departments, and others to share test results.

UMLS

The U.S. National Library of Medicine **Unified Medical Language System (UMLS)** is a reference database of medical vocabularies. While originally developed to suggest translations among terminologies, today it also serves as the major thesaurus of medical terms. The UMLS contains over one hundred separate information sources. By grouping alternative terms from different vocabularies together by concept, UMLS make it easier for health professionals and researchers to retrieve and integrate relevant information from different sources. The website for the UMLS (http://www.nlm.nih.gov/research/umls/umlsmain.html.) appears in Figure 2-5.

Unified Medical Language System (UMLS) major thesaurus database of medical terms.

CLASSIFICATION SYSTEMS

While vocabulary systems encompass the entire subject field and support detailed descriptions, **classification systems** organize related terms into categories for easy retrieval. For example, a classification system might organize terms by major categories, alphabetically, chronologically, or numerically. Classification systems are considered broad ways of organizing information and are not the most appropriate tool for describing the clinical aspects of patient care. Such systems are used primarily for administrative functions, such as billing and reimbursement, resource utilization, and statistical reporting.

classification systems systems that organize related terms into categories.

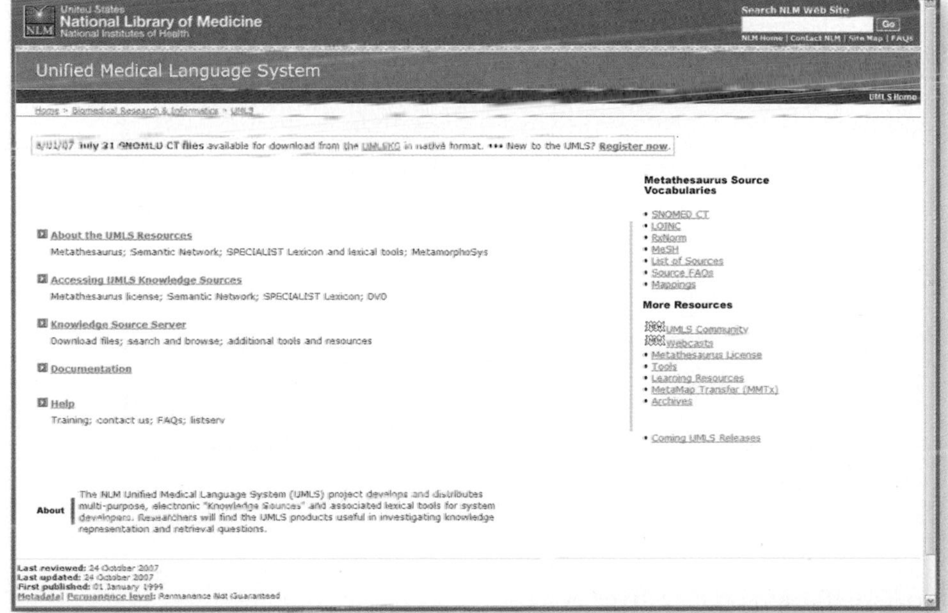

Figure 2-5
The website for the UMLS.

ICD-9 and ICD-10

International Classification of Diseases, Ninth Revision standard that categorizes diseases.

The **International Classification of Diseases, Ninth Revision** (ICD-9) is a standard developed by the World Health Organization (WHO) to categorize diseases. In the United States, a modified version—the International Classification of Diseases, Ninth Revision, Clinical Modification (ICD-9-CM)—is used. Volumes 1 and 2 of ICD-9-CM contain diagnosis codes that are used in all health care settings, including physician offices, hospitals, long-term care facilities, and home health agencies. Volume 3 includes procedure codes which are used by hospitals to code inpatient procedures. In the United States, ICD-9-CM is the basis not only for disease and illness classification, but also for establishing medical necessity for health insurance reimbursement.

In 1993, WHO released ICD-10 as a replacement for ICD-9. While many countries already use ICD-10, the United States currently uses it only for coding death certificates. A gradual mandated transition to ICD-10 is expected to take place in the next decade.

ICD-10 has already been modified to produce ICD-10-CM to replace ICD-9-CM Volumes 1 and 2. A new standard, ICD-10-PCS (ICD-10, Procedure Classification System), has been developed to replace the current Volume 3. In contrast to the ICD-9-CM system, which uses three- to five-digit codes, ICD-10-PCS is based on a seven-character alphanumeric code that uses the digits 0 through 9 and the letters A to H, J to N, and P to Z. This system provides greater specificity than does ICD-9, and as a result, information can be captured at a very detailed and thorough level.

The timely transition to the ICD-10-CM (diagnoses) and ICD-10-PCS (procedures) is supported by a number of organizations, including the American Hospital Association and the American Health Information Management Association (AHIMA). Figure 2-6 compares the two standards.

ICD-9-CM, ICD-10-CM / ICD-10-PCS Comparisons

	ICD-9-CM	ICD-10-CM	ICD-10-PCS
Diagnosis Usage	Inpatient and Outpatient	Inpatient and Outpatient	
Number of Characters	3–5 Alphanumeric	3–7 Alphanumeric	
Number of Codes	13,000	120,000	
Procedure Usage	Inpatient*		Inpatient†
Number of Characters	3–4 Numeric		7 Alphanumeric
Number of Codes	4,000		200,000

*Some hospitals currently dual code outpatients with ICD–9–CM procedure codes for internal management purposes.
†Some hospitals may, in the future, choose to dual code outpatients with ICD–10–PCS for internal management purposes.

Figure 2-6

Comparison of ICD-9-CM to ICD-10-CM and ICD-10-PCS.

CPT

The **Current Procedural Terminology (CPT),** developed and maintained by the American Medical Association (AMA), is a listing of descriptive terms and identifying codes for reporting medical services and procedures performed by health care providers in outpatient settings. CPT codes provide a standard method of communicating treatment services among doctors, insurance companies, and patients. CPT Category I codes, for example, group medical procedures into six sections. Procedures within each section are assigned numeric codes.

Current Procedural Terminology (CPT) classification system for reporting medical services and procedures performed by physicians.

SECTION	CODE RANGE
Evaluation and Management	99201–99499
Anesthesia	00100–01999
Surgery	10021–69990
Radiology	70010–79999
Pathology and Laboratory	80047–89356
Medicine	90281–99607

HCPCS

The **Healthcare Common Procedure Coding System (HCPCS), Level II** contains codes for products, supplies, and certain services not included in CPT. The HCPCS codes are maintained by the Centers for Medicare and Medicaid Services (CMS). Level II codes consist of a letter followed by four numbers, such as J7630. The codes are grouped into more than twenty sections, which each cover a related group of items. For example, codes from A4000 through A8999 contain codes for medical and surgical supplies. HCPCS codes are used in much the same way as CPT, such as provider billing and data collection for reporting purposes.

Healthcare Common Procedure Coding System (HCPCS), Level II classification codes for products, supplies, and certain services not included in Current Procedural Terminology (CPT).

MESSAGING STANDARDS

In addition to clinical vocabularies and classification systems, **messaging standards** play a crucial role in providing interoperability among information systems. Messaging standards make it possible to transfer data from systems such as laboratory or pharmacy systems to an electronic health record system. They are also used to exchange information between different EHR systems.

messaging standards standards that allows data transfer to an electronic health record system.

Messaging standards enable data to be exchanged by establishing the order and sequence of data during transmission. For example, a standard might require the first block of data to include the patient's name and birth date. Later blocks might transmit the results of a complete blood count, communicating one result (for example, hemoglobin) per block.

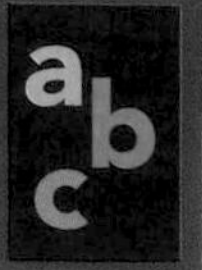

Systematized Nomenclature of Medicine Clinical Terms (SNOMED-CT)

Description

- A comprehensive clinical vocabulary designed to encompass all the terms used in medicine

Developed by

- The College of American Pathologists (CAP; www.cap.org)

Logical Observation Identifiers Names and Codes (LOINC)

Description

- A set of universal terms and codes used for the electronic exchange of laboratory results and clinical observations

Maintained by

- The Regenstrief Institute, Inc. (www.regenstrief.org)

Unified Medical Language System (UMLS)

Description

- A reference database of medical vocabularies that was originally developed to suggest translations among terminologies, but today also serves as the major thesaurus of medical terms

Maintained by

- U.S. National Library of Medicine (www.nlm.nih.gov)

Examples of messaging standards include HL7, DICOM, NCPDP, and IEEE1073.

HL7

Health Level Seven (HL7) messaging standard used to send data from one application to another.

Health Level Seven (HL7) is a messaging standard that is used to send data from one application (such as a laboratory system) to another (such as the EHR). HL7 messaging standards allow separate health information systems to communicate with one another.

The HL7 standard prescribes messages for the transmission of patient demographic and registration information as well as for clinical orders, observations, and results data. The standard is thus well suited for transmitting data between integrated clinical information systems and systems dedicated to the support of specific clinical services, such as laboratory and radiology.

DICOM

Digital Imaging and Communications in Medicine (DICOM) standards that enable information exchange between imaging systems.

Digital Imaging and Communications in Medicine (DICOM) standards enable the exchange of information between imaging systems

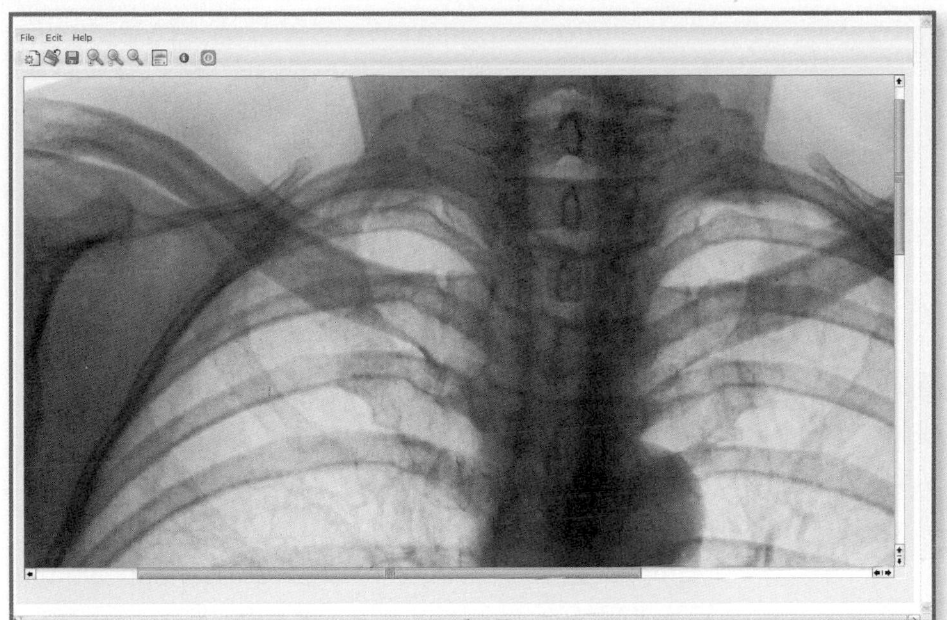

Figure 2-7

Image viewed on a computer using a PACs system.

and allow access to the images from remote locations, such as a physician office. Images come from different diagnostic equipment and techniques, including angiography, computed tomography, magnetic resonance, nuclear medicine, ultrasound, and X-ray procedures (see Figure 2-7). Images acquired on the devices are transmitted to workstations or to a picture archiving and communication system. A **picture archiving and communication system (PACS)** is an image management system for capturing, transmitting, archiving, and displaying medical images.

picture archiving and communication system (PACS) image management system.

NCPDP

National Council for Prescription Drug Program (NCPDP) standard transactions are used for exchanging prescription information, including pharmacy claims, eligibility, and coordination of benefits. The Health Insurance Portability and Accountability Act (HIPAA) of 1996 required the use of NCPDP code sets in the retail pharmacy environment.

National Council for Prescription Drug Program (NCPDP) standard for exchanging prescription information.

IEEE1073

The Institute of Electrical and Electronics Engineers 1073 (IEEE1073) standard was developed to provide communication between medical devices at a patient's bedside, such as cardiac monitors, and provides clinicians with access to the information via a computer network. These standards make it easy to obtain data from multiple bedside devices and efficiently collect patient data.

Institute of Electrical and Electronics Engineers 1073 (IEEE1073) standard that provides communication among medical devices at a patient's bedside.

ELECTRONIC HEALTH RECORD CONTENT STANDARDS

Content standards specify the functional content of an information system. In the case of electronic health record systems, Health

content standards standards that specify the functional content of an information system.

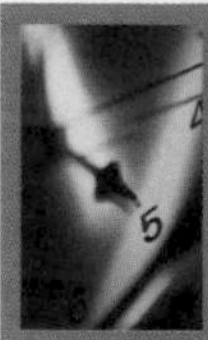

Making It Real

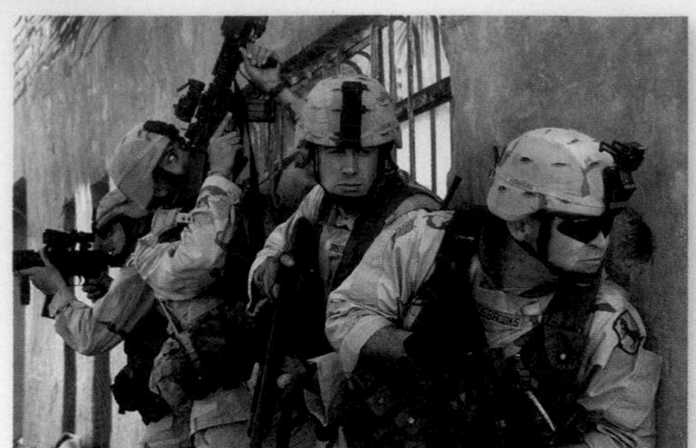

Veterans Benefits Delayed

In 2006, about 806,000 military veterans filed disability cases, compared with just 579,000 in the year 2000. The numbers have been rising in recent years, largely due to the Iraq and Afghanistan wars. More than a quarter of military veterans with disability cases before the Department of Veterans Affairs wait six months or longer to find out whether their cases are approved. In March 2007, 115,000 of 401,000 pending disability cases were not resolved within six months due to delays in the system. Military veterans and their families go without monthly payments during that time, often causing financial hardship.

One problem causing serious delay is the transfer of electronic medical records for veterans from the Department of Defense (DoD) to the Department of Veterans Affairs (VA). While on active duty, service members' records are maintained by DoD; once they are no longer active-duty personnel, their records must be transferred to the VA. The two departments are still unable to share electronic health records through their computer systems even though work began on the project in 1998. Efforts to standardize the sharing of health information across the Department of Defense and the Department of Veterans Affairs are more than two years behind schedule. The high level of disability claims entering the system is expected to continue through 2011.

Level Seven (HL7) has released Electronic Health Record System Functional Model (EHR-S-FM; see Figure 2-8). The standard, which has been approved by the American National Standards Institute (ANSI), lists critical features and functions contained in an EHR system. There are approximately a thousand criteria across 130 functions, including problem lists, clinical decision support, and privacy and security.

All functions do not apply to a single EHR system; the model contains profiles that specify functions for particular care settings and uses. Profiles define how the EHR functions are used and whether there are any setting-specific functions. Examples of profiles include acute inpatient care and long-term care. The EHR-S-FM standard was used as the framework for the Certification Commission for Health Information Technology (CCHIT) development of EHR product certification criteria.

Direct Care	DC.1	Care Management
	DC.2	Clinical Decision Support
	DC.3	Operations Management and Communication
Supportive	S.1	Clinical Support
	S.2	Measurement, Analysis, Research and Reports
	S.3	Administrative and Financial
Information Infrastructure	IN.1	Security
	IN.2	Health Record Information and Management
	IN.3	Registry and Directory Services
	IN.4	Standard Terminologies & Terminology Services
	IN.5	Standards-based Interoperability
	IN.6	Business Rules Management
	IN.7	Workflow Management

Figure 2-8

Structure of the Electronic Health Record System Functional Model (EHR-S-FM).

Voluntary Versus Mandatory Standards

Some standards are mandated by the federal government, while the use of others is voluntary. ICD-9 and CPT classifications were first mandated by the Centers for Medicare and Medicaid Services (CMS) for use in medical billing and insurance claims. When the HIPAA code set standards were announced following the law's passage in 1996, ICD-9-CM and CPT/HCPCS became mandatory for all electronic billing and claims, not just those administered by government programs. The HIPAA legislation also set mandatory standards for the electronic exchange of health care transactions, including claim and encounter information, payment and remittance advice, and claim status and inquiries.

The Medicare Prescription Drug and Modernization Act of 2003 mandated the use of clinical vocabularies and messaging standards in federal agencies. Selected by the Consolidated Health Informatics Initiative (CHI), the standards must be used by all federal agencies as they develop and implement new information technology systems. About twenty government departments and agencies are affected, including the Department of Health and Human Services (HHS), the Department of Veterans Affairs, the Department of Defense, and the Social Security Administration (SSA). The adoption of these standards will enable all federal agencies to easily share clinical health information electronically.

The standards all federal agencies are required to use as they develop and implement new information technology systems are listed in Table 2-1 on page 64.

TABLE 2-1 **Clinical Standards Adopted for Use by all Federal Agencies**

CONTENT	DESCRIPTION	STANDARD
Laboratory results names		Logical Observation Identifiers Names and Codes (LOINC)
Messaging standards	Scheduling, medical record and image management, patient administration, observation reporting, financial management, public health notification, and patient care	Standard: Health Level Seven (HL7) Version 2.3+
Messaging standards	Retail pharmacy transactions	National Council for Prescription Drug Programs (NCPDP) SCRIPT
Messaging standards	Device-device connectivity	Institute of Electrical and Electronics Engineers, Inc. 1073
Messaging standards	Image information to workstations	Digital Imaging and Communications in Medicine (DICOM)
Demographics		HL7 Version 2.4+
Lab result contents		Systematized Nomenclature of Medicine Clinical Terms (SNOMED CT)
Units of measure		HL7 Version 2.x+
Immunizations		HL7 Version 2.3.1, specifically the Vaccines Administered (CVX) and Manufacturers of Vaccines (MVX) external code sets maintained by the Centers for Disease Control and Prevention (CDC) National Immunization Program (NIP).
Medications		Federal Drug Terminologies: (Subdomain: Standard Adopted): • *Active Ingredient:* FDA Established Names and Unique Ingredient Identifier (UNII) codes • *Manufactured Dosage Form:* FDA/CDER Data Standards Manual • *Drug Product:* FDA's National Drug Codes (NDC) • *Medication Package:* FDA Standards Manual • *Label Section Headers:* LOINCClinical Structured Product Labeling (SPL) • *Special Populations:* HL7 Version 2.4 and greater • *Drug Classifications:* Department of Veterans Affairs National Drug File Reference Terminology (NDF–RT) for mechanism of action and physiologic effect • *Clinical Drug:* The National Library of Medicine's RxNorm
Interventions/procedures (Part A): Lab test order names		LOINC
Interventions/procedures (Part B): Nonlaboratory		SNOMED CT
Anatomy		SNOMED CT and the National Cancer Institute (NCI) Thesaurus
Diagnosis/problem lists		SNOMED CT
Nursing		SNOMED CT
Financial/payment		HIPAA Transactions and Code Sets
Genes		Human Genome Nomenclature
Clinical encounters		HL7 Version 2.4 and greater
Text-based reports		HL7 and Clinical Document Architecture (CDA) Version 1.0–2000
Chemicals		Environmental Protection Agency Substance Registry System

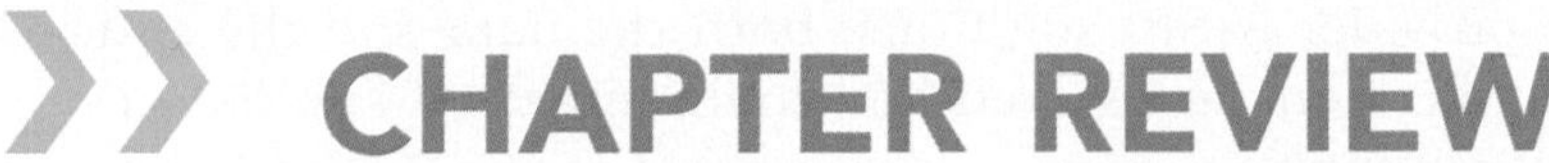

CHAPTER REVIEW

CHAPTER SUMMARY

1. There are a number of strategies for converting paper-based charts to electronic health records. The major advantage of the total conversion strategy is that all data are converted at once and are available in the EHR. The incremental approach offers significant cost savings since the conversion is done internally by the office administrative staff members who are simultaneously converting the data and learning the new system. A combination of the two approaches is known as a hybrid system, in which some records may be outsourced and others converted in-house.

2. The four primary methods of entering live patient data into EHR are dictation and transcription, clinical templates, voice recognition, and scanning. Dictation remains the most traditional and familiar method of documenting patient encounters. Clinical templates have the advantage of providing the most consistent data. Voice recognition can potentially eliminate transcription costs. Document scanning is an efficient way to enter text and images.

3. Desktop, laptop, and tablet computers are all examples of computer workstations. The desktop computer is a fixed, hardwired computer that stays in one location and cannot be moved from room to room. A laptop computer is a fully functioning computer that is small enough to be portable. The tablet computer, or tablet PC, is a third type of workstation that contains built-in handwriting and voice recognition software.

4. Wireless networks offer a number of advantages compared to wired networks. With a wireless network, portable computers, such as laptops and tablet PCs, can be transported from room to room and still maintain a network connection. This offers major advantages in the health care environment. A wireless network makes it possible for physicians to access medical reference tools in the examination room and at a patient's bedside. Other tasks, such as basic charge capture, prescription writing, clinical documentation, and messaging, are all more convenient with a wireless network.

5. Medical facilities can choose whether to house hardware and software on-site (traditional model) or off-site at an external vendor's location (ASP model). The core differences between the traditional locally hosted model and the ASP model are where the data are stored and who maintains the hardware and software. In a locally hosted model, the hardware and software required to run an electronic health record program are located on-site at the provider's location. In application

service provider (ASP) solutions, both the data and the software applications are stored and maintained off-site by an external company.

6. The clinical information in a patient record must be recorded in standard ways so its meaning can be shared among individuals and organizations in the health care system. The use of different terms to indicate the same condition or treatment complicates retrieval and reduces the consistency of patient care data. Developing standards capable of addressing the enormous complexity of clinical processes is a major challenge for the health care field.

7. Clinical vocabularies are sets of common definitions for medical terms that facilitate communication by minimizing ambiguity. A shared vocabulary leads to consistent descriptions of a patient's medical condition regardless of where the data were created. While vocabulary systems encompass the entire subject field and support detailed descriptions, classification systems organize related terms into categories for easy retrieval. Classification systems are considered broad ways of organizing information.

8. Messaging standards make it possible to transfer data from systems, such as laboratory or pharmacy systems, to an electronic health record system. They are also used to exchange information between different EHR systems. Examples of messaging standards are HL7, DICOM, NCPDP, and IEEE1073.

9. The Medicare Prescription Drug and Modernization Act of 2003 mandated the use of clinical vocabularies and messaging standards in federal agencies. Selected by the Consolidated Health Informatics Initiative (CHI), the standards must be used by all federal agencies as they develop and implement new information technology systems. About twenty government departments and agencies are affected.

CHECK YOUR UNDERSTANDING

Part 1. Write *T* or *F* in the blank to indicate whether you think the statement is true or false.

_____ **1.** When considering the transition of paper records to an EHR, it is important to determine how much historical information in the patient record should be converted.

_____ **2.** The total conversion approach to converting paper records to an EHR risks converting unnecessary data.

_____ **3.** Clinical templates are structured progress notes that physicians use to document patient encounters in an EHR.

_____ **4.** Voice recognition offers the promise of reducing the need for keyboard entry while providing a cost-effective alternative to traditional transcription.

_____ 5. A personal digital assistant is a type of workstation.

_____ 6. The desktop computer can function independently or can share data with other devices in a network.

_____ 7. Tablet PCs offer physicians a workflow that is similar to traditional dictation methodology.

_____ 8. A client is a powerful computer that houses software applications and data.

_____ 9. Wireless networks, also known as "Wi-Fi," allow multiple computers to access a server or the Internet without using cables.

_____ 10. In a locally hosted model, the programs and information on the server are accessed from client computers located throughout the office.

_____ 11. In an ASP environment, the practice is responsible for hardware and software maintenance.

Part 2. Match each term below with its correct definition.

_____ 12. application service provider (ASP)

_____ 13. classification systems

_____ 14. clinical templates

_____ 15. clinical vocabularies

_____ 16. content standards

_____ 17. Health Level Seven (HL7)

_____ 18. incremental conversion

_____ 19. locally hosted

_____ 20. messaging standards

_____ 21. network

_____ 22. scanning

_____ 23. Systematized Nomenclature of Medicine Clinical Terms (SNOMED-CT)

_____ 24. total conversion

_____ 25. voice recognition

a. A messaging standard that is used to send data from one application to another.

b. Sets of common definitions for medical terms that facilitate communication by minimizing ambiguity.

c. Standards that specify the functional content of an information system.

d. A hosting model in which the hardware and software required to run a program are housed on-site at the provider's location.

e. A method of entering information in which providers dictate using a microphone connected to a desktop or laptop computer equipped with special voice recognition software, and the recording is converted into an electronic text file.

f. Systems that organize related terms into categories for easy retrieval.

g. Structured progress notes that physicians use to document patient encounters in an EHR.

h. The equipment required to enable computers and other types of hardware to exchange information electronically.

i. A method of capturing electronic text or images from paper documents.

j. Comprehensive clinical vocabulary designed to encompass all the terms used in medicine.

k. A paper to electronic document conversion process in which records are converted gradually, beginning with patients with scheduled appointments.

l. Standards that make it possible to transfer data from systems, such as a laboratory or pharmacy systems, to an electronic health record system.

m. A hosting model in which an external company houses the software and data on servers at its site.

n. A paper to electronic document conversion method in which the conversion process is outsourced to an external company.

THINKING ABOUT THE ISSUES

Part 3. In the space provided, write a brief paragraph describing your thoughts on the following issues.

26. Despite the lower start-up costs, why have some physicians been resistant about moving to ASP solutions in comparison to locally hosted models?

____

____

27. While there are a number of ways to enter patient information into an EHR, dictation and transcription remain the most popular. Why do you think this is so, and how do you think this might change in the future? Are there any drawbacks to using dictation and transcription?

____

____

28. Why is creating standards for clinical medical information such a major challenge for the health care field?

____

____

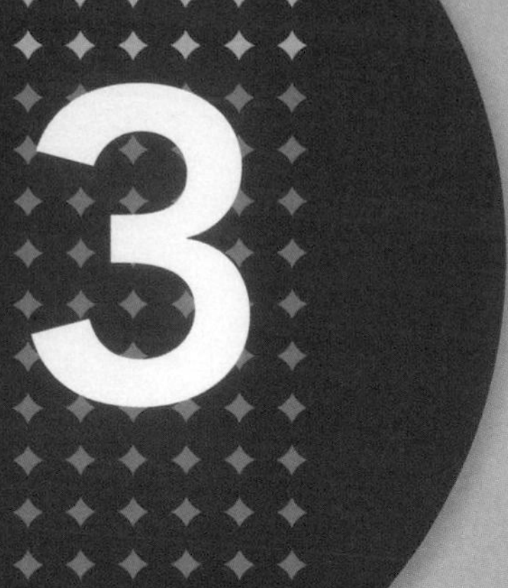

3 Electronic Health Records in the Physician Office

CHAPTER OUTLINE

Patient Flow in the Physician Practice
Step 1. Pre-Visit: Appointment Scheduling and Information Collection
Step 2. Patient Check-in and Payment Collection
Step 3. Rooming and Measuring Vital Signs
Patient Examination and Documentation
Step 4. Patient Checkout
Step 5. Post-Visit: Coding and Billing
Post-Visit: Reviewing Test Results
Coding and Reimbursement in Electronic Health Records
Computer-Assisted Coding
Clinical Tools in the Electronic Health Record
Decision-Support Tools
Tracking and Monitoring Patient Care
Screening for Illness or Disease
Identifying at-Risk Patients
Managing Patients with Chronic Diseases
Improving the Quality and Safety of Patient Care with Evidence-Based Guidelines
E-Prescribing and Electronic Health Records
Keeping Current with Electronic Drug Databases
Increasing Prescription Safety
Saving Time and Money

LEARNING OUTCOMES

After completing this chapter, you will be able to define key terms and:

1. List the five steps of the office visit workflow in a physician office.
2. Discuss the advantages of pre-visit scheduling and information collection for patients and office staff.
3. Describe the process of electronic check-in.
4. Explain how electronic health records make documenting patient exams more efficient.
5. Explain what occurs during patient checkout.
6. Explain what two events take place during the post-visit step of the visit workflow.
7. Describe the advantages of computer-assisted coding.
8. List three decision-support tools the EHRs contain to provide patients with safe and effective health care.
9. List four important safety checks that an EHR's e-prescribing feature can perform when a physician selects a new medication for a patient.

KEY TERMS

chronic diseases
clinical guidelines
computer-assisted coding
decision-support tools
disease management (DM)
formulary
point-of-care

Why This Chapter
Is Important to You

The information in this chapter will enable you to:

- Understand the ways in which EHR enhances each step of the office visit.
- Understand how clinical tools, a feature of EHRs, assist physicians in making medical decisions and managing patients with chronic diseases.
- Understand how electronic documentation leads to more timely reimbursement for the practice.
- Understand how using EHR tools to monitor patients' compliance with recommended wellness guidelines can improve the quality of patient care.

The transition from paper records to electronic health records (EHRs) represents a fundamental change in the way a physician office operates and interacts with patients. Everyone who works in the office, whether in a clinical or an administrative position, in the front office or the back office, will have to learn a new way of doing things. All tasks related to providing health care to patients will be entered, stored, and maintained in a computer-based EHR. Consider how a few common tasks are different in an office that has fully implemented an EHR:

- There is no need to pull a patient's chart the day before an appointment. *All the information that was stored on the paper chart is in the computer and can be accessed instantly.*
- There is no need to print a superbill for a patient on the day of the appointment. *The provider will document the office visit in the computer, which will generate preliminary codes based on the electronic documentation.*

- There is no need to handwrite a patient's vital signs on paper. *Vital signs will be automatically entered in the computer by digital medical devices.*
- There is no need to manually enter procedures and diagnoses from a superbill into the office billing system. *Procedure and diagnosis codes generated during the office visit will be reviewed and finalized by a coding specialist and will automatically become part of the billing module of the EHR.*
- There is no need to handwrite most prescriptions. *Prescriptions will be entered in the computer and electronically transmitted to a pharmacy, with a few exceptions.*
- There is no need to wait for a patient's test results to arrive via a fax machine or in the mail. *Laboratory and radiology results are transmitted electronically to the physician and become part of the patient's EHR.*

In this chapter, we will compare and contrast patient flow in a paper-based office and in an office that has an electronic health record (EHR). The processes described in this chapter reflect an office that has a fully implemented EHR. In reality, many practices are using a combination of electronic and paper systems, known as hybrid systems. Eventually, almost all practices are expected to make the shift to a completely electronic environment. In addition to describing differences in the patient flow, the chapter also focuses on three key features of EHRs: electronic documentation and coding, clinical tools that make it easier for the physician to provide patients with the highest quality of care, and electronic prescribing of medications, referred to as e-prescribing. While the examples in the chapter refer to a physician practice, they are also relevant for an outpatient clinic at a hospital and other ambulatory care settings.

Patient Flow in the Physician Office

Patient flow refers to the progression of patients from when they enter the practice's system by scheduling an appointment until they exit the system by leaving the office after a physician visit. Between entering and exiting, many clinical and administrative events take place, including checking the patient in, collecting payment for services, rooming the patient, examining the patient, prescribing medications, ordering tests, and checking the patient out at the end of the visit. The following steps occur before, during, and after an office visit, regardless of whether the office is using an EHR or paper for record-keeping (see Figure 3-1).

Step 1. Pre-visit: Appointment scheduling and information collection

Step 2. Patient check-in and payment collection

Step 3. Rooming, measuring vital signs, and patient examination and documentation

Step 4. Patient checkout

Step 5. Post-visit: Coding and billing, and reviewing test results

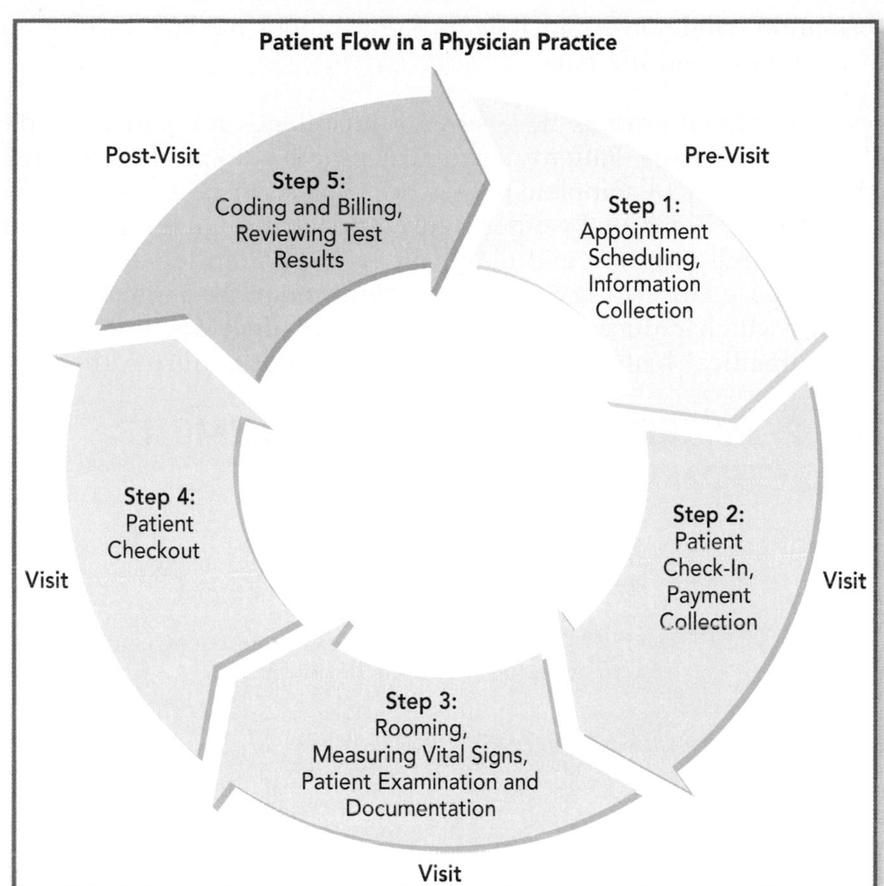

Figure 3-1
The flow of activity in a physician office.

STEP 1. PRE-VISIT: APPOINTMENT SCHEDULING AND INFORMATION COLLECTION

PAPER	ELECTRONIC
1. Patient calls for appointment.	1. Patient schedules appointment on the Internet.
2. Front desk staff member schedules appointment and confirms insurance information.	2. Patient completes information forms online.

In a practice with an EHR, patients may have the option of making appointments on the office's website or using the traditional method of telephoning the office. The ability to make appointments online reduces the amount of time the front desk staff must spend scheduling patients, since appointments are made without their assistance. On the practice website, patients view a calendar with available openings and select a time slot. This information is transmitted to the office and if approved, the patient receives an e-mail conformation.

Medical office websites also offer new ways to collect patient information. Patients have the option of entering information about themselves before their scheduled office visits. The amount of information collected varies greatly. Some websites collect only demographic and insurance information, while others include questions about medical history, current condition, and lifestyle.

These automated options have several advantages for patients, office staff, and physicians. Patients new to the practice do not have to arrive at the office early to complete paperwork. The front desk staff member does not have to manually enter information from handwritten forms into the billing program and file forms in the patient chart. The physician has a chance to review information about the patient prior to the visit, which reduces the amount of time spent documenting the patient's medical history and preventive care status during the visit.

STEP 2. PATIENT CHECK-IN AND PAYMENT COLLECTION

PAPER	ELECTRONIC
1. Staff member pulls patient chart and prints superbill for today's appointment.	1. Patient arrives and checks in electronically at a computer in the waiting room.
2. Patient arrives and signs in.	2. Patient confirms demographics and billing information on a computer.
3. Front desk verifies demographics and billing information with patient.	3. EHR checks insurance eligibility.
4. Patient returns to waiting room.	4. Patient enters copayment via computer or pays at front desk.
5. Front desk checks eligibility by Internet or telephone.	5. Medical assistant (MA) sees alert on EHR screen that patient is ready to be roomed.
6. Patient called to front desk to make copayment.	6. MA rooms the patient.
7. Patient returns to waiting room.	
8. Front desk notifies the medical assistant (MA) that the patient is ready to be roomed; places the chart, superbill, and labels in a tray.	
9. MA takes the papers from the tray and rooms the patient.	

Some physician practices with EHRs offer electronic check-in. Electronic check-in allows patients access to a computer in a private area of the waiting room. When patients arrive for their visits, they sit at the computer and confirm address, phone number, and billing and other information. Since the computer is linked to the Internet, the EHR checks insurance eligibility in real time. Once eligibility is verified, patients are prompted to enter their copayments online, using credit or debit cards or checking accounts. Patients who are not comfortable paying online have the option of paying at the front desk. Once the patient checks in on the computer, the front desk is notified that the patient has arrived and is ready to see the doctor (see Figure 3-2).

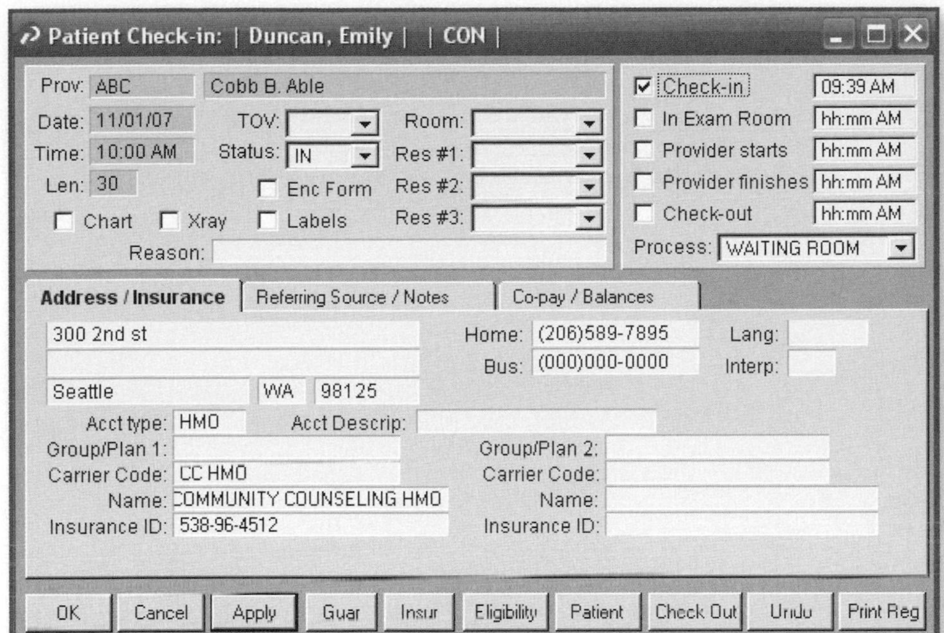

Figure 3-2

A patient check-in screen.

Electronic check-in offers several benefits, including:

- Shorter waiting times for patient check-in
- No need to file paper forms in a patient chart
- Fewer errors, since information is entered once by the patient, rather than by the patient plus by the person who inputs the information in the billing program

STEP 3. ROOMING AND MEASURING VITAL SIGNS

PAPER	ELECTRONIC
1. MA checks vital signs.	1. MA checks vital signs.
2. MA asks the reason for the visit.	2. MA asks the reason for the visit.
3. MA verifies medications and allergies.	3. MA verifies medications and allergies.
4. MA documents findings on face sheet in chart.	4. MA documents findings in EHR via computer in exam room.
5. MA leaves the room and places patient chart in pocket on exam room door, flips colored flag on wall.	5. EHR sends an alert to physician that patient is ready for exam.
6. Physician walks down hallway and notices that patient is ready to be seen.	

After the patient is escorted to an exam room, a member of the clinical team, such as a medical assistant, checks the patient's vital signs. Some offices use digital devices that measure the vital signs and transmit them directly into the EHR (see Figure 3-3 on page 76).

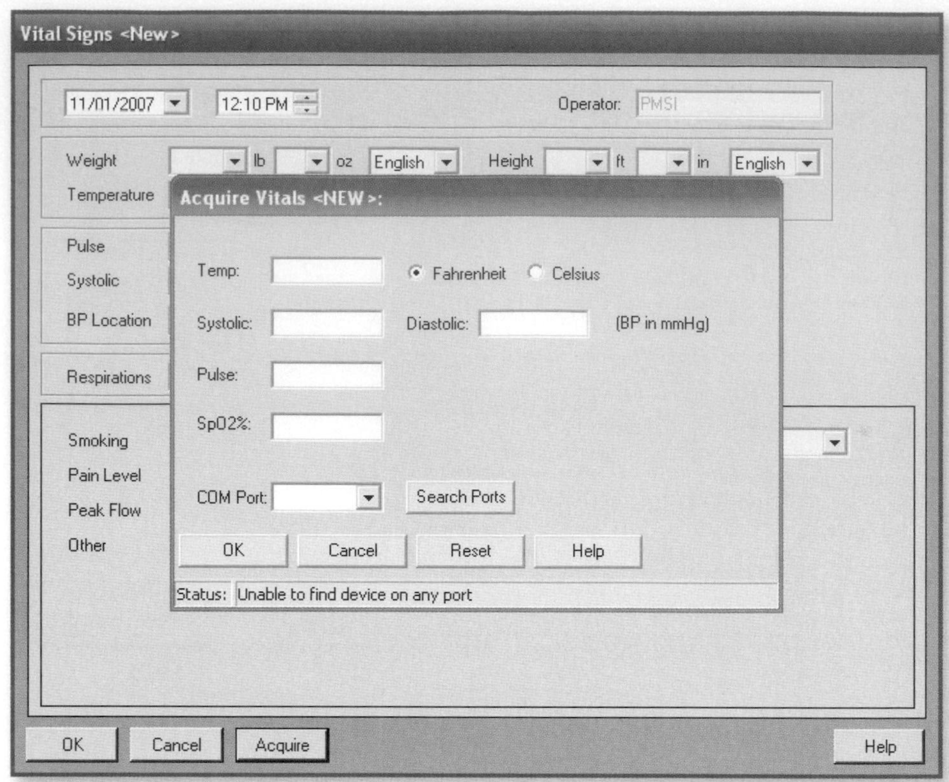

Figure 3-3

A screen where a patient's vital signs are entered, with options to acquire data directly from digital measuring devices.

The MA also gathers information relevant to the day's visit, including the chief complaint, medical history, and information about allergies and medication. The MA enters this information in the EHR while in the room with the patient. Once the MA is finished entering the data, the provider is notified that the patient is ready and can review information about the patient from his or her desk before entering the exam room.

STEP 3. PATIENT EXAMINATION AND DOCUMENTATION

PAPER	ELECTRONIC
1. Provider reviews face sheet in paper chart on door.	1. Provider reviews patient record in EHR.
2. Provider enters exam room.	2. Provider enters exam room.
3. Provider reviews MA documentation.	3. Provider examines patient.
4. Provider examines patient.	4. Provider documents visit in EHR.
5. Provider jots visit notes on superbill.	5. Provider enters needed prescriptions and requisitions for tests in EHR.
6. Provider writes needed prescriptions and requisitions for tests.	
7. Provider hands the patient orders, prescriptions, and superbill.	

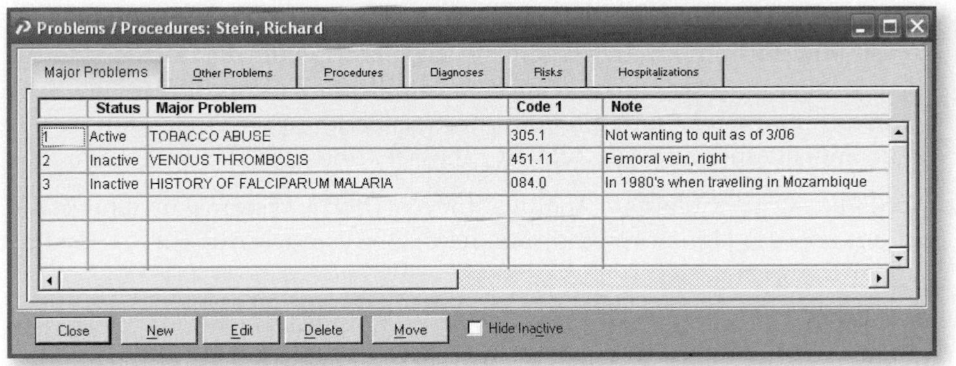

Figure 3-4

Summary of a patient's major medical problems.

During an office visit, the provider may want to see a summary of the patient's past problems, history, visits, tests, procedures, and medications, all while in the exam room with the patient. The EHR provides easy access to each of these major content areas, usually all from one screen (see Figure 3-4). Trying to review this information with a paper chart that contains many pages and forms would be difficult and time-consuming. The EHR lets the provider locate and review specific information in seconds.

Clinical Documentation Components

The clinical information contained in documentation of a patient visit is the same as with a paper-based system. EHRs contain areas in which a provider details the clinical components of an examination, including the following information:

Vital signs: Measurements of a patient's temperature, respiratory rate, pulse, and blood pressure.

Chief complaint: A brief description of the patient's current problem in his or her own words.

Progress notes: Notes documenting the care delivered to a patient, and the medical facts and clinical thinking relevant to diagnosis and treatment.

Past medical history (PMH): The patient's history of medical problems, including chronic conditions, surgeries, and hospitalizations. This should include any illness (past or present) for which the patient has received treatment.

Family history (FH): The medical events among members of the patient's family, including the ages, living status, and diseases of siblings, children, parents, and grandparents. This includes diseases related to the chief complaint as well as any hereditary diseases.

Social history (SH): Information about the patient's tobacco use, alcohol and drug use, sexual history, relationship status, and other significant social facts that may contribute to the care of the patient.

Allergies: A list of the patient's known allergies, including reactions to each one.

Medication list: Includes all currently prescribed medications as well as over-the-counter and nontraditional therapies. Dosage and frequency should be noted.

HPI (history of present illness): A description of the course of the present illness, including how and when the problem began, up to the present time. It includes everything related to the illness or condition, including aggravating and alleviating factors, associated symptoms, previous treatment and diagnostic tests, related illnesses, and risk factors.

ROS (review of systems): An inventory of body systems in which the patient reports signs or symptoms he or she is currently having or has had in the past.

Diagnosis and assessment: The physician's thinking about the cause of patient's problem as well as any tests performed to come to this determination.

Plan and treatment: The physician's thinking about the intervention that will be necessary to cure or manage the patient's condition, including medications, procedures, and lifestyle changes.

Documenting a Patient Encounter

In a traditional paper-based office, providers often document patient encounters in between seeing patients or at the end of the day. Electronic health records contain tools that make documenting patient encounters more efficient for clinicians. While these tools vary from one program to another, most EHRs offer the option of documenting the visit at the point-of-care. The **point-of-care** is the setting in which a physician makes decisions about the nature of a patient's illness and the best course of treatment.

point-of-care setting in which a physician makes decisions about a patient's illness and treatment.

Most EHRs offer several options for documenting patient visits. Providers enter data during the patient visit by typing in free text, using voice recognition software, or by responding to templates that contain commonly used clinical words, phrases, and symptoms. With a template, the physician responds to prompts on the computer during the patient examination. The EHR then uses these responses to create a clinical note. The templates are specific to the type of visit (routine physical, immunization) or to the specific disease (hypertension, diabetes). Figure 3-5 illustrates a sample list of templates, while Figure 3-6 shows a template inserted in a progress note.

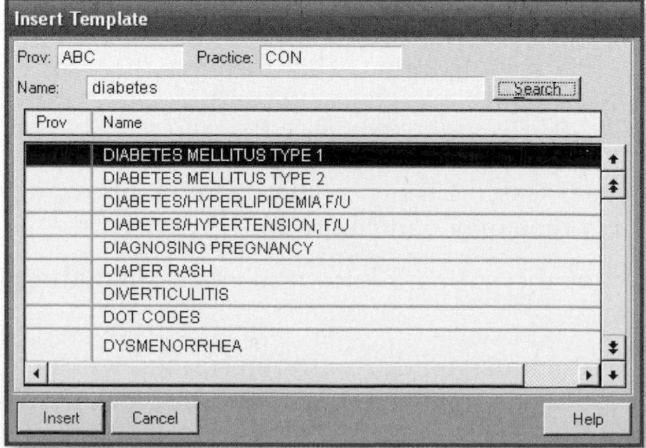

Figure 3-5

Screen with a list of templates for documenting a patient encounter.

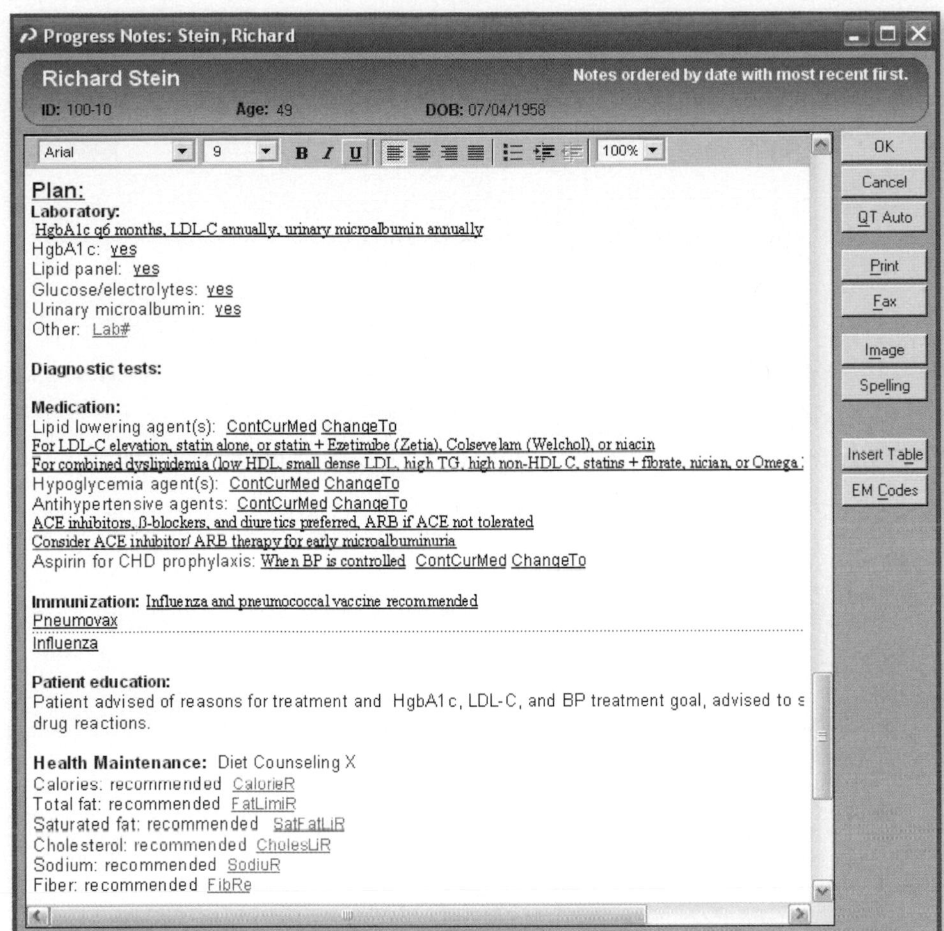

Figure 3-6

A partial view of a template for documenting an encounter for a patient with diabetes mellitus type 2.

Documenting encounters in EHRs offers several advantages over paper-based techniques. Since the provider enters the data while with the patient, information is less likely to be left out or forgotten, as sometimes happens when doctors record their observations and findings later. In addition, without paper chart pulls and filing and without the need for transcription of physician notes, costs are reduced. Another advantage is that physician notes are available as soon as the office visit has ended, instead of twenty-four to forty-eight hours after the visit. This makes it possible to include a complete, up-to-date patient record when referring a patient to another provider, such as a specialist.

Clinical Tools

EHRs offer a number of features that make it easier for the clinician to provide patients with quality care. These clinical tools allow doctors to access electronic databases that summarize the latest evidence-based research, detail national treatment and screening guidelines, and make overseeing care of patients with chronic diseases easier. Clinical tools allow physicians to manage large quantities of rapidly changing health information, bringing data to the providers at the time of medical decision making. The tools are becoming more and more important because the amount of information in clinical medicine is growing so quickly that providers are hard-pressed to stay current in their field. You will learn more about these tools later in this chapter.

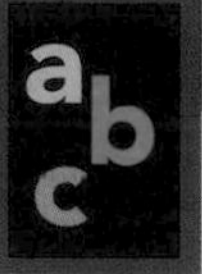

Clinical Documentation

FH—Family History

The medical events among members of the patient's family, including the ages, living status, and diseases of siblings, children, parents, and grandparents.

H&P—History and Physical

Documentation of the clinical components of an examination.

HPI—History of Present Illness

A description of the course of the present illness, including how and when the problem began, up to the present time.

PMH—Past Medical History

The patient's history of medical problems, including chronic conditions, surgeries, hospitalizations, and so on.

ROS—Review of Systems

An inventory of body systems in which the patient reports signs or symptoms he or she is currently having or has had in the past.

SH—Social History

Information about the patient's tobacco use, alcohol and drug use, sexual history, relationship status, and other significant social facts that may contribute to the care of the patient.

SOAP—Subjective, Objective, Assessment, Plan

A documentation format in which patient encounter information is grouped into subjective, objective, assessment, and plan categories.

Physician Order Entry

Once a physician is finished examining a patient, it may be necessary to order tests or medications as part of diagnosing or treating the patient's condition. EHRs allow doctors to order tests without the use of traditional paper forms (see Figure 3-7). Some EHRs include built-in standard order sets based on the provider's specialty or on a specific disease.

Prescriptions can also be ordered electronically. Instead of writing a prescription on a separate prescription pad and then documenting the medication in a patient's chart, the prescription is entered in the EHR and transmitted to the patient's pharmacy. As a result, the prescription is ready when the patient arrives at the pharmacy. EHRs contain additional prescribing features that are intended to prevent errors and enhance patient safety (see "e-Prescribing and Electronic Health Records" later in this chapter).

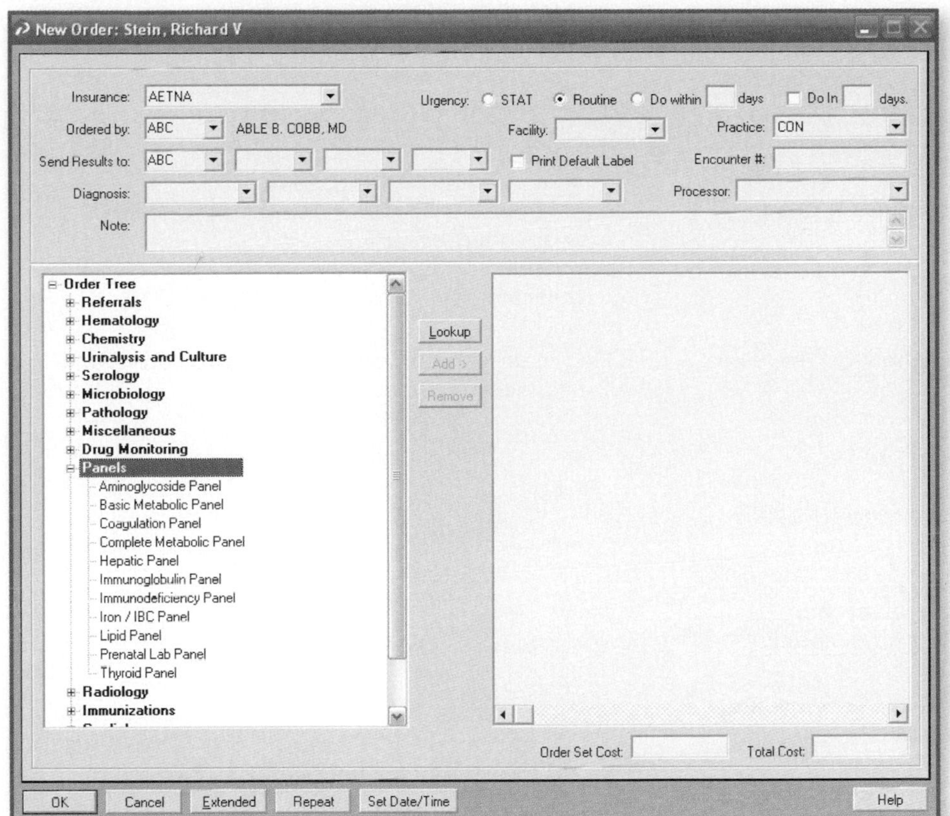

Figure 3-7

An order entry screen showing a list of built-in orders.

STEP 4. PATIENT CHECKOUT

PAPER	ELECTRONIC
1. Patient hands superbill to front desk staff member.	1. Patient stops at front desk to pick up copies of orders, prescriptions, and educational materials.
2. Staff member verifies the charges and collects any payment due.	2. Front desk staff member reviews EHR and collects any payment due.
3. Staff member schedules any follow-up appointments.	3. Staff member schedules any follow-up appointments.
4. Patient leaves the office.	4. Patient leaves the office.

In an office with an EHR, all test orders, prescriptions, and educational materials are waiting for the patient at the checkout desk. The front desk staff member reviews the billing screen in the EHR to see if any additional payment is due and schedules any follow-up appointments before the patient leaves.

STEP 5. POST-VISIT: CODING AND BILLING

PAPER	ELECTRONIC
1. Provider returns to office and dictates notes on patient visit.	1. Coder reviews procedure, visit, and diagnosis codes assigned by EHR based on provider documentation; after review, codes are automatically sent to billing module of EHR.
2. Outside agency transcribes dictation and sends to physician's office.	2. Billing staff member reviews visit information and submits electronic claim.
3. Physician reviews transcribed visit notes.	
4. Patient chart and superbill forwarded to billing staff.	
5. Coder reviews provider documentation and assigns procedure, visit, and diagnosis codes.	
6. After review, coder writes codes on superbill and places it in tray for billing staff.	
7. Billing staff member enters visit information in practice management system and submits electronic claim.	

In a paper-based environment, the coding staff member reads and evaluates the provider's documentation to determine the procedures performed by the provider and the patient's diagnoses. Coders translate words in the documentation into HIPAA-mandated codes that are then submitted to third-party payers for reimbursement. The payers review the claims and decide reimbursement for services based on the codes, looking for a logical relationship between diagnosis and procedure to justify the medical necessity of the services billed.

Most EHRs have a feature that automates one or more aspects of the coding process. The level of coding assistance varies from one program to another. The basic systems include searchable electronic versions of coding references, while the more sophisticated programs automatically assign codes based on information in the provider's electronic documentation (see Figure 3-8). These codes are then checked for accuracy by a coding specialist and included in electronic claims.

The billing staff member creates electronic claims and transmits them to payers for reimbursement. Some practices use a practice management system (PMS) that is linked to the EHR; others use a comprehensive EHR that includes billing features. There is more information about how electronic systems are used for coding and billing later in this chapter.

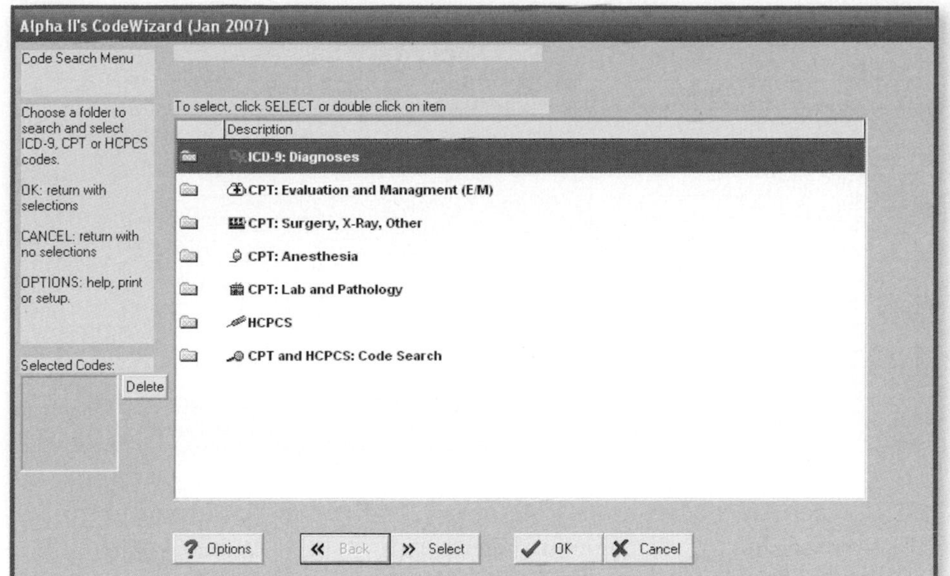

Figure 3-8

Searchable electronic database of codes accessed from an EHR.

STEP 5. POST-VISIT: REVIEWING TEST RESULTS

PAPER	ELECTRONIC
1. Locate patient's chart.	1. Alert appears on MA screen that patient's lab results have arrived; if results are abnormal, physician is sent an immediate alert.
2. Attach lab results sheet to top of chart.	2. Physician reviews results, electronically signs them, and forwards to MA.
3. Route chart to physician for review.	3. MA telephones patient with follow-up instructions.
4. Physician reviews, signs, and adds note for follow-up request.	4. MA documents phone call in EHR.
5. Chart placed in physician outbox, waits to be routed to MA inbox.	
6. MA telephones patient with follow-up instructions.	
7. MA documents phone call in patient chart.	
8. Chart with added lab results and physician's notes filed.	

Incoming results from labs and radiology facilities are received by the practice EHR (see Figure 3-9 on page 84). Clinical staff, such as the medical assistant, nurse, and physician, are notified that the results have been received even if there are no abnormal values. Any abnormal results are flagged, and the provider automatically receives an alert on the

Figure 3-9
Screen displaying laboratory results in an EHR.

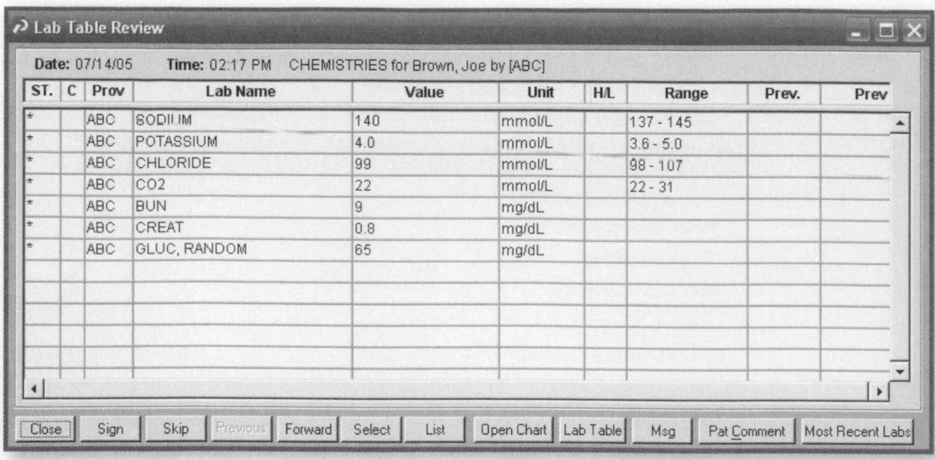

Lab Table Review
Date: 07/14/05 Time: 02:17 PM CHEMISTRIES for Brown, Joe by [ABC]
ST. C Prov Lab Name Value Unit H/L Range Prev. Prev
* ABC SODIUM 140 mmol/L 137 - 145
* ABC POTASSIUM 4.0 mmol/L 3.6 - 5.0
* ABC CHLORIDE 99 mmol/L 98 - 107
* ABC CO2 22 mmol/L 22 - 31
* ABC BUN 9 mg/dL
* ABC CREAT 0.8 mg/dL
* ABC GLUC, RANDOM 65 mg/dL
Close Sign Skip Previous Forward Select List Open Chart Lab Table Msg Pat Comment Most Recent Labs

EHR screen. The current and historical results can be viewed in graphical format, making it easier to see trends in the values over time.

Electronically entering and tracking laboratory and radiology tests has several advantages:

› There is no need to pull a patient chart to file the result and then to route the chart to the physician. This saves time and money, since no staff members are locating, routing, and filing paper charts.
› Physicians can view the results when and where they are needed, which can result in quicker diagnosis and treatment of the medical problem.
› Electronic test ordering and results management also reduces the number of duplicate tests, since physicians can determine whether a test has already been ordered. This helps lessen the costs and inconvenience associated with redundant testing.

Coding and Reimbursement in Electronic Health Records

Every service submitted for payment must be documented in the patient's medical record, including medical care, diagnostic tests, consultations, surgeries, and other services eligible for payment. Documentation is directly linked to the financial health of the practice. To be reimbursed, providers must document each service provided to the patient. If a treatment is given to a patient and the provider fails to document it, the service should not be billed. Incomplete or inaccurate records may result in claim denials or may even lead to an investigation as the federal government steps up its efforts to identify and reduce fraud.

Coding is the process of applying the mandatory HIPAA code sets—CPT (Current Procedural Terminology, Fourth Edition), HCPCS (Healthcare Common Procedure Reporting System), and ICD-9-CM (International Classification of Diseases, Ninth Revision, Clinical Modification)—to diagnostic and procedural information in the medical record for reporting on health care claims. Whether physicians are reimbursed for the services they provide is directly linked to the codes submitted to the payer on the insurance claim. When a payer receives a claim, the codes are reviewed.

Case Study

A PATIENT OFFICE VISIT

Note to the student: This is one of a number of case studies illustrating the differences between a paper-based medical office and an electronic medical office. These case studies will take you through many of the everyday events in a medical office. This particular case focuses on chart preparation in a large cardiology practice.

Susan is a medical assistant working in a large, busy cardiology practice in suburban Philadelphia. The practice consists of eleven individual sites scattered throughout the Philadelphia area. Susan works at the main site in the hospital's medical office building. Her responsibilities include taking patients to exam rooms on arrival, taking and recording vital signs and weight, ensuring that the proper documentation is on the chart and available at the time of the visit, performing ECGs, and assisting with prescription refills.

Until recently, the practice "drop-filed" chart documents. This means that when paperwork came into the practice, the document was simply dropped into the chart without regard to what type of document it was or where in the chart it belonged. The transcription of dictation was performed in India and was sent via secure messaging to a database housed at the main practice site. Errors occurred when the dictation was indexed in a database, including missing dictation, dictation going to the wrong patient's chart, and typographical errors in the dictation itself.

Six months ago, the practice implemented an EHR. After about three months of upheaval, the practice has now stabilized.

Today, Susan is assisting in the care of Clara Baker. Ms Baker is a sixty-eight-year-old woman who recently had an angioplasty procedure to open a partially blocked coronary artery. She is here today for follow up.

Susan uses the stylus on her tablet PC to double click on Clara Baker's name in the schedule, and Ms. Baker's chart automatically appears, open to the summary page. The summary page includes an updated problem list, an updated medication list, a list of all the documentation in Ms. Baker's chart by type of document, and a flow sheet with all pertinent lab studies listed by type. The summary sheet is updated in real time when the provider documents the visit, so it is current.

West Side Medical Associates

About the Clinic

Clinic name: Suburban Philadelphia Cardiology

Specialty: Cardiology

Location: Main Line, PA

About the poviders: 58 physicians, 5 nurse-practitioners

The physicians perform invasive and noninvasive diagnostic testing and intervention as well as electrophysiology and vascular procedures and surgeries.

Susan takes Ms. Baker's pulse, blood pressure, and temperature using a Welch Allyn vital signs machine, and the readings are automatically transferred to the office visit chart note for today. Susan also weighed Ms. Baker on a digital scale that automatically transferred the measurement to the chart. Susan was able to chat with Ms. Baker and congratulate her on the five pounds she has lost, and Ms. Baker said that her best friend at church had just gone through the same procedure and was experiencing a poor outcome. Susan added this to an alert note, which Dr. Mary Baird read before she came into the room.

When asked how EHR has changed her work life, Susan said, "Six months ago I had to spend my time between 3 and 5 P.M. preparing charts for the next day. I had to first find them, then make sure everything needed for the visit was available: lab results, ECGs, and the rest. Now I spend that time returning patient phone calls and doing work from today, like completing referral forms and helping patients make appointments for studies requested by the doctor. I am happier, the doctor is happier, and most importantly the patient is happier." The EHR and the digital devices for taking vital signs allow Susan to chat with patients and learn about social issues that may affect their well-being. The office is so efficient now that there are three more office visit appointments on each provider's schedule. Susan also states that patients seem happier and that there are fewer complaints.

—continued

—continued from page 85

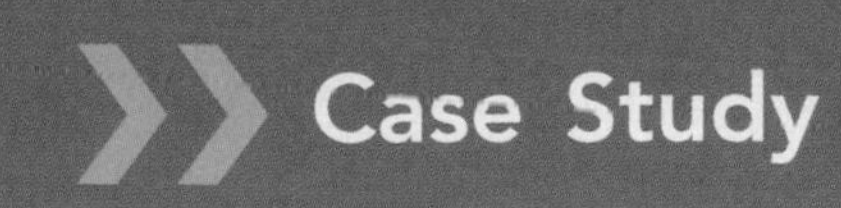

Case Study

Preparing for a Patient Visit in a Paper-Based Office

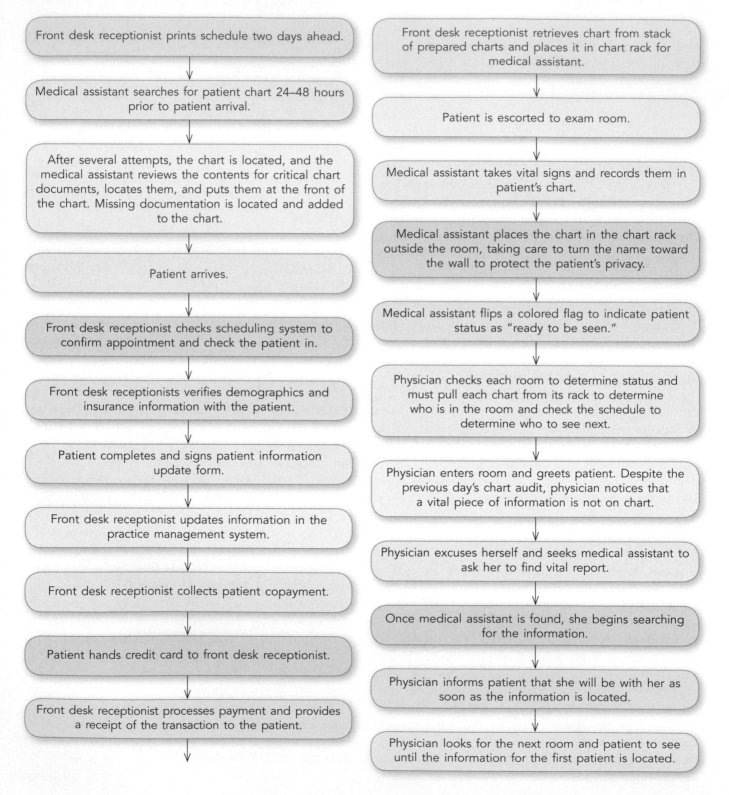

Front desk receptionist prints schedule two days ahead.

↓

Medical assistant searches for patient chart 24–48 hours prior to patient arrival.

↓

After several attempts, the chart is located, and the medical assistant reviews the contents for critical chart documents, locates them, and puts them at the front of the chart. Missing documentation is located and added to the chart.

↓

Patient arrives.

↓

Front desk receptionist checks scheduling system to confirm appointment and check the patient in.

↓

Front desk receptionists verifies demographics and insurance information with the patient.

↓

Patient completes and signs patient information update form.

↓

Front desk receptionist updates information in the practice management system.

↓

Front desk receptionist collects patient copayment.

↓

Patient hands credit card to front desk receptionist.

↓

Front desk receptionist processes payment and provides a receipt of the transaction to the patient.

↓

Front desk receptionist retrieves chart from stack of prepared charts and places it in chart rack for medical assistant.

↓

Patient is escorted to exam room.

↓

Medical assistant takes vital signs and records them in patient's chart.

↓

Medical assistant places the chart in the chart rack outside the room, taking care to turn the name toward the wall to protect the patient's privacy.

↓

Medical assistant flips a colored flag to indicate patient status as "ready to be seen."

↓

Physician checks each room to determine status and must pull each chart from its rack to determine who is in the room and check the schedule to determine who to see next.

↓

Physician enters room and greets patient. Despite the previous day's chart audit, physician notices that a vital piece of information is not on chart.

↓

Physician excuses herself and seeks medical assistant to ask her to find vital report.

↓

Once medical assistant is found, she begins searching for the information.

↓

Physician informs patient that she will be with her as soon as the information is located.

↓

Physician looks for the next room and patient to see until the information for the first patient is located.

Preparing for a Patient Visit in an Office with Electronic Health Records

Front desk receptionist prints the day's schedule and distributes copies to the clinical staff.

↓

Patient arrives and checks herself in electronically, using a computer in the waiting room. Patient verifies demographics and insurance information and submits a copayment using the computer.

↓

The system notifies the front desk and the medical assistant of the patient's arrival and displays the patient's status as ready to be placed in an examination room.

↓

Patient is escorted to exam room.

↓

Medical assistant wraps the blood pressure cuff on the patient's arm and activates the machine, which is integrated with the electronic medical record. Vital signs are automatically recorded within the office visit documentation in the electronic record.

↓

Medical assistant changes the patient status in the electronic medical record, indicating to the physician that the patient is ready to be seen.

↓

Physician is flagged that the patient in room 1 is ready to be seen.

↓

Physician enters room, greets patient, and completes the office visit with all relevant information available at the point of service because there are interfaces for laboratory and diagnostic study reports. Orders are signed and messaged to the staff in real time.

↓

The office visit is completed; if payment was not collected at check-in, it is collected now; the diagnosis, impression, and plan are documented; and prescriptions, including refills, are electronically sent to the pharmacy.

↓

The patient proceeds to checkout to schedule follow-up appointments and/or diagnostic testing that has been ordered. The checkout clerk prints educational materials and/or referrals and gives them to patient.

What Do You Think?

1. How many steps are saved in the electronic office?
2. How many steps must the medical assistant/front desk receptionist complete in the paper-based office? In the electronic office?
3. What steps must the patient perform in the electronic office that the medical assistant does in the paper-based office?
4. What is the greatest advantage for the patient in an electronic office? For the staff? For the physician?

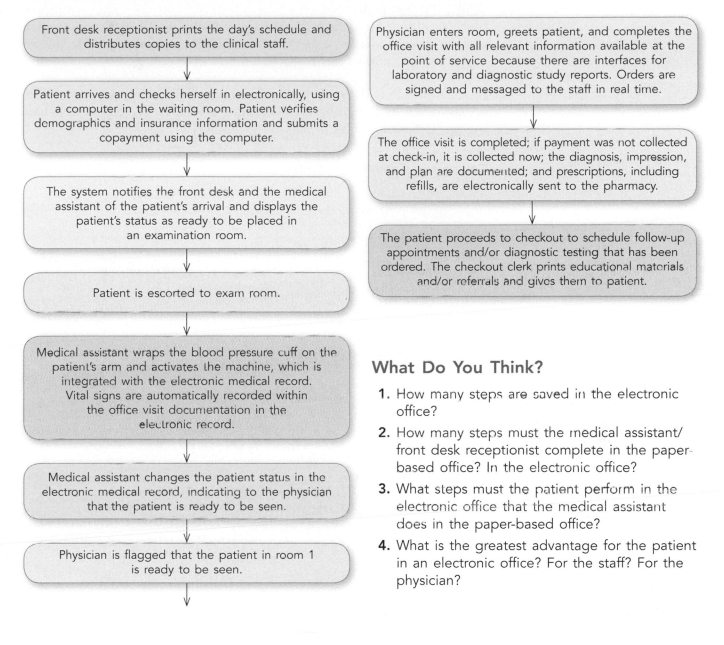

Payers want to know whether the service provided was appropriate for the patient's condition and whether the treatment was necessary. If an asthmatic patient diagnosed with an upper respiratory infection receives a chest X-ray to rule out pneumonia, the payer probably will not question the claim. However, if the same patient receives an ankle X-ray, the claim will probably be rejected, since there is not a clear relationship between the diagnosis and the service provided. And while a chest X-ray would be common for the asthmatic patient, its medical necessity might be questioned if it was performed on a twenty-year-old with the same symptoms but no asthma. Since the codes assigned to diagnoses and services play a major role in whether a physician is paid, it is important to document and code as accurately as possible.

In an office that does not use software in the coding process, codes are assigned by a member of the coding staff. The typical sequence of the paper-based coding process is as follows:

Coding in a Paper-Based Office

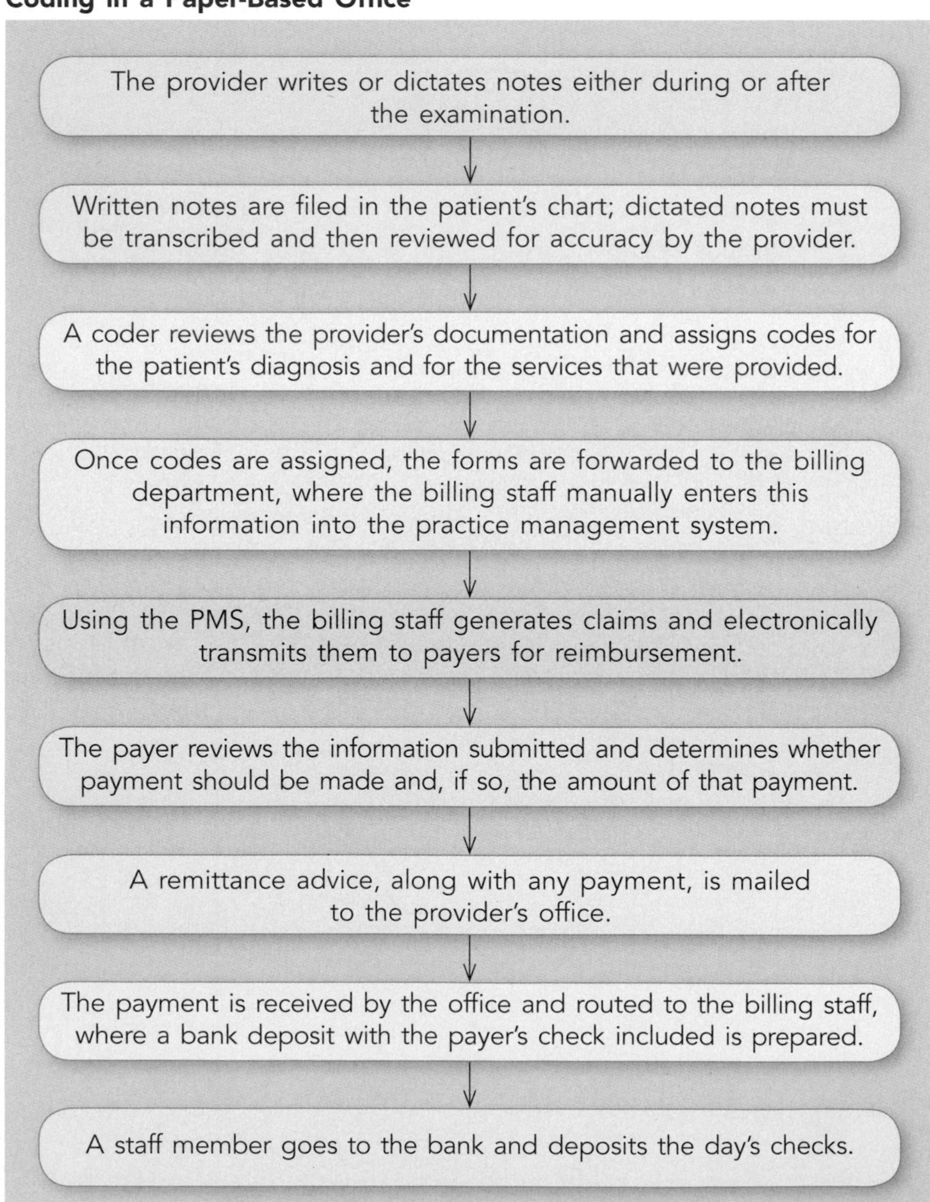

The provider writes or dictates notes either during or after the examination.
Written notes are filed in the patient's chart; dictated notes must be transcribed and then reviewed for accuracy by the provider.
A coder reviews the provider's documentation and assigns codes for the patient's diagnosis and for the services that were provided.
Once codes are assigned, the forms are forwarded to the billing department, where the billing staff manually enters this information into the practice management system.
Using the PMS, the billing staff generates claims and electronically transmits them to payers for reimbursement.
The payer reviews the information submitted and determines whether payment should be made and, if so, the amount of that payment.
A remittance advice, along with any payment, is mailed to the provider's office.
The payment is received by the office and routed to the billing staff, where a bank deposit with the payer's check included is prepared.
A staff member goes to the bank and deposits the day's checks.

In a paper-based office, the coding, billing, and reimbursement cycle normally takes anywhere from three to fourteen days. As a result, there is an extra time lag between when the service was provided and when the provider receives reimbursement. Also, it has been estimated that physicians lose as much as 10 percent of potential revenue as a result of forgetting to bill for services, losing patients' paperwork, making errors when preparing claims, and other reasons.

COMPUTER-ASSISTED CODING

In an effort to minimize the problems with paper-based coding and billing, some offices are using software that automates part of the coding process (see Figures 3-10 and 3-11). The process of coding

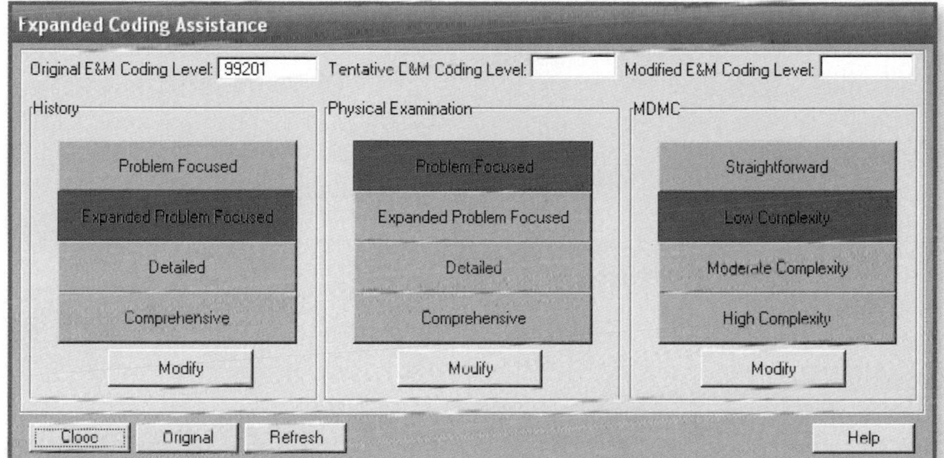

Figure 3-10

An evaluation and management visit tool in an EHR.

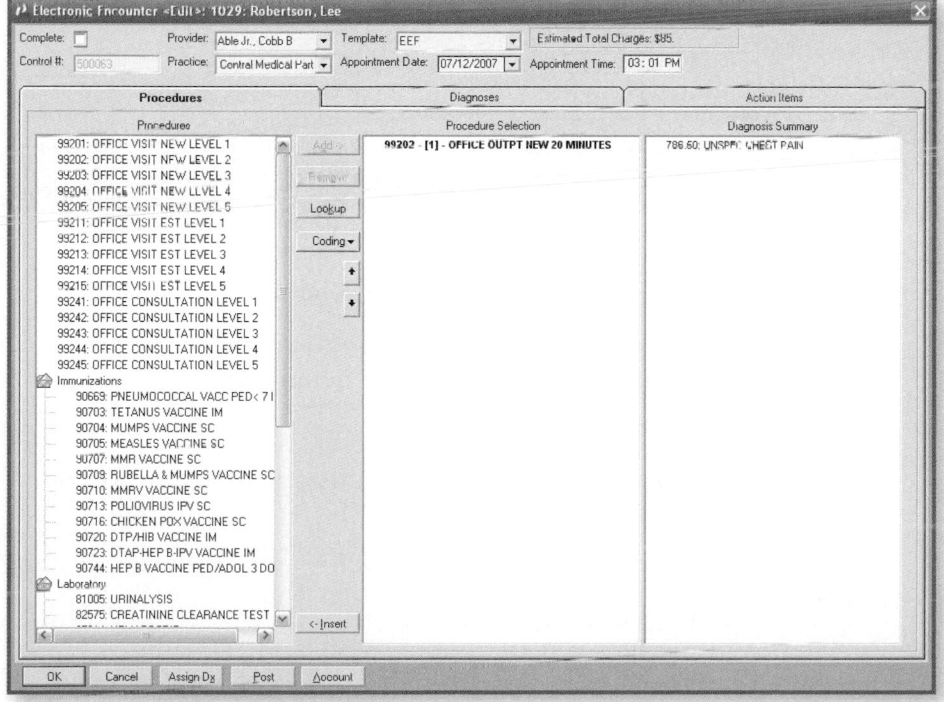

Figure 3-11

An electronic encounter form.

computer-assisted coding software that automates part of the coding process.

with software is known as **computer-assisted coding.** These software programs work in a variety of ways. Some assign codes based on keywords that are included in the template the provider uses when documenting the visit in the EHR. Other programs analyze words, phrases, and sentences in the electronic documentation to determine the appropriate codes. Once the codes have been suggested by the software, they are reviewed and verified by a professional coder. If the coder wants to review the documentation before finalizing the codes, the EHR provides fast access to the patient's chart. Once the codes are finalized, they are used by the billing staff to generate claims. The integration of automated coding with the billing system facilitates claim processing.

The coding process in an electronic office consists of the following steps:

Coding in a Electronic Office

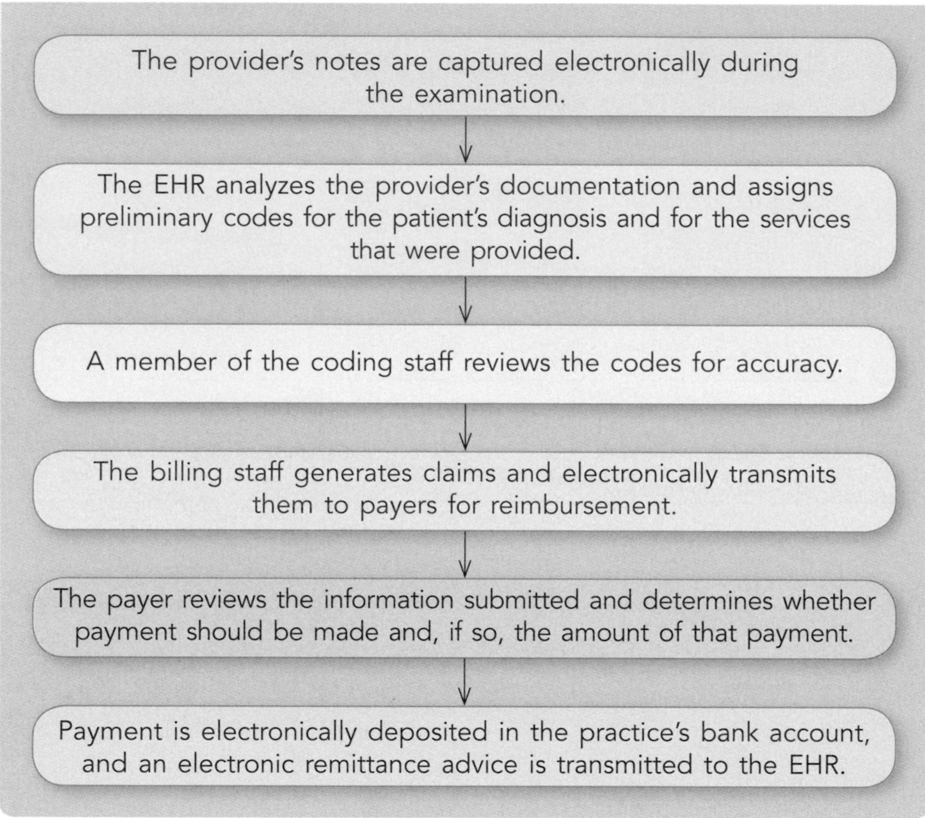

The provider's notes are captured electronically during the examination.
The EHR analyzes the provider's documentation and assigns preliminary codes for the patient's diagnosis and for the services that were provided.
A member of the coding staff reviews the codes for accuracy.
The billing staff generates claims and electronically transmits them to payers for reimbursement.
The payer reviews the information submitted and determines whether payment should be made and, if so, the amount of that payment.
Payment is electronically deposited in the practice's bank account, and an electronic remittance advice is transmitted to the EHR.

Among the advantages of computer-assisted coding are that it:

- Ensures that documentation exists for services billed, since codes were assigned based on electronic documentation
- Aids in selection of appropriate codes
- Reduces the number of unbilled procedures due to lost or forgotten procedures
- Automatically enters codes in the practice management system (PMS) or EHR
- Reduces the time between the patient visit and the submission of the claim for payment, leading to more timely reimbursement

Clinical Tools in the Electronic Health Record

Electronic health records are much more than a computerized form of a paper medical record. In addition to streamlining the workflow in a physician practice, EHRs contain features that aid clinicians in providing patients with safe, effective health care. Some of the more common features are access to current clinical information while making a diagnosis, identifying patients at risk for a specific disease, and monitoring patients' compliance with prevention guidelines and recommended treatments.

To provide effective treatment to patients, providers need up-to-date information about diseases and their treatment options. This information is not static; it changes on a regular basis. At the same time it is changing, the volume of information is also expanding. Researchers are working on developing new treatments, and the availability of inexpensive computing facilities makes it easy to collect and process large amounts of data.

Today, physicians are faced with an overload of clinical information. This is especially true for family care and internal medicine providers, who require knowledge about a broad range of diseases. Since a provider cannot possibly read and retain such a large amount of clinical information, there is a significant lag between the time research discoveries are made and the time they are applied in clinical practice. The care given to patients is not always as effective as it would be if the latest scientific evidence were applied.

DECISION-SUPPORT TOOLS

Deciding on the best treatment for a patient requires not just information about the patient's current and past condition, but also access to the latest medical knowledge. **Decision-support tools,** a feature of many EHRs, make the latest clinical information available to providers at the point-of-care. While these tools are no replacement for the judgment of an experienced physician, their use may lower the number of medical errors and result in better patient outcomes.

decision-support tools computer-based program that make the latest clinical information available.

Consider an example of how a decision-support tool can assist a physician and lead to a more timely diagnosis. When a physician enters a patient's age, signs, and symptoms into the EHR, the software provides additional questions to ask the patient. Based on the patient's answers to these questions, the software offers a list of possible diagnoses, with the more likely ones listed first. Once the physician selects a diagnosis, the program lists the tests that should be performed to confirm or rule out the diagnosis as well as the latest advances in treatment options.

TRACKING AND MONITORING PATIENT CARE

In outpatient settings such as a physician practice, it is not always possible to know what actually happens once a patient leaves the office.

Often the doctor does not know whether the patient followed the care instructions. Did he get an X-ray of his left shoulder? Did she pick up the prescription? Did he go for a colonoscopy? While offices try to follow up on patients and determine whether they followed the care plan laid out by the doctor, it is difficult to follow up on all patients all the time. The electronic health record provides doctors with a greater ability to manage and track patients' care, since information from external sources is also available in electronic form. For example, radiology and laboratory facilities can send electronic reports to the physician office, and the reports become part of the EHR. Some pharmacies electronically alert a physician office when a prescription has not been filled within a certain amount of time.

SCREENING FOR ILLNESS OR DISEASE

A clinician can use an EHR to search patient records and determine whether individuals have received recommended preventive screenings for breast cancer, heart disease, and other conditions (see Figure 3-12). Patients who are not current with wellness screenings can be called or contacted by mail or e-mail with reminders to schedule the overdue tests. In an office with paper-based records, it is much more difficult to determine which patients are up-to-date with screenings and which are not, since it requires pulling and searching each patient's chart.

IDENTIFYING AT-RISK PATIENTS

Electronic health records (EHRs) are being used to help identify patients who are at risk for certain diseases. If individuals can be identified before they develop a disease, they may be able to take preventive measures to avoid developing the illness. In an office without an EHR, a provider would have to spend many hours reading patient charts to determine who might be at risk for certain

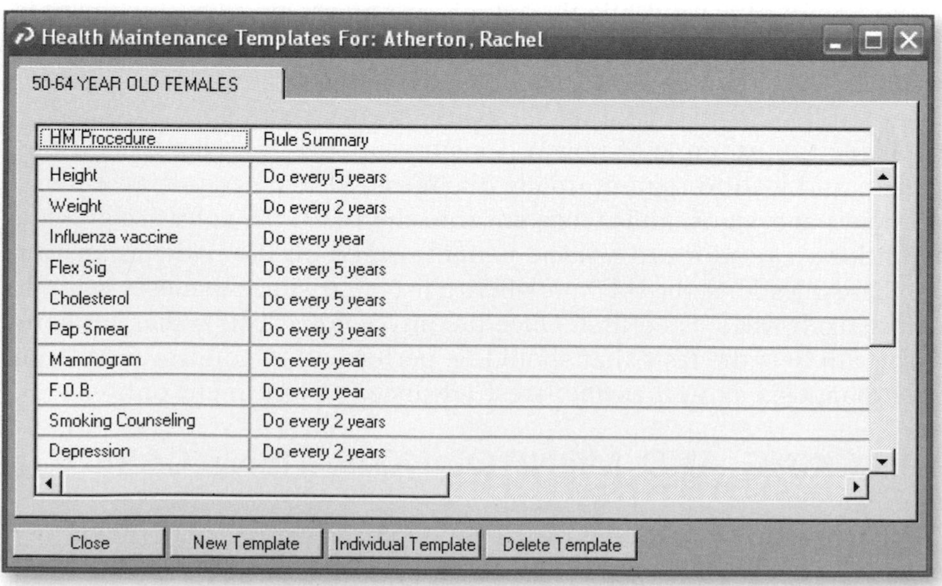

Figure 3-12

A list of recommended health maintenance screenings for a 50-64 year-old female.

Making It Real

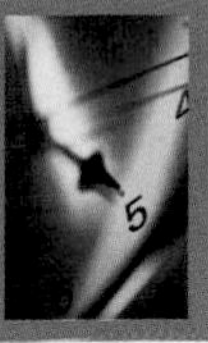

Screening for Cancer

While most Americans are aware that screening tests are available for a number of different cancers, they are not sure when they should be tested or, in some cases, which particular test is best.

Breast

The most common screening for breast cancer is a mammogram, which is an X-ray of the breast used to detect breast changes in women.

By the numbers:

› 57 percent of American women are not aware that age forty is the recommended age to start getting mammograms.

› 73 percent know that they should get mammograms every one to two years after screening has begun.

› 75 percent of women over age thirty-five report that their health care provider has recommended a mammogram for breast cancer screening within the past year.

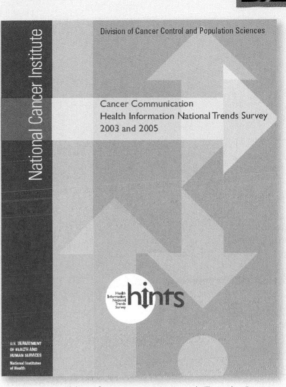

Source: Health Information National Trends Survey (HINT), hints.cancer.gov

Colon and Rectum

A number of screening methods are available to detect colorectal cancer, including fecal occult blood tests (FOBT), double contrast barium enema, sigmoidoscopy, and colonoscopy. By giving patients a choice, physicians hope to increase the number of patients who get screened.

By the numbers:

› 54 percent know that screening for colorectal cancer should start at age fifty.

› 53 percent of respondents over age forty-five say that their health care provider has recommended screening for colorectal cancer.

› When asked to name tests that detect colorectal cancer, 40 percent of respondents were unable to come up with the name of one of the tests.

conditions. With an EHR, it is much easier to develop a list of patients at risk for developing a specific disease. Taking into account factors such as a patient's age, gender, and family history as well as clinical examination results, the EHR identifies these patients and notifies the person responsible for scheduling appointments as well as the patients' providers.

For example, women with osteoporosis are at greater risk of fractures due to falls. To reduce that risk, a practice decided that all women at risk for osteoporosis should receive bone density scans every two years. Women who had not had bone density screenings in the last two years were sent letters and received telephone calls suggesting that they schedule the test. If a test showed signs of bone thinning, the patient was given medication to halt the progression of the disease. In this practice, the EHR plays a key role in identifying and treating potential problems before they become serious health issues.

MANAGING PATIENTS WITH CHRONIC DISEASES

chronic diseases prolonged conditions that rarely improve and often cannot be cured.

disease management (DM) systematic approach to improving health care for people with chronic diseases.

Diseases such as diabetes, depression, congestive heart failure, obesity, and asthma are considered chronic diseases. **Chronic diseases** are prolonged conditions that rarely improve and that often cannot be cured. **Disease management (DM)** is a systematic approach to improving the health of people with chronic diseases. Research has demonstrated that patient compliance with regular tests and treatments can reduce future complications and help delay progression of the disease.

In the physician practice, EHR contains tools that facilitate the ongoing management of chronic diseases, including alerts and reminders. Disease management requires tracking patients over time to monitor the course of the disease and the patients' compliance with treatment. An EHR can be set up to track individuals with chronic diseases, including sending a reminder to the patient when an appointment is near and alerting the provider when patients miss an appointment or a procedure such as a blood test.

IMPROVING THE QUALITY AND SAFETY OF PATIENT CARE WITH EVIDENCE-BASED GUIDELINES

clinical guidelines recommended patient care based on the best available scientific evidence.

The EHR makes it easy for physicians to identify all patients diagnosed with a specific disease and ensure that their care follows recommended clinical guidelines. **Clinical guidelines** are descriptions of recommended patient care for a given condition based on the best available scientific evidence. The content of a guideline is based on a systematic review of clinical evidence and is developed with consensus among experts in the field. For example, research has shown that patients with congestive heart failure respond well to treatment with beta blocker and ACE inhibitor medications. With an EHR in place, an alert can be set up to send a message to the provider with a list of all patients whose current treatment is not in compliance with the guideline.

For example, one of the clinical guidelines for the management of diabetes is that optimal care for patients ages eighteen to seventy-five requires meeting all of the following:

- Annual screening for LDL with LDL less than 100 mg/dL
- HbA1C screening within the last six months with a value less than 7 percent
- Last recorded systolic blood pressure less than 130 mm
- Documentation in the medical record that the patient does not use tobacco
- Documentation that the patient regularly takes aspirin (if age forty or older)

The goal of a practice is to increase the number of diabetic patients who meet all requirements. To do this, the office must identify and monitor where their patients stand on each of the requirements. Using an EHR system, this would entail the following steps:

1. Search for all patients who have been diagnosed with diabetes.
2. Examine laboratory results in the EHR, and determine which patients' lab values do not meet the standards.
3. Contact these patients to schedule lab tests followed by office visits.

Some insurers and government programs offer physicians pay for performance incentives to increase the number of patients who meet care standards. One example is Medicare's voluntary Physician Quality Reporting Initiative (PQRI). Medicare-eligible providers who elect to participate and who meet quality measures receive a bonus payment of 1.5 percent of total allowed charges for covered Medicare physician fee schedule services. There is a maximum allowable bonus payment per year.

The Centers for Medicare and Medicaid Services developed a list of seventy-four quality measures. For example, Measure 56, Vital Signs for Community-Acquired Bacterial Pneumonia, looks at the percentage of patients eighteen or older diagnosed with community-acquired bacterial pneumonia whose vital signs have been documented in the medical record and reviewed by the clinician. To be eligible for the bonus, a provider must report on at least three of the seventy-four measures.

E-Prescribing and Electronic Health Records

According to *Preventing Medication Errors: Quality Chasm Series* (Institute of Medicine, 2006), errors in prescribing or taking medication harm 1.5 million Americans each year. Examples of errors include prescribing a drug that could interact with another medication the patient is taking, dispensing the wrong medication because the handwriting

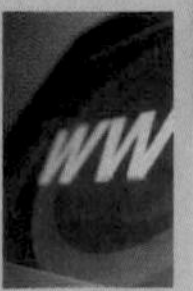

Chapter 3 Online Discovery

The National Guideline Clearinghouse™ (NGC) is an online clearinghouse of evidence-based clinical guidelines that is updated on a weekly basis. The site contains more than two thousand documents created and updated by such leading health care organizations as the American Academy of Family Physicians, the American Academy of Pediatrics, the American Cancer Society, and the American Heart Association. Open a web browser and go to www.guideline.gov.

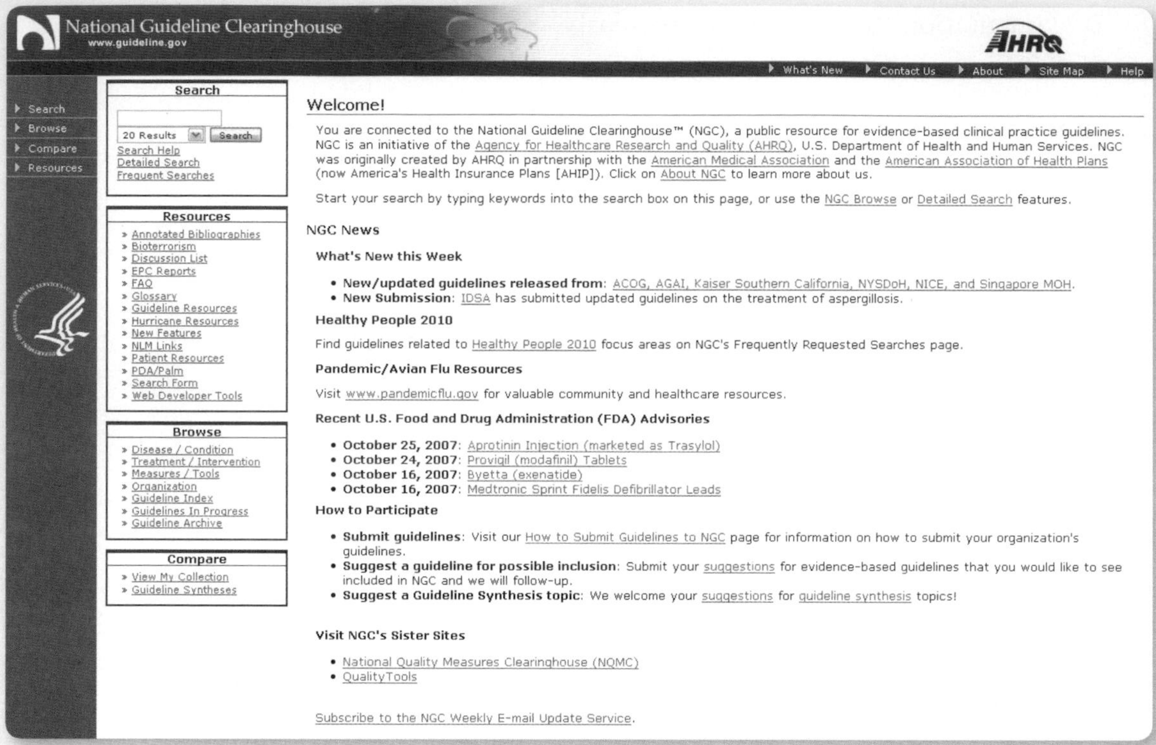

In the Search box on the left side of the window, enter *migraine* and click the Search button. Select a guideline from the list that appears, and read it by clicking the underlined words. After you have reviewed the guideline answer the questions below.

Thinking About It

1. Describe the type of information provided in the guideline you selected.

   ____

2. What group or organization wrote the guideline?

   ____

3. Is evidence listed to support the guideline? What type of evidence?

   ____

When you are finished viewing the website and answering the questions, close your web browser.

on the prescription was misread, and prescribing the wrong dose of a drug for a very young or very old patient. The IOM report suggests that many of these errors could be avoided if e-prescribing were adopted on a widespread basis and recommends the use of e-prescriptions by all providers and pharmacies by 2010.

The e-prescribing functions vary from one EHR to another, yet the ability to write a prescription and electronically transmit it to a pharmacy is a feature of most EHRs (see Figure 3-13). By writing prescriptions electronically, providers can avoid many of the mistakes that occur with handwritten prescriptions. Once a provider selects a drug for a patient, the EHR checks for drug allergies, drug-drug interactions, and other potential conflicts, using information in the patient's medical record, including past history, allergies, and a complete medication list.

The EHR also checks that the medication is in the formulary of the patient's health plan. A **formulary** is a list of pharmaceutical products and dosages deemed by a health care organization to be the best, most economical treatments for a condition or disease. Health plans reimburse patients for drugs listed in the formulary only, so it is essential for the provider to have this information before the patient leaves the office (see Figure 3-14 on page 98). If a medication is not in the formulary, the EHR can suggest an alternative drug. Since the medications in formularies change from time to time, the formulary data in the EHRs are updated regularly.

formulary pharmaceutical products and dosages deemed the best, most economical treatments.

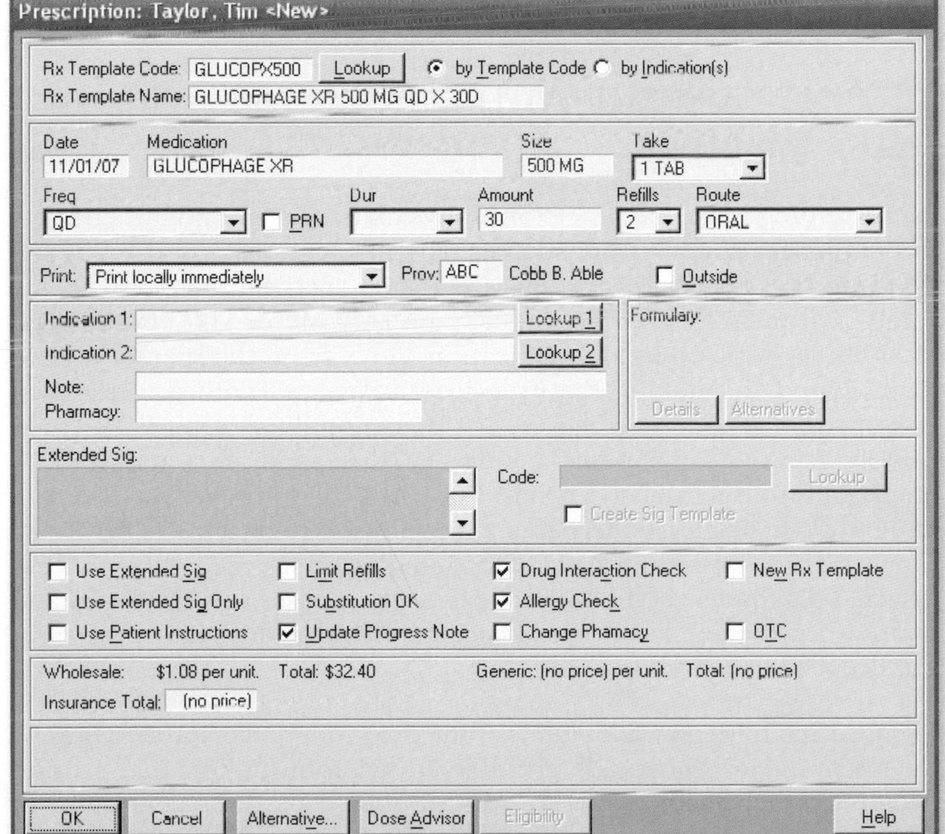

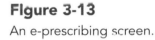

Figure 3-13

An e-prescribing screen.

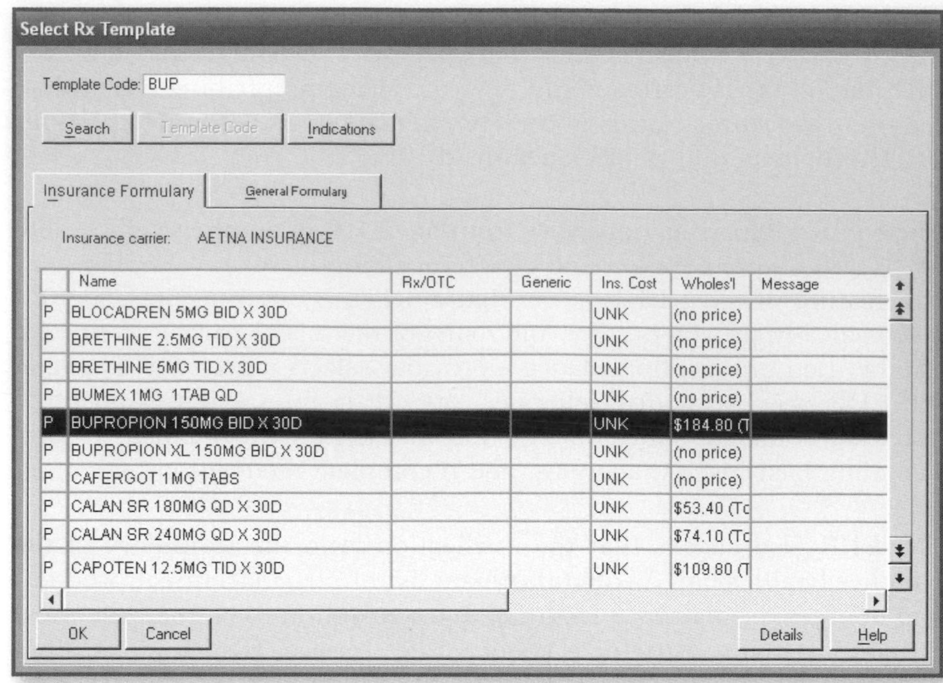

Figure 3-14
Partial list of medications available in a patient's health plan formulary.

Some EHRs even check whether the medication is in stock at the patient's preferred pharmacy. It is much better to know that a drug is in stock before the patient goes to pick it up at the pharmacy. E-prescribing also gives the pharmacy time to prepare the prescription so the patient will not have to wait once he or she arrives.

KEEPING CURRENT WITH ELECTRONIC DRUG DATABASES

E-prescribing makes it easier for a physician to keep up with changes in the pharmaceutical field, such as new medications approved by the Food and Drug Administration (FDA) and medications recalled for safety reasons. The pharmaceutical company Merck voluntarily withdrew its arthritis and pain medication Vioxx from the market after a study found that taking the drug was associated with an increased risk of serious cardiovascular events. In a case like this, an EHR could rapidly identify all patients taking the drug and alert the staff to quickly notify them of the recall. The EHR also provides access to a database that suggests alternate medications to replace recalled drugs. Some EHRs have built-in medication databases, but most access external databases via the Internet. These databases are developed and maintained by companies that specialize in providing up-to-the minute drug information.

Because an EHR provides up-to-date drug reference information at the point-of-care, providers are able to get information that aids in deciding which medications to prescribe for a patient's condition. In

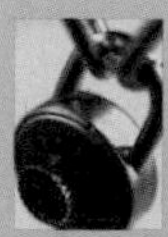

Privacy and Security Alert

Prescription Information Found in Dumpsters

In 2006, NBC-TV affiliate WTHR in Indianapolis visited the garbage dumpsters of sixty-five local pharmacies, including major chains such as CVS and Walgreens. While some were secured by locking mechanisms, most had no security in place. Investigators from the station collected plastic bags full of trash from each of the dumpsters and looked at the contents. Among other things, they found medications, prescriptions, and prescription labels. Investigators were able to find names addresses, and even phone numbers of people who take medication for depression and for genital herpes. Someone used information obtained from discarded records to enter the home of one woman and steal pain medication.

As a result of the investigation, the Indiana Board of Pharmacy filed complaints against thirty pharmacies. Several of the major pharmacy chains have already taken measures to comply with state and federal laws that require drugstores and health care providers to protect patient privacy. Walgreens is requiring locking dumpsters, while CVS employees must keep trash from the pharmacy in a certain area in the store, from where it will be picked up and taken to a regional facility for appropriate disposal.

The U.S. Department of Health and Human Services Office for Civil Rights, as well as the Indiana attorney general's office, have launched independent investigations as a result of WTHR's prescription privacy investigation to determine whether pharmacies featured in the reports should face fines or other penalties for improperly disposing of patient information.

addition to information about dosage, side effects, interactions, and other data, these databases offer the latest clinical evidence on drug effectiveness.

The steps required to refill a patient prescription in a paper-based office and in an electronic office illustrate the advantages of e-prescribing:

Prescription Refill—Paper-Based

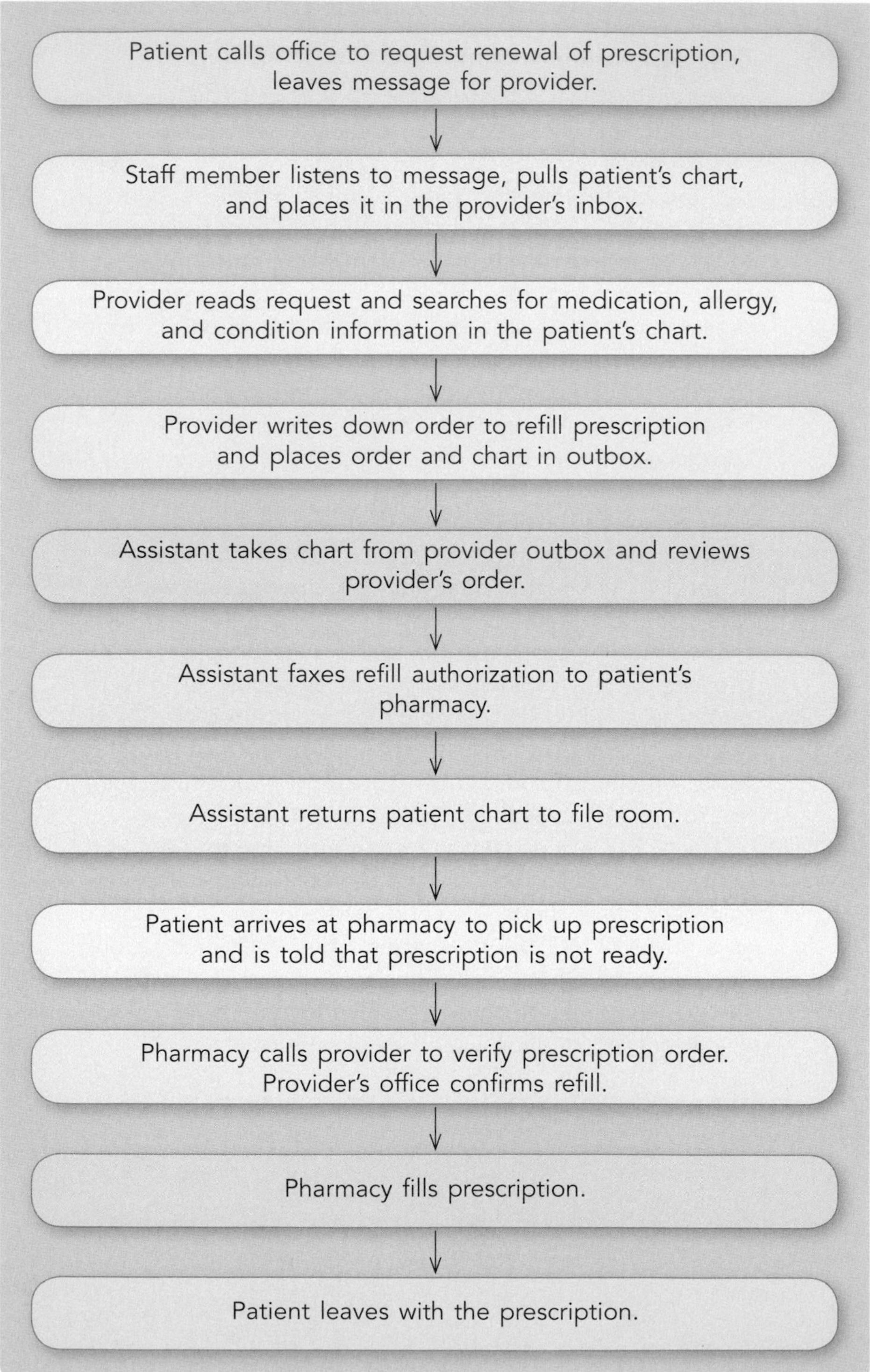

Patient calls office to request renewal of prescription, leaves message for provider.
Staff member listens to message, pulls patient's chart, and places it in the provider's inbox.
Provider reads request and searches for medication, allergy, and condition information in the patient's chart.
Provider writes down order to refill prescription and places order and chart in outbox.
Assistant takes chart from provider outbox and reviews provider's order.
Assistant faxes refill authorization to patient's pharmacy.
Assistant returns patient chart to file room.
Patient arrives at pharmacy to pick up prescription and is told that prescription is not ready.
Pharmacy calls provider to verify prescription order. Provider's office confirms refill.
Pharmacy fills prescription.
Patient leaves with the prescription.

Prescription Refill—Electronic

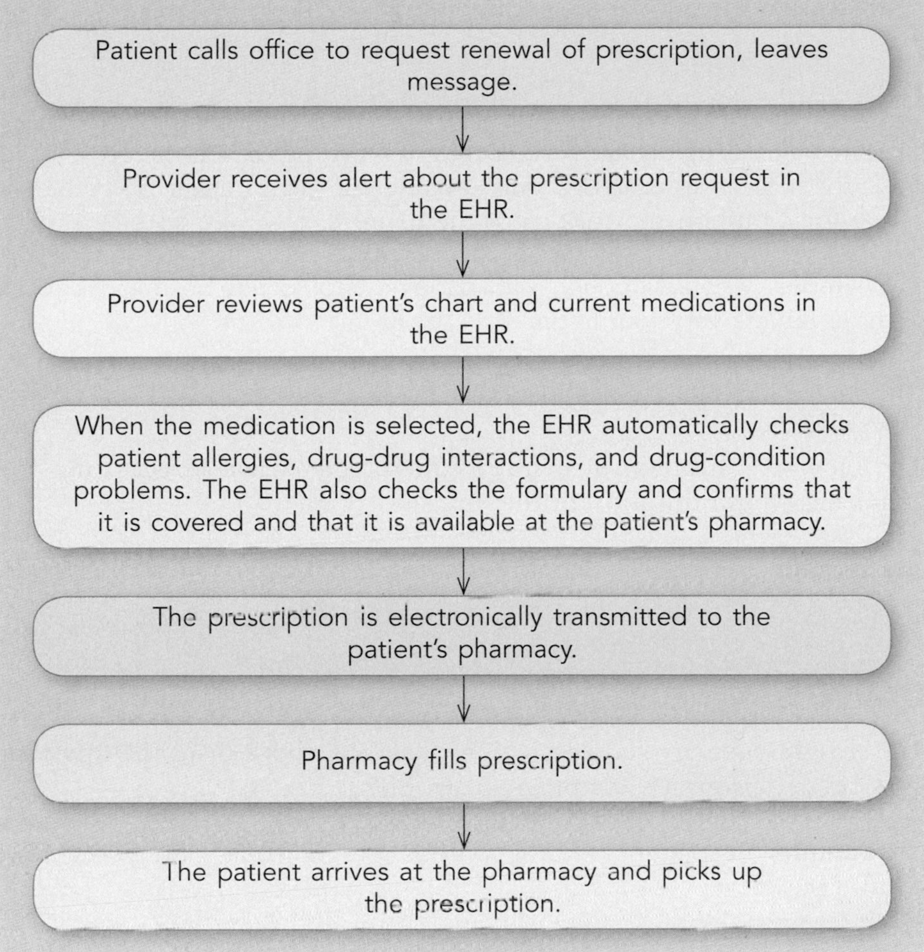

Patient calls office to request renewal of prescription, leaves message.
Provider receives alert about the prescription request in the EHR.
Provider reviews patient's chart and current medications in the EHR.
When the medication is selected, the EHR automatically checks patient allergies, drug-drug interactions, and drug-condition problems. The EHR also checks the formulary and confirms that it is covered and that it is available at the patient's pharmacy.
The prescription is electronically transmitted to the patient's pharmacy.
Pharmacy fills prescription.
The patient arrives at the pharmacy and picks up the prescription.

INCREASING PRESCRIPTION SAFETY

One of the main advantages of e-prescribing is its ability to rapidly perform important safety checks. As the provider selects a new medication, the EHR provides real-time alerts about potential problems. Medication safety screenings performed by an e-prescribing module include drug-allergy conflict, drug-disease conflict, incorrect dosage, incorrect duration, drug-pregnancy conflict, drug-age conflict, drug-gender conflict, and drug-drug interaction.

Drug-Allergy Conflict

The drug-allergy screen identifies and creates warnings associated with the use of target drugs in patients with a history of hypersensitivity to the target drug or drug class.

Example A patient who is allergic to penicillin should not be prescribed the drug.

Drug-Disease Conflict

The drug-disease screen creates warnings about the use of select target drugs in patients with specified medical conditions.

Example A patient diagnosed with an eating disorder should not be prescribed the antidepressant Bupropion.

Incorrect Dosage

The incorrect drug dosage screen creates warnings when the prescribed dose for select target drugs falls outside the usual adult or pediatric range for common indications of the drug.

Example Acetaminophen with codeine should not be prescribed as three tablets very four hours.

Incorrect Duration

The incorrect duration of therapy edit screens select target drugs for usual maximum duration of therapy.

Example Amoxicillin should not be prescribed for more than fourteen days.

Drug-Pregnancy Conflict

The drug-pregnancy screen creates warnings about drug therapy that may be inappropriate for pregnant women.

Example A patient who is pregnant should not be prescribed tetracycline.

Drug-Age Conflict

The drug-age screen creates warnings on select target drug use in pediatric or geriatric patients.

Example A patient under the age of two should not be prescribed acetaminophen with codeine.

Drug-Gender Conflict

The drug-gender screen creates warnings about specific drug use in males or females. This screen identifies prescriptions submitted for target drugs labeled for use by one sex only.

Example A male patient should not be prescribed the oral contraceptive Depo-Provera.

Drug-Drug Interactions

Drug-drug interactions are potential adverse medical effects that occur when patients receive two or more specific drugs together.

Example A patient taking Warfarin should not be prescribed the antibiotic ciprofloxacin.

SAVING TIME AND MONEY

In addition to increasing the safety of prescribed medications, e-prescribing saves the medical practice time and money. Consider the steps required to complete a typical prescription refill request in a paper system and in an electronic system, as shown on pages 100–101.

The use of e-prescribing also saves the provider and the support staff time. Since the EHR checks for most potential medication incompatibilities before the prescription reaches the pharmacy, there are fewer calls from the pharmacy to clarify a prescription. There is also no need for a staff member to pull a patient chart when a request is made, since the patient's record is stored in the EHR, not on paper. Before formularies were available electronically, the support staff was required to manually check whether a drug was in a particular health plan's formulary.

CHAPTER REVIEW

CHAPTER SUMMARY

1. Regardless of whether an office is using EHR or paper-based records, the office visit workflow consists of five steps: pre-visit, pre-exam, exam, post-exam, and post-visit. While paper-based offices accomplish the same tasks, offices that use an EHR complete the tasks in less time, often with increased patient safety and health care quality.
2. During Step 1, pre-visit, a patient schedules an appointment and completes patient information forms online. This takes the place of filling out paper forms in the waiting room and saves time, since the office staff does not have to manually enter the patient's information into the billing program and file the paper forms.
3. Step 2 is completed at a computer in the waiting room. The patient confirms the demographic and insurance data he or she has already entered. The EHR checks insurance eligibility, and the patient has the option of making a copayment via computer or paying at the front desk. The medical assistant then escorts the patient to an exam room.
4. Step 3 consists of two parts. During the first phase, the medical assistant checks the patient's vital signs and gathers information relevant to the current visit as well as allergy and medication information. The MA enters this information in the EHR while the exam is taking place. In the second phase, the physician reviews the patient's chart in the EHR and examines the patient. The physician documents the visit by typing in free text or responding to templates that contain commonly used clinical words and phrases. Since data are entered while the physician is with the patient, it is less likely for information to be left out or forgotten, as sometimes happens when doctors wait until after the exam to record their observations and findings. Using an EHR allows the doctor to order tests and medications electronically, without the use of paper forms.
5. In Step 4, the patient stops at the front desk to pick up radiology or laboratory test orders, prescriptions, and educational materials. The front desk reviews the billing module of the EHR to see whether additional payment is due and schedules follow-up appointments before the patient leaves.
6. In Step 5, post-visit, two different tasks are completed. The coding staff reviews the codes assigned by the EHR, makes any required changes, and finalizes the codes. A member of the billing department uses the coding and visit information to prepare and submit an electronic claim to the patient's health plan. Reimbursement is electronically deposited into the practice's bank account. Also during Step 5, reports from radiology and

laboratory facilities arrive in electronic form and are reviewed by the physician. Any abnormal results are indicated by a special alert that appears on the physician's EHR screen.

7. Every service submitted for payment must be documented in the patient's medical record, including medical care, diagnostic tests, consultations, surgeries, and other services eligible for payment. To be reimbursed for services, the provider must document each service provided to the patient. Electronic health records contain tools that make it easier for clinicians to document patient encounters. With an EHR, physicians can efficiently document all the services they provide at the point-of-care, using structured templates, unformatted text, or a number of other choices. As a result, documentation is completed sooner, and the elimination of physician dictation means that there is no transcription expense.

Whether physicians are reimbursed for the services they provide is directly linked to the codes submitted to the payer on the insurance claim. When a payer receives a claim, the codes are reviewed. Payers want to know whether a service was appropriate for the patient's condition and whether the treatment was necessary. In a paper-based office, the coding, billing, and reimbursement cycle normally takes anywhere from three to fourteen days. The process of coding with software is known as computer-assisted coding. Initial codes are suggested by the software and are later reviewed and verified by a professional coder. The integration of automated coding with the billing system ensures documentation of services billed, aids in the selection of appropriate codes, reduces number of unbilled procedures, and shortens the time between a patient visit and receipt of reimbursement.

8. Electronic health records are much more than a computerized form of a paper medical record. In addition to streamlining the workflow in a physician practice, EHRs contain features that aid clinicians in providing patients with safe, effective health care. Some of these features include access to current clinical information at the point-of-care, decision-support tools that help confirm or rule out a diagnosis, ability to track patient compliance with care plans, ability to ensure that patients receive appropriate wellness screenings, identification of patients at risk for a specific disease, management of patients with chronic diseases, and evidence-based clinical guidelines to improve the quality of care.

9. The ability to write a prescription and transmit it to a pharmacy electronically, known as e-prescribing, is a feature of most EHRs. By writing prescriptions electronically, providers can avoid many of the mistakes that occur with handwritten prescriptions. E-prescribing also makes it possible to determine ahead of time whether a medication is included in the formulary of the patient's health plan. One of the main advantages of e-prescribing is its ability to rapidly perform important safety checks. As the provider selects a patient's new medication, the EHR provides real-time alerts about potential problems, including drug-allergy conflicts, drug-drug conflicts, and incorrect dosages. In addition to increasing the safety of prescribed medications, e-prescribing saves the provider and the support staff time, with fewer calls from pharmacies to clarify prescriptions and no need to pull a patient chart when a refill request is made.

CHECK YOUR UNDERSTANDING

Part 1. Write *T* or *F* in the blank to indicate whether you think the statement is true or false.

_____ **1.** Some EHRs offer patients the option of making appointments on a website.

_____ **2.** With electronic check-in, the EHR verifies insurance eligibility without the assistance of the staff at the front desk.

_____ **3.** After the patient is escorted to the exam room, the medical assistant checks the patient's vital signs, gathers information relevant to the current visit, and enters this information in the EHR while the exam is taking place.

_____ **4.** The electronic entering and tracking of laboratory and radiology tests eliminates the need to pull a patient chart, file the result, and route the chart to the physician.

_____ **5.** With computer-assisted coding, a coder must still review documentation and finalize procedure and diagnosis codes.

_____ **6.** Disease management is a method of screening to determine which patients are at-risk for a certain disease.

_____ **7.** A formulary's main function is to check for interactions between the patient's current medication and the newly prescribed medication.

_____ **8.** Clinical guidelines are based on scientific evidence.

_____ **9.** Templates enable providers to document patient encounters more efficiently.

_____ **10.** The history of present illness (HPI) is an inventory of body systems in which the patient reports any symptoms experienced.

_____ **11.** Clinical tools help physicians manage large amounts of information.

_____ **12.** Most EHRs offer more than one method of documenting a patient encounter.

Part 2. In the space provided, write a definition of the term.

13. Chronic diseases

____

____

14. Clinical guidelines

____

____

15. Computer-assisted coding

16. Decision-support tools

17. Disease management

18. Formulary

19. Point-of-care

THINKING ABOUT THE ISSUES

Part 3. In the space provided, write a brief paragraph describing your thoughts about the following issues.

20. In practices using EHR, websites offer new ways to collect patient information. Patients complete such information as demographic and insurance information, medical history, current condition, and lifestyle. This offers several advantages to the patient, the office staff, and the physicians. However, many patients are reluctant to enter data on the website. Why do you think this is the case?

21. EHRs contain features that aid clinicians in providing patients with safe, effective health care. Some of the more common features include access to current clinical information when making a diagnosis, identifying patients at risk for a specific disease, and monitoring patients' compliance with prevention guidelines and recommend treatments. Yet many physicians have been slow to take advantage of these features. Why do you think this is the case?

Electronic Health Records in the Hospital

CHAPTER OUTLINE

The Need for Clinical Information Systems
The Complexity of Hospital Information Systems
Components of an Inpatient EHR System
Clinical Documentation
Computerized Physician Order Entry
Decision-Support Tools
Medication Management in Hospitals
Technology and Medication Ordering
Electronic Medication Administration Records (eMAR)
Results Reporting
Digital Images and the Electronic Health Record
Advantages of Electronic Results Reporting

LEARNING OUTCOMES

After completing this chapter, you will be able to:

1. Explain the functions of an EHR in an acute care hospital.
2. List the primary benefits of a hospital EHR.
3. List the uses of clinical documentation in an inpatient setting.
4. Discuss the advantages of computerized physician order entry (CPOE).
5. Explain how decision-support tools improve the quality of patient care.
6. Describe how CPOE and electronic medication administration records (eMAR) work together to reduce medication errors.
7. Describe the advantages of electronic results reporting over traditional paper-based reporting systems.

KEY TERMS

adverse drug event (ADE)
computerized physician order entry (CPOE)
electronic medication administration records (e-MARs)
five rights
medication administration record (MAR)
medication reconciliation
order sets
transition points

Why This Chapter Is Important to You

The information in this chapter will enable you to:

- Understand the advantages of electronic health records (EHR) in a hospital.
- Understand the role of documentation in quality improvement efforts.
- Understand how CPOE reduces medication errors.
- Understand how eMAR systems are used to check the five rights when administering medication to a patient.

In an acute care setting, an electronic health record (EHR) integrates electronic data from multiple clinical systems to provide a single access point for information about a patient's health care. These systems commonly include data for ancillary services such as laboratory, radiology, and pharmacy systems, among others. If the information in each of these systems is not integrated by the EHR, caregivers will not have a complete picture of a patient's condition.

In addition, an EHR captures and stores patient information of its own flow of care, such as progress notes and care plans. An EHR makes a person's health information available at the place and time that it is needed by health care professionals and enhances communication among them. The primary function of an inpatient EHR is to assist in managing the transactions involved in a patient's care, such as ordering diagnostic tests, viewing lab results, and administering medications, with the goal of improving quality and increasing patient safety.

The Need for Clinical Information Systems

While hospitals have used information technology (IT) for billing and administrative functions for a long time, the widespread use of IT in clinical functions is a fairly recent development. A number of factors are responsible for the increased adoption of EHRs and other clinical systems in acute care hospitals.

Major studies report that medical errors are still a serious problem. According to a report by the Institute of Medicine (IOM) released in 2006, the incidence of medication errors is higher than previously estimated, and a HealthGrades study released in 2007 found that medical errors actually rose 3 percent from 2003 to 2005 (Institute of Medicine,

"Preventing Medication Errors: Quality Chasm Series," July 20, 2006; "HealthGrades Patient Safety in American Hospitals Study," www.healthgrades.com). At the same time, a number of studies have suggested that information technology can play a key role in reducing the number of errors.

Furthermore, the amount of medical information available has become unmanageable. It is difficult for physicians, nurses, and other health care practitioners to keep up with the latest developments, which makes it difficult to ensure that patients receive the highest quality care.

Another factor in the increased adoption of EHRs is that, more and more, Medicare and other payers are basing payment on hospitals' ability to achieve certain quality standards. One way hospitals can meet standards is to encourage clinicians to follow evidence-based treatment plans. At the same time, hospitals must be able to document clinicians' performance. This requires complete, accurate documentation, which is easier to capture and store in an electronic system.

The Complexity of Hospital Information Systems

Information technology is even more complex in a hospital setting than in a physician office. In the physician office, the EHR contains all the clinical information about patients. It may also contain administrative and billing information, or this may reside in a separate billing program. In either case, the EHR is largely self-contained and functions as the sole clinical system.

Hospitals, in contrast, have a number of clinical systems that capture and store specialized information. Hospitals require multiple systems because of the number of functions they perform. Blood samples are drawn and sent to the hospital laboratory for analysis. Patients are transported to radiology for CT scans, ultrasounds, and MRIs. Tissues are sent from the operating room to the pathology department for analysis. Cardiology procedures such as ECGs are administered at the patient's bedside, while angiograms are conducted in the cardiology catheterization laboratory. The pharmacy fulfills orders for medication. Each these departments has its own system, designed to meet the specific needs of that function. The components of a typical hospital information system (HIS) consist of the following separate systems:

- *Financial information systems* manage the business needs of a hospital, including payroll, billing and claim management, accounts receivable and payable, and others.
- *Laboratory information systems* manage information for all the laboratory units in the hospital, such as chemistry and hematology. Laboratory systems capture and track orders and store test results.

- *Pharmacy information systems* manage the pharmacy practice within the hospital, including medication orders, inventory, and reports.
- *Picture archiving and communication systems (PACS)* facilitate the archiving, processing, viewing, and storage of digital radiological images and reports, such as CT scans and ultrasounds.
- *Radiology information systems* facilitate the storing, tracking, and reporting of the results of radiological examinations such as CT scans and ultrasounds.
- *Clinical information systems* provide information about the patient's condition, diagnosis, and treatment that is intended to help physicians and other health care practitioners improve the quality, safety, and efficiency of clinical care.

Components of an Inpatient EHR System

In an inpatient setting, physicians and other clinicians use the system to document patient care; record observations of the patient's condition; place orders for tests, medications, and treatments; and review and interpret results. The major components of an inpatient EHR that this chapter will focus on include:

- Clinical documentation
- Computerized physician order entry
- Clinical decision support
- Electronic prescribing and electronic medication administration records
- Electronic results reporting

These areas are all interrelated. For example, when a physician is selecting a medication for a patient using computerized physician order entry, clinical decision support tools help the physician select the most appropriate medication. Similarly, orders for blood work or radiology examinations are placed using electronic order systems, while the results of the tests are reported by the electronic results reporting feature. Electronic reporting of test results is the natural outcome of computerized order entry. Figure 4-1 on page 112 shows a screen from an inpatient EHR.

The primary benefits of hospital EHRs include:

- Immediate access to complete, up-to-date information about patients, including progress notes, results of laboratory tests and imaging studies, medication administration, and responses to treatment
- Decreased turnaround times for medication delivery and completion of diagnostic tests due to electronic delivery of orders and results
- Increased efficiency by standardizing work processes and by integrating information from different departments

Figure 4-1

Screen from an inpatient EHR.

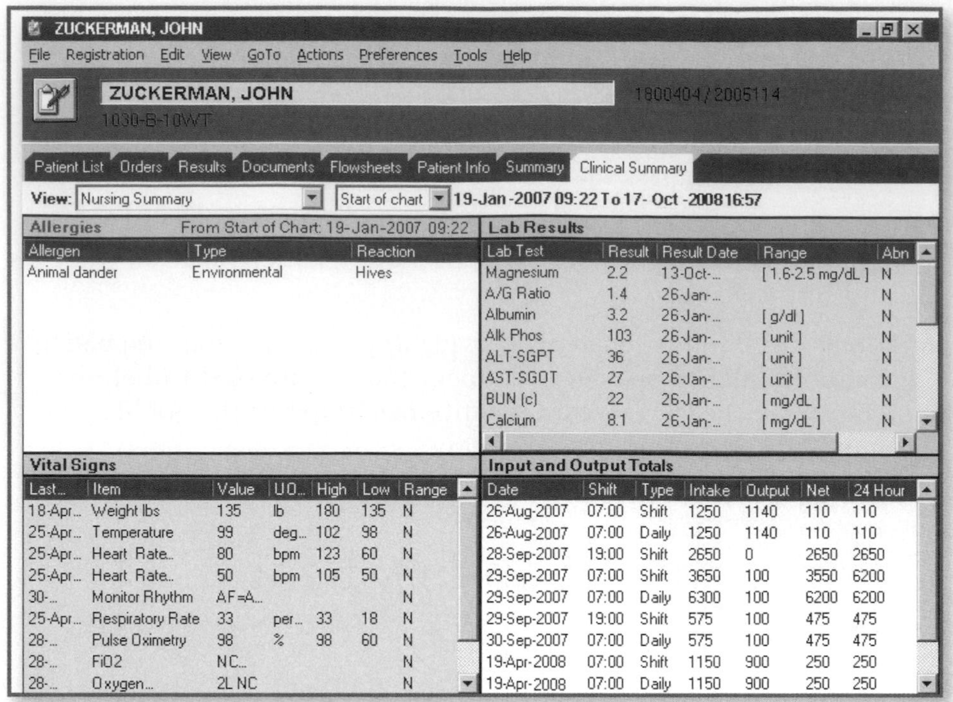

Allergen	Type	Reaction
Animal dander	Environmental	Hives

Lab Test	Result	Result Date	Range	Abn
Magnesium	2.2	13-Oct-...	[1.6-2.5 mg/dL]	N
A/G Ratio	1.4	26-Jan-...		N
Albumin	3.2	26-Jan-...	[g/dl]	N
Alk Phos	103	26-Jan-...	[unit]	N
ALT-SGPT	36	26-Jan-...	[unit]	N
AST-SGOT	27	26-Jan-...	[unit]	N
BUN (c)	22	26-Jan-...	[mg/dL]	N
Calcium	8.1	26-Jan-...	[mg/dL]	N

Last...	Item	Value	UO...	High	Low	Range
18-Apr...	Weight lbs	135	lb	180	135	N
25-Apr...	Temperature	99	deg...	102	98	N
25-Apr...	Heart Rate...	80	bpm	123	60	N
25-Apr...	Heart Rate...	50	bpm	105	50	N
30-...	Monitor Rhythm	AF=A...				N
25-Apr...	Respiratory Rate	33	per...	33	18	N
28-...	Pulse Oximetry	98	%	98	60	N
28-...	FiO2	NC...				N
28-...	Oxygen...	2L NC				N

Date	Shift	Type	Intake	Output	Net	24 Hour
26-Aug-2007	07:00	Shift	1250	1140	110	110
26-Aug-2007	07:00	Daily	1250	1140	110	110
28-Sep-2007	19:00	Shift	2650	0	2650	2650
29-Sep-2007	07:00	Shift	3650	100	3550	6200
29-Sep-2007	07:00	Daily	6300	100	6200	6200
29-Sep-2007	19:00	Shift	575	100	475	475
30-Sep-2007	07:00	Daily	575	100	475	475
19-Apr-2008	07:00	Shift	1150	900	250	250
19-Apr-2008	07:00	Daily	1150	900	250	250

The main benefit of EHRs, however, is not their ability to provide fast access to current and complete patients' records. The most significant contribution of EHRs is that they offer decision-support tools that help physicians make diagnosis and treatment decisions that provide patients with the safest, most effective care.

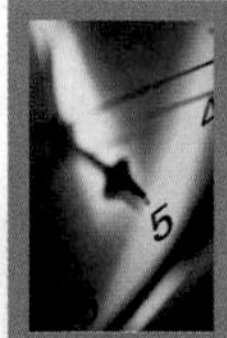

Making It Real

A Day in the Life of a Medical Record

What happens to a paper-based medical record during a day in a hospital? Where does it go? Who has access to it? A representative from the National Alliance for Health Information Technology visited a typical hospital that used paper records and tracked the movements of a record throughout the day.

The report follows the case of a woman who is being escorted in a wheelchair for a variety of tests. She has symptoms that suggest she might have had a stroke. Her chart is placed in a pocket on the back of the wheelchair, and before 3:00 P.M. it changes hands seventeen times.

The full report is available for download at www.nahit.org/dl/A_Day_in_the_Life.pdf.

TIME	CHART LOCATION	ACCESS
7:00am	Chart arrives in nurses' station with the patient from the ER – various elements from the ER (lab tests and observations) are being compiled by the unit clerk – *unit clerk has access to entire record*	1
7:20am	Hospital transport arrives to take patient to get EEG – chart given to porter – *porter has access to entire record*	2
7:25am	Chart placed in wheelchair pocket – wheeled through waiting area to EEG lab – chart left on desk in EEG room for 5 minutes	
7:30am	EEG technician looks at chart – *EEG technician has access to entire record*	3
8:00am	EEG completed – chart left on desk in EEG room for 5 minutes	
8:05am	Hospital transport arrives to take patient to cardiology lab for enchocardiogram – chart given to porter – *porter has access to entire record*	4
8:05am	Chart placed in wheelchair pocket – wheeled down corridor to cardiology lab – chart left on desk outside cardiology lab	
8:07am	Cardiology technician looks at chart and closes door – chart left on desk outside cardiology lab for 40 minutes – *cardiology technician has a ccess to entire record*	5
8:47am	Echocardiogram completed – door opens and technician flips through chart next to door	
8:50am	Hospital transport arrives to take patient to radiology department – chart given to porter – *porter has access to entire record*	6
8:50am	Chart placed in wheelchair pocket – wheeled down corridor to radiology lab and patient left in hallway by porter – chart left in wheelchair pocket in corridor for 5 minutes	
8:55am	Radiology technician arrives to take patient into x-ray room – chart taken into x-ray room – *radiology technician has access to entire record*	7
9:20am	Test is completed and patient is returned to wheelchair – chart placed on chair in hallway, then returned to wheelchair pocket	
9:25am	Hospital transport arrives to take patient back to hospital room – chart given to porter – *porter has access to entire record*	8
9:25am	Chart placed in wheelchair pocket – wheeled down corridor to nursing unit and wheeled into room – chart left at nursing station	
9:30am	Chart inspected at nursing unit by physical therapist – *physical therapist has access to entire record*	9
9:30am	Physical therapist and occupational therapist enter patient room – chart left on counter at nursing station – *occupational therapist has access to entire record*	10
10:00am	Visitor makes phone call at nursing station standing over chart that was left on the nursing station counter – *visitor potentially has access to record*	*
10:10am	Items added to chart at nursing station by physical therapist – a second physical therapist looks over at open chart while items are added – *second physical therapist can view all information in record*	11
10:12am	Nurse takes chart from physical therapist and works with it on nursing station – *nurse has access to entire record*	12
	Chart placed on shelf before noon	
1:45pm	Chart pulled from shelf to order CT scan	
2:15pm	Hospital transport arrives to take patient to radiology department for CT scan – chart given to porter – *porter has access to entire record*	13
2:15pm	Chart placed in wheelchair pocket – wheeled downstairs and to radiology department	
2:20pm	Chart delivered to radiology technician and left on the computer desk	
2:25pm	Radiology technician flips through chart as prepares for scan – *radiology technician has access to entire record*	14
2:35pm	Second radiology technician flips through chart at request of the first technician – *second radiology technician has access to entire record*	15
2:45pm	Hospital transport arrives to take patient back to hospital room – chart given to porter – *porter has access to entire record*	16
2:48pm	Chart placed in wheelchair pocket – wheeled down corridor to nursing unit and wheeled into room – chart left at nursing station – *nurses and unit clerk have access to the entire record*	17

Clinical Documentation

Clinical documentation contains all pertinent data collected in the course of providing care during a patient's hospital stay. It provides an accurate account of what happened and when it happened. Health care professionals record information chronologically on patient status, interventions provided, and the impact of the interventions on the patient's condition. Discharge planning, including instructions for the patient and any necessary follow-up, is also documented. Figure 4-2 illustrates a screen for entering patient documentation in an EHR.

In an inpatient setting, documentation is used to:

- Assist in patient care planning and continuity of care
- Provide evidence of the course of the patient's care and treatment during the hospital stay
- Facilitate communication among members of the patient care team
- Serve as a legal record to protect the interests of the patient, the hospital, and the clinician
- Supply data for research purposes
- Supply data for utilization review and quality improvement analysis and reporting
- Provide information that enables coders to determine the appropriate diagnosis and procedure codes to substantiate patient billing

Complete, up-to-date information is required to make the best treatment decisions, which is difficult when information is missing from patent documentation. If such information as a patient's lab results is not available, it is difficult to make a diagnosis, choose a course of treatment, and manage medications. In addition, staff members waste time and resources

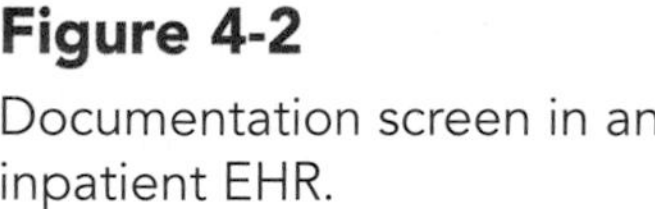

Figure 4-2

Documentation screen in an inpatient EHR.

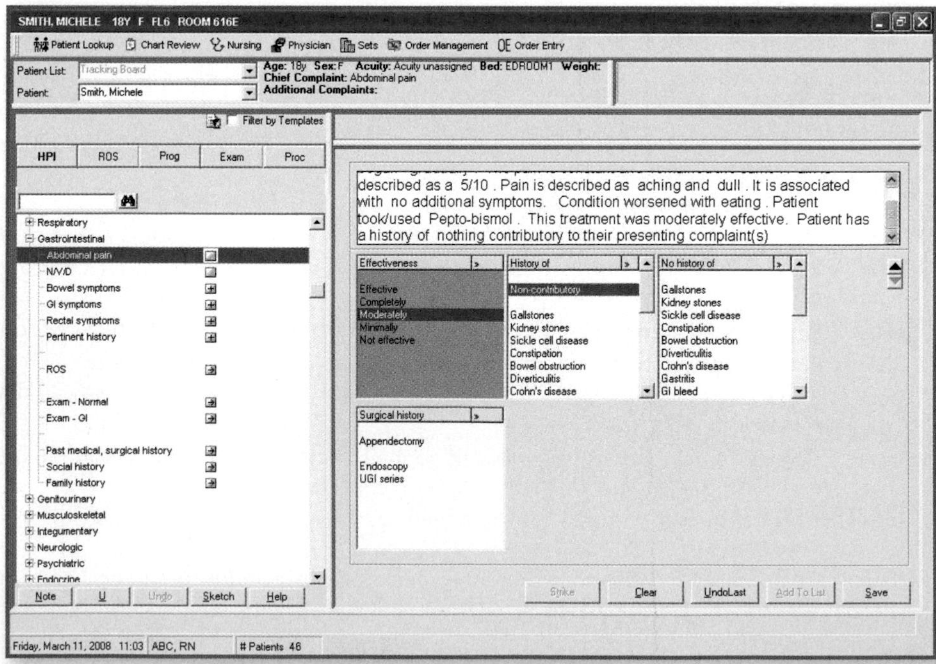

searching for the information. When orders for testing or treatment are illegible, errors are more likely to occur. Documentation that is of poor quality cannot be used as data for quality improvement efforts and outcomes reporting. The lack of accurate, timely data can lead to medication errors, duplicate testing, and less than optimal care.

Electronic documentation can eliminate many problems associated with paper documentation systems, including missing and incorrect data, duplication of patient records, and illegible entries. Electronic health records contain tools that make it easier to document care, such as preconfigured documentation templates, flow sheets, summaries, and care plans for common patient conditions. Templates may be based on best practice guidelines to assist caregivers in providing optimal care to patients. While documenting care, the EHR provides electronic prompts that alert the caregiver to required actions.

Computerized Physician Order Entry

Patient safety has been the subject of many articles and books, with a major focus on the frequency and costs of medical errors. A number of major health care organizations are looking for ways to reduce medical errors. One of the most promising developments to come from these studies is the use of computerized physician order entry (CPOE). **Computerized physician order entry (CPOE)** is an application used by physicians and other health care providers to enter patient care orders, including blood work, laboratory tests, radiology examinations, medication, and therapies. CPOE has the potential to reduce medication errors, standardize patient care, improve the efficiency of care delivery, and eliminate the need for paper ordering. Figure 4-3 illustrates a screen for entering orders in an inpatient EHR.

computerized physician order entry (CPOE) application for health care providers to enter patient care orders.

Physicians' orders are important elements of a patient's diagnosis and treatment. Prior to the use of CPOE systems, physicians' orders were generally

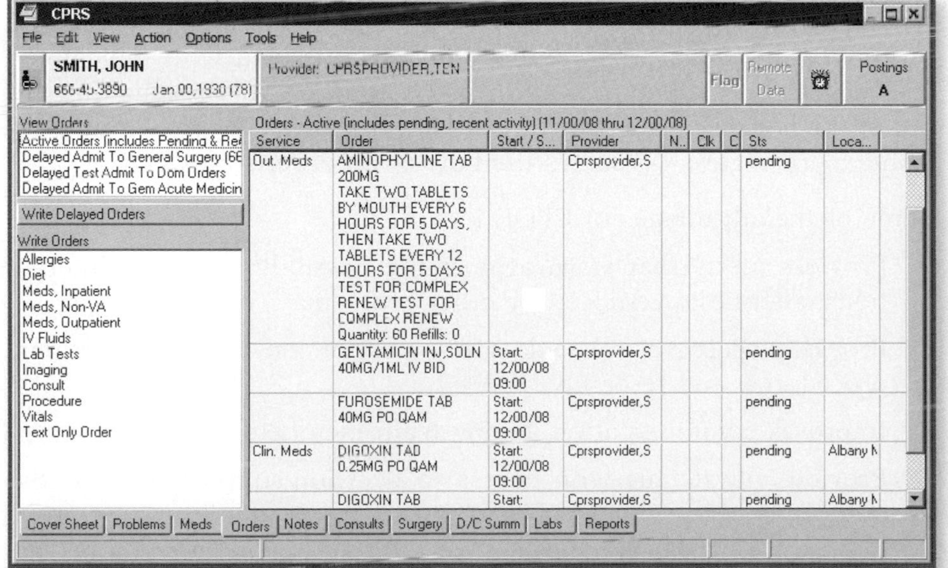

Figure 4-3

A screen for entering orders in an inpatient EHR.

handwritten and were later transcribed by a staff member. Once transcribed, orders were faxed to the appropriate department. Results from tests and procedures were faxed from the various departments to the patient's nursing unit. Problems could occur at each step of the process.

Handwritten orders were not always legible, and the physician had to be contacted for clarification. Even though the order was placed in the fax machine and went through, the department that was supposed to perform the test never received it. When results were faxed to the patient's floor, the physician who ordered the test was not always there to read them. These examples have one thing in common: delays in providing the patient with the appropriate treatment.

In addition, the system did little to provide checks that would prevent such errors as these:

- The physician was not aware of the most appropriate test or medication.
- The test results arrived late or could not be located.
- The physician was not notified quickly of critical test results that posed a danger to a patient's health.

CPOE systems replace handwriting orders with entering orders in a computer. During the order selection process, tools assist clinicians in selecting medications, tests, and other patient care. These decision-support tools incorporate best practice guidelines and evidence-based medicine. The system performs checks in the background while the clinician is placing the order, such as whether the medication dose is within range.

Once entered in the computer by the clinician, orders are communicated over a computer network to the personnel responsible for carrying them out. For example, orders for blood work are sent to the laboratory, orders for medication to the pharmacy, and orders for CT scans to radiology. Orders for patient care, such as respiratory therapy or physical therapy, are sent to the appropriate departments. When an order is received by the department responsible for filling the request, an electronic confirmation message is sent back to the ordering clinician, making it possible to track orders. Then, when the test has been completed or the therapy provided, the clinician is notified of the results. In the EHR, orders already placed are listed with indications of what has been completed and what is pending. Any results that are out of the normal range are marked, and the physician is sent an electronic alert. Figure 4-4 shows the flow of an order in a CPOE.

Some of the advantages of CPOE include:

- Provides alerts that warn against the possibility of drug interactions, allergies, overdoses, or other problems
- Provides accurate, up-to-date information on new medications, procedures, and research
- Improves communication among team members
- Provides physicians with access to decision-support tools at the point-of-care
- Reduces the amount of time it takes to fill physician orders

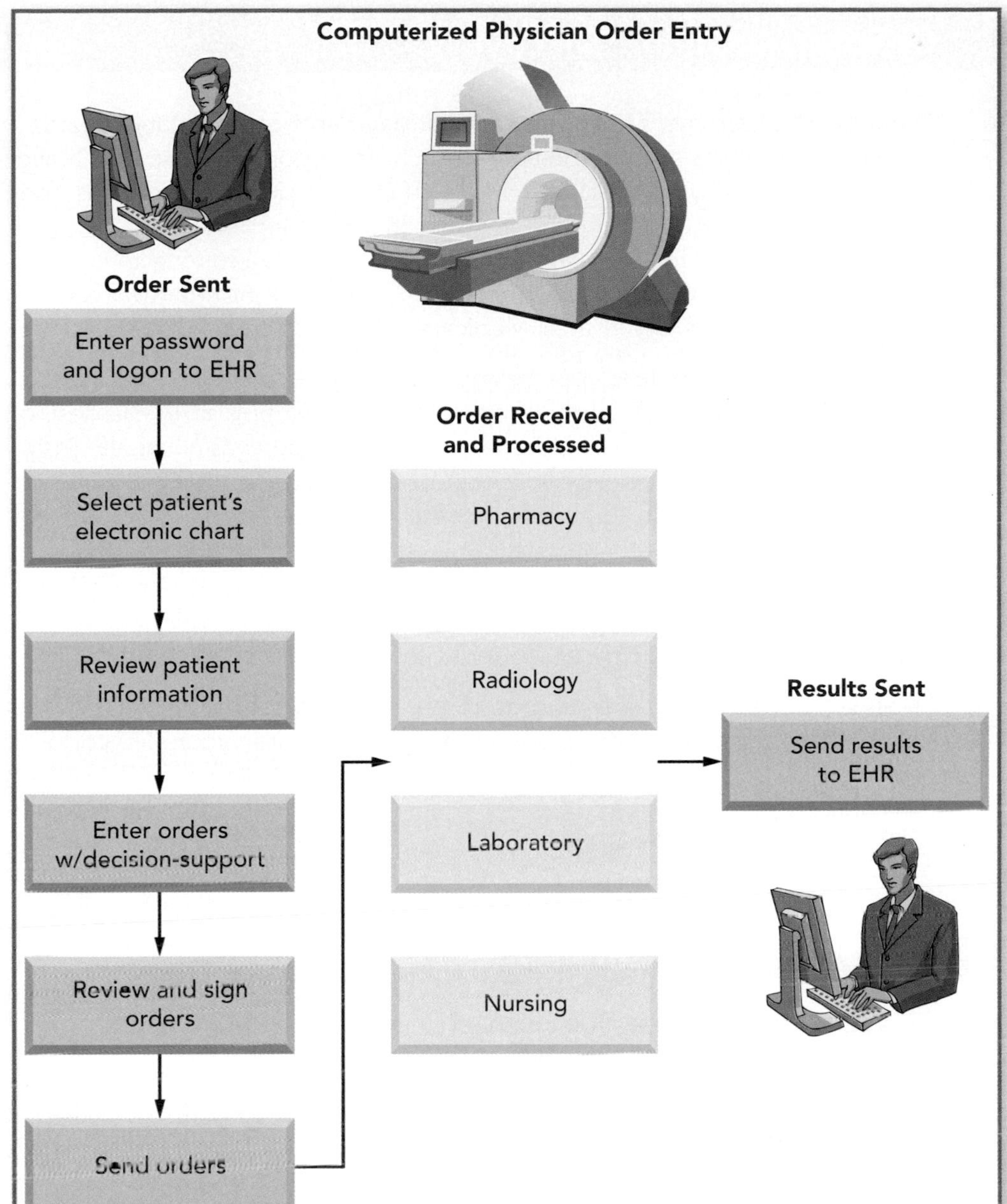

Figure 4-4
The flow of an order from entry to completion in a CPOE.

- Eliminates the chance of an order's being misplaced or lost
- Eliminates errors resulting from illegible handwriting
- Enables orders to be entered from any location with computer access—in the hospital or off-site
- Provides easier access to data for reporting and quality assessment purposes
- Reduces costs by improving efficiency, eliminating duplicate tests, and reducing the number of lawsuits due to medication errors

DECISION-SUPPORT TOOLS

Electronic health records with CPOE provide computerized decision-support tools to the physician. These tools allow physicians to select medications, diagnostic tests, and treatments that result in improved

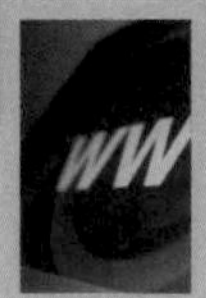

Chapter 4 Online Discovery

The federal government is linking hospital payments to voluntary reporting on quality measures through initiatives such as Reporting Hospital Quality Data for Annual Payment Update (RHQDAPU). The program provides consumers with quality of care information to make more informed decisions about their health care, while encouraging hospitals to improve the quality of inpatient care. Hospitals that do not participate in the program will receive a reduction of 2 percent in their Medicare Annual Payment Update.

Businesses are using their purchasing power to encourage hospitals to improve the quality and safety of patient care. Leapfrog is the largest of these business initiatives, with member companies purchasing health insurance for 37 million Americans at a cost of $67 billion annually. Businesses that join Leapfrog must agree to purchase health care from hospitals that show significant improvements in quality, safety, and affordability. Each year, hospitals can choose to participate in the Leapfrog Group Hospital Quality and Safety Survey. The survey examines hospital performance based on four practices that have been shown to reduce preventable medical errors.

Open your Internet browser, and go to www.leapfroggroup.org/cp. To see survey results for hospitals in your town or city, enter your Zip code. If

THELEAPFROGGROUP
Informing Choices. Rewarding Excellence.
Getting Health Care Right.

Site Map
Contact Us
Search Site
E-mail This Page

Home | About Us | For Consumers | For Members | For Hospitals | For Data Partners | News & Events

Welcome to the Leapfrog Hospital Quality and Safety Survey Results

Each year, Leapfrog gathers and reports information on hospital quality and patient safety efforts to help patients make informed decisions about where to receive hospital care. Use the search function below to get information on hospitals in your area.

1 **Find Hospitals by** (choose one):
Zip Code

2 **Find hospitals by Zip Code:**
Your Zip Code:
and search within a radius of:
1 mile | 50 miles
5 miles | 100 miles
10 miles | 200 miles

3 **List Results:**
Click "GO!" to perform your hospital search.
GO!

Please note: The information on this site is derived from hospitals' voluntary submissions of The Leapfrog Hospital Quality and Safety Survey and Leapfrog Hospital Insights data. This data is derived from third parties, and accordingly Leapfrog disclaims any and all warranties with respect to this data and the Survey and the Leapfrog Hospital Insights initiative. Hospitals that implement these quality, safety, and/or efficiency practices have reported that their internal processes of care include safeguards that may decrease a patient's probability of receiving poor quality and/or inefficient care. However, no specific representation is made, nor should be implied, nor shall Leapfrog be liable for any and all damages or costs with respect to the use of the data, including but not limited to for any individual patient's potential or actual outcome by having a procedure performed at these hospitals. A hospital's placement score does not convey whether its risk-adjusted mortality rate is statistically significantly different from (a) the statewide average or (b) the risk-adjusted mortality rate of any hospital with its score or any other score.

Home + About Us + For Consumers + For Members + For Hospitals + For Data Partners + News & Events
Site Map + Contact Us + Search Site + E-mail This Page + Print This Page
© The Leapfrog Group (2007)

your area is not yet part of the Leapfrog initiative, enter the Zip code 02114, and select a search radius of 5 miles. Click the Go button.

A page appears with survey results from hospitals within five miles of the Zip code you entered. Not all hospitals participate in the survey, so not all will be listed.

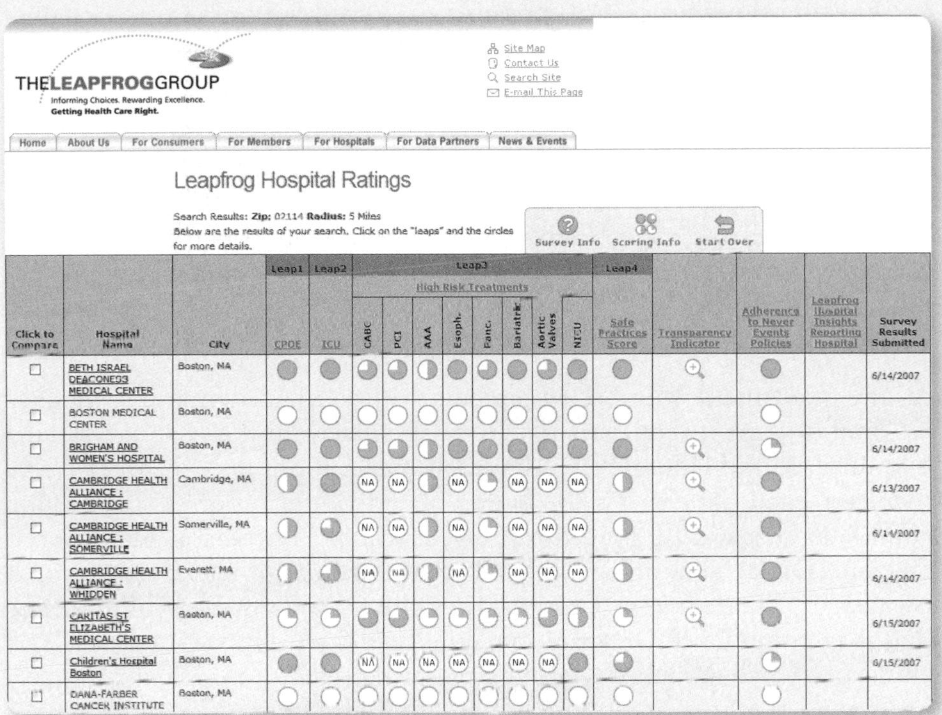

Click on one of the green, underlined column headings—CPOE, ICU, or High Risk Treatments. A second window will open with information on the types of information included in the survey. After reading this information, close the second window so you can see the survey results. Study the results, and then answer the questions below. (Be sure to scroll down the page to the section "What Do the Results Mean" to understand the symbols used in the chart.)

Thinking About It

1. What does a solid blue circle in the CPOE column indicate?

____

2. What is the Leapfrog Safe Practices score?

____

3. Based on the survey results, which hospital in your area would you go to? Why?

____

When you are finished answering the questions, close your web browser.

quality of care and patient outcomes. Examples of the capabilities of decision-support tools include:

- Recommending the most appropriate test to confirm or rule out a diagnosis
- Recommending the best medication for a patient
- Providing access to best practices and evidence-based guidelines
- Incorporating electronic order sets based on clinical research
- Alerting the physician to possible drug interactions, improper dosages, and allergy conflicts during the ordering process

Some decision-support tools are automatic and occur without any action on the part of the physician. For example, if a physician selects a medication dose that is higher than the standard dose, the system automatically provides an alert. In other instances, the tools activate at the request of the physician, such as when a physician queries the system for information on recommended tests to rule out a specific diagnosis.

Order Sets

At any one time, a number of patients with similar symptoms, diagnoses, and treatment requirements are hospitalized. In the past, physicians had to place individual orders for each medication, test, or other treatment for each patient. The grouping of individual orders for a specific condition, disease, or procedure into sets makes ordering much more efficient. **Order sets** are predefined groupings of standard orders for a condition, disease, or procedure. They are based on medical evidence that is in compliance with national quality and regulatory standards and clinical practice guidelines. Given the ever-increasing complexity of diagnostic and therapeutic options for treating patients, order sets make it easier for physicians to deliver quality patient care. Hospitals usually have hundreds of order sets organized by condition (fever, heart failure), disease (diabetes, asthma), and procedure (coronary artery bypass graft, total knee replacement). An order set is illustrated in Figure 4-5.

order sets predefined groupings of standard orders for a condition, disease, or procedure.

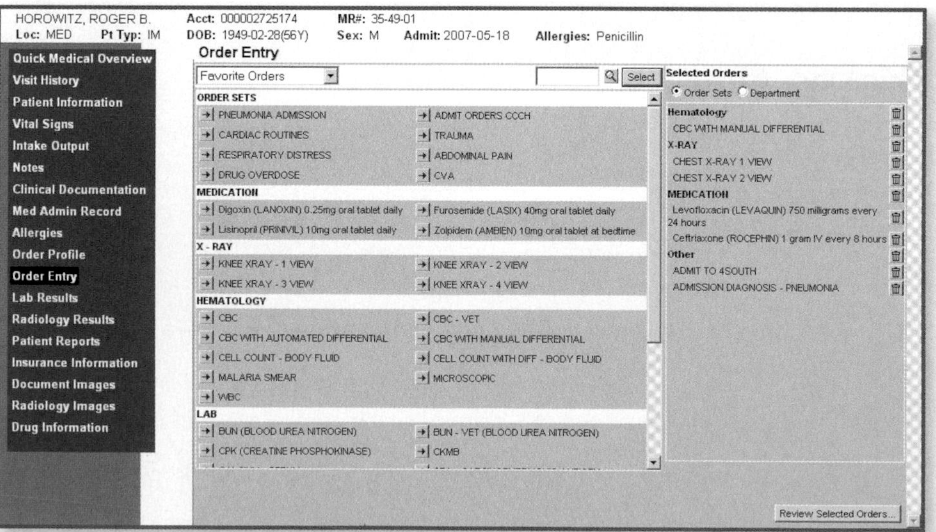

Figure 4-5

Order sets in an inpatient EHR.

The use of order sets reduces unnecessary variation in patient care by encouraging adherence to clinical practice guidelines. Through the use of predefined templates and order sets, physicians are encouraged to incorporate these practices into their care plans. Practice guidelines are based on sound clinical research and the consensus of professionals in the field. While order sets are not rules that must be followed to the letter, they do provide a set of practices that have been found to lead to quality patient care.

In addition to making the order writing process more efficient for physicians, order sets eliminate errors that result from memory lapses or lack of current clinical knowledge, and they provides fast, easy access to clinical content that would normally require time-consuming research.

The benefits of using order sets include:

- Encouraging the adoption of evidence-based standards and guidelines
- Enabling clinicians to work more efficiently
- Improving the quality of care received by patients
- Maintaining compliance with quality and safety standards

Medication Management in Hospitals

Medication errors are the most frequent source of preventable medical errors in the hospital setting. The 1999 Institute of Medicine (IOM) report, *To Err is Human*, noted both the seriousness and the extent of medical errors. A 2006 report by the IOM indicates that while progress has been made, there is still a long way to go in improving patient safety (*Preventing Medication Errors: Quality Chasm Series*, Institute of Medicine, 2006). The report estimates that a hospitalized patient is exposed to a medication error each day of his or her stay. Examples of drug errors include:

- Selecting the wrong drug for a condition
- Selecting the wrong dose, route, interval, or duration
- Overlooking drug allergies
- Overlooking drug-drug interactions
- Overlooking drug-disease interactions

The frequency of medication errors is partly a result of the nature of medication management in an inpatient setting. The process requires accurate information from patients, physicians, nurses, and pharmacists. The medication use process contains many steps—diagnosing, prescribing, preparing, dispensing, administering, and monitoring—tasks performed in different departments by different people:

1. Physicians diagnose patients and write prescriptions.
2. Nurses or aids transcribe the prescription order into the **medication administration record (MAR),** a log that contains information about the prescription order and is used to document the administration of the medication to the patient.

medication administration record (MAR) log with information about a medication order.

3. The order is faxed to the in-house pharmacy.
4. A pharmacist or pharmacy technician interprets the order, checks for contraindications, prepares the medication, labels the medication, and routes it back to the inpatient unit.
5. A nurse or aid checks the medication against the information in the MAR, administers the drug to the patient, and documents it in the MAR.
6. The nursing staff monitors the patient's condition after the medication has been given.

adverse drug event (ADE) side effect or complication from a medication.

This complex multistep process is a source of frequent medical errors and adverse drug effects. An **adverse drug event (ADE)** is a side effect or complication from a medication. ADEs that could have been prevented are classified as medical errors. ADEs are the most commonly occurring injuries to hospitalized patients.

transition points times when patients move from one setting to another.

medication reconciliation process of obtaining and updating an accurate list of all of a patient's medications.

According to the Institute for Healthcare Improvement (IHI), numerous studies have indicated that poor communication of medical information at transition points is responsible for almost half of all medication errors and up to one-fifth of ADEs in hospitals. **Transition points** are times when patients move from one setting to another—from home to hospital, from operating room to recovery room, from recovery room to patient room, from patient room to a lab for tests, and finally from hospital to home. As a consequence of this discovery, the Joint Commission initiated a program designed to reduce the risk of errors during transition points through medication reconciliation. **Medication reconciliation** is the process of obtaining and continually updating an accurate list of all medications a patient is taking and then using this list to ensure that patients are given the correct medications. A medication reconciliation screen is displayed in Figure 4-6.

In a hospital inpatient setting, the list of medications provided by the patient at admission must be compared against the medications ordered during the patient's hospital stay. If there is a question or conflict, the differences must be reconciled before a drug is administered to the patient; if that does not happen, an ADE may occur. The goal of medication reconciliation is to provide patients with the correct medications at all transition points in the hospital.

For example, consider a patient who was transferred from an intensive care unit (ICU) to a standard room on a nursing floor. The patient's medication administration record (MAR) did not travel with the patient, so it was not immediately available to the nurses on the floor. The MAR did eventually arrive, but not until after the patient was given a duplicate dose of heparin. The nurse had no way of knowing that the medication had been given in the ICU before the patient was transferred. This is an example of an error that occurred during a transition because information was not available when needed.

Medication errors can occur at any stage of the medication delivery system. The majority, however, occur during the first stage, physician ordering (39 percent), and the last stage, medication administration

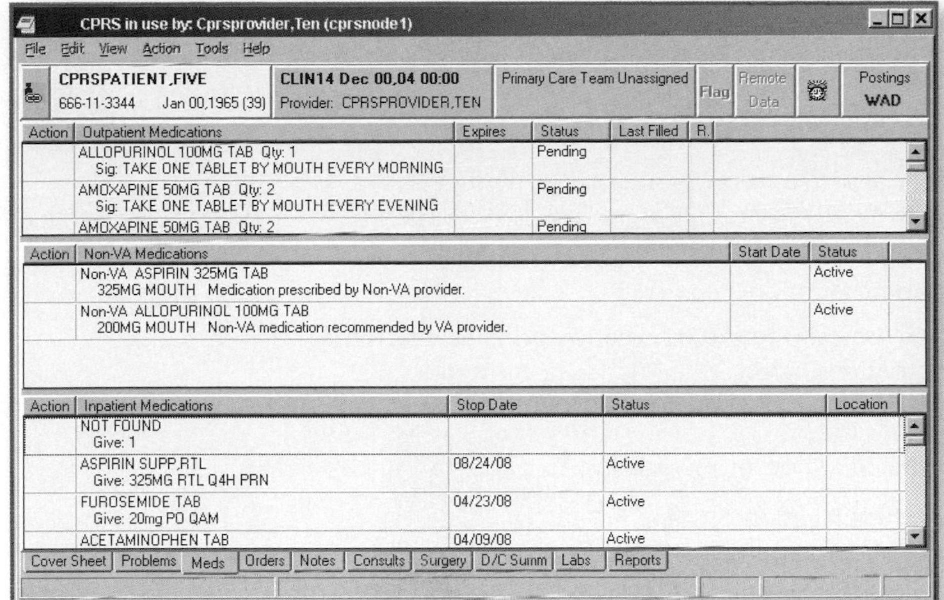

Figure 4-6

Medication reconciliation screen in an EHR.

(38 percent) (Leape L.L., D.W. Bates, D.J. Cullen, J.W. Cooper, H.J. Demonaco and T. Gallivan et al. 1995. "Systems Analysis of Adverse Drug Events." ADE Prevention Study Group. *Journal of the American Medical Association*, 274: 35-43.). The two most common causes of medication errors are lack of knowledge about the drug and lack of information about the patient. Information technology can be effective in reducing errors during both stages.

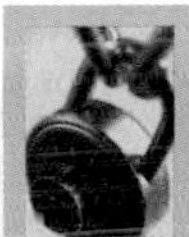

Privacy and Security Alert

Questions About Hospital Security

In March 2007, the Office of the Inspector General (OIG) of the Department of Health and Human Services (HHS) asked officials at Piedmont Hospital in Atlanta for information on its compliance with HIPAA security requirements. Some of the information requested included:

- Procedures for establishing and terminating access to electronic medical records
- Information about physical access to information systems and the buildings they are located in
- Procedures for logging security violations
- Procedures for handling violations of internal security rules by employees
- Procedures for logging and auditing user activities in information systems

Source: Computerworld, June 19, 2007, www.computerworld.com/action/article.do?command=viewArticleBasic&articleId=9025253.

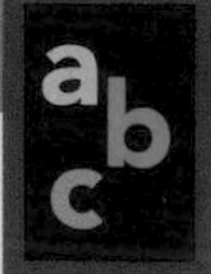

Hospital Information Systems

CPOE—Computerized Physician Order Entry

An application used for entering patient care orders, such as laboratory tests, radiology examinations, and medication.

eMAR—Electronic Medication Administration Record

A computerized system that electronically tracks medication administration and uses barcode technology to increase patient safety.

MAR—Medication Administration Record

A log used to document the administration of medication to patients.

PACS—Picture Archiving and Communication System

A computer system that facilitates the archiving, processing, viewing, and storage of digital radiological images and reports, such as CT scans and ultrasounds.

TECHNOLOGY AND MEDICATION ORDERING

Electronic health records that incorporate CPOE reduce errors by automating the ordering of medication and by providing built-in error checks. During the ordering process, the system checks the order for accuracy and completeness and uses clinical decision-support rules to evaluate the medication order. A typical decision-support tool:

- Checks for all safety conflicts, including drug-allergy, drug-drug, drug-disease, and so on
- Checks for duplicate orders
- Provides information on the range of doses for each medication
- Displays relevant laboratory results during the ordering process
- Evaluates order against evidence-based medicine and best practice guidelines

For example, when a medication is ordered electronically, the order is compared against standards for dosing and is checked for interactions with other medications and patient allergies. The physician placing the order is alerted to potential problems and must resolve the issues before finalizing the order.

A study at Brigham and Women's Hospital in Boston found that when a CPOE system was instituted, medication-related preventable adverse events were reduced by 17 percent, while serious medication errors went down 55 percent. (Bates, D. W., Leape, L. L., and Cullen, D. J., et al. 1998. "Effect of Computerized Physician Order Entry and a Team Intervention on Prevention of Serious Medication Errors." *Journal of the American Medical Association*, 28015: 1311-1316).

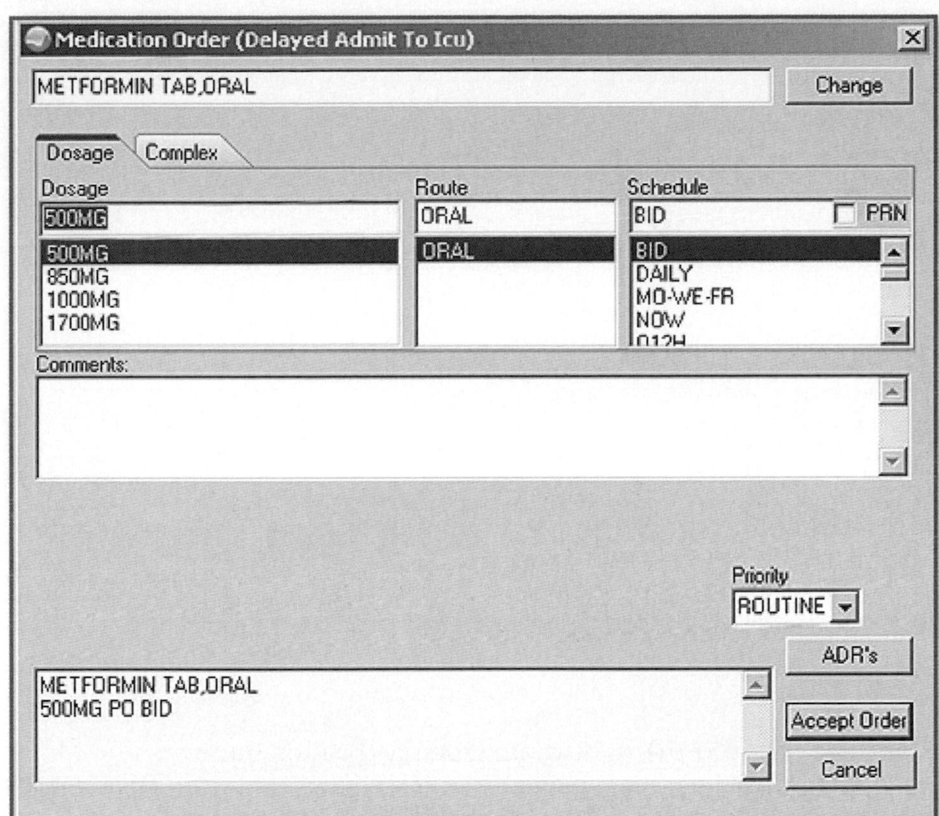

Figure 4-7
Medication order in an inpatient EHR.

Another benefit is a reduction in costs. By reducing medication order turnaround times, reducing duplicate orders, and prompting the ordering of appropriate less-expensive medications, CPOE can reduce the overall costs of patient care. In addition, CPOE reduces the incidence of medication errors that can lead to costly lawsuits. Figure 4-7 illustrates a medication order for a patient.

ELECTRONIC MEDICATION ADMINISTRATION RECORDS (EMAR)

Electronic medication administration records (e-MARs) work with CPOE systems to increase patient safety by enabling electronic tracking of medication administration at the bedside. When a physician enters a medication order in the CPOE, the order is automatically transmitted to the pharmacy, the billing office, and the eMAR system. Electronic ordering takes the place of transcribing the physician's orders into the paper MAR, eliminating mistakes due to illegible handwriting. In addition, eMAR systems eliminate the problems of lost or misplaced pages of a paper MAR (see Figure 4-8 on page 126 for example of an eMAR screen).

electronic medication administration records (e-MARs) enable electronic tracking of medication administration at the bedside.

An eMAR system utilizes barcode technology to verify that medication administration is performed in compliance with the five rights of medication management. The **five rights** are safety rules followed during the administration of medication in an attempt to reduce errors. They are (1) the right patient, (2) the right medication, (3) the right dose, (4) the

five rights safety rules followed during the administration of medication.

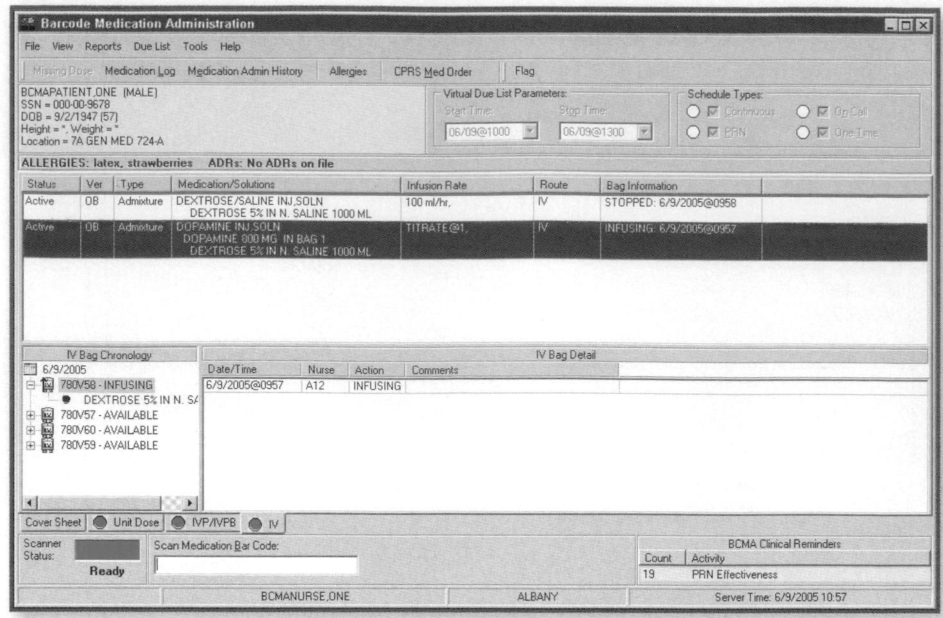

Figure 4-8

A barcode medication administration screen.

right time, and (5) the right route (such as oral or intravenous). Many professional organizations believe the five rights do not go far enough, and have expanded the rights to include (6) the right documentation and (7) the right technique (for administering the medication).

In a hospital that has implemented eMAR, all patients admitted to the hospital receive a wristband that contains an identifying barcode. When a medication is ordered, the order is electronically transmitted to the pharmacy. The pharmacist dispenses the prescribed medication with a barcode label that references the physician, the patient, the drug, and the dose. Once the medication arrives on the patient's floor, the nurse scans the barcode on the medication and on the patient's wrist to check the five rights before administering the medication.

Results Reporting

Electronic results reporting is another significant component of an inpatient EHR. The results of tests ordered by a clinician are often key factors in determining a patient's diagnosis and in planning treatment. Diagnostic testing includes a range of tests, from imaging tests such as ultrasound, CT scans, and MRIs, to laboratory analysis of urine and blood specimens.

In the past, the results of diagnostic tests were transmitted from the testing department to the ordering physician on paper, usually via a fax machine. Even in the best of circumstances, the time from when the doctor ordered the test, to when the test occurred, to when the physician received the results was often longer than desirable. Test results provide practitioners with information to make critical decisions about a patient's diagnosis and treatment at the point-of-care. This is especially true in emergency medicine. Consider a patient who

Case Study

WEST COAST COMMUNITY HOSPITAL

West Coast Community Hospital (WCCC) is a 300-bed hospital serving the communities to the south of Portland, Oregon. Like most hospitals, WCCC installed "best of breed" information technology systems in the pharmacy, lab, and radiology departments at least 10 years ago. In the last three years, it implemented an EHR for physicians, and a system for nursing documentation including flow sheets and electronic medication administration.

West Coast Associates in Obstetrics and Gynecology (WCAOG) is a large, busy OB/Gyn practice, consisting of 55 OB/GYN physicians and Certified Nurse Midwives. The group has nine individual sites scattered throughout the Portland area.

West Coast Community Hospital

About the Hospital

Name: West Coast Community Hospital

Units:

- Medical/Surgical
- Obstetrics
- ICU
- OR
- PACU
- Cardiac Cath Lab
- Radiology
- Pharmacy
- Lab
- Cardiac Step-down

Location: Suburban Portland, Oregon

Beds: 300

THE PATIENT

Rose Turner is a 27 year-old Caucasian female in the 35th week of her pregnancy. Rose has had an uneventful pregnancy, but this morning she received a phone call from her OB/Gyn practice. In addition to the spike in her blood pressure noted at her visit late yesterday, she has large amounts of protein in her urine. Rose is asked to report to the labor and delivery unit at West Coast Community Hospital as soon as possible.

Since the OB/Gyn practice is using an EHR that is linked to the local hospitals, the Labor and Delivery team at the hospital have been notified to expect Rose. When Rose arrives at WCCC, the monitoring room is ready, and as a result of a secure interface between the practice and the hospital, the staff has immediate access to Rose's past medical, surgical, and social histories, as well as progress on this pregnancy. The hospital staff also has access to all lab and ultrasound results from this pregnancy through the PACS system that is integrated with the EHR.

Soon after Rose's arrival, orders are entered in the EHR to start an IV, place maternal and fetal monitors, and obtain an ultrasound. The team also wants to obtain basic lab work in case an emergency delivery is necessary. Since the hospital EHR contains order sets, the orders do not have to be entered individually. Once entered, the orders are electronically sent to the nursing staff, the lab, and the radiology department.

The neonatologists are automatically informed of Roses arrival and are prepared to intervene as necessary. The midwife arrives to find all the needed data to assist in medical decision-making in one place, documented legibly and in a format that makes for easy analysis. The midwife also has instant access to the obstetrician and neonatologists for consultation, and the team can collaborate around Rose's lab, ultrasound, and fetal monitoring results.

Initially there is no concern, but the team decides to keep Rose over night. On day two, the midwife, obstetrician, and neonatologists hold an online collaboration session. Rose's blood pressure is dangerously high and refuses to yield to bed rest. Her kidney function is deteriorating, and the baby is showing signs of distress.

THE LABOR AND DELIVERY NURSE

Rachael Smith checks her employee web portal every morning before going to work. This day was no different. Rachael began to prepare for a 12-hour shift.

—*continued*

—continued from page 127

Case Study

When she logged in, she had a message waiting from the hospital scheduling system, alerting her to report to her per diem job at the local hospital labor and delivery unit. The message was based on computerized decision support supplied by the hospital information system that forecast eight deliveries before noon.

Rachael noted that in addition to two other patients in early labor, Rose Turner was on her work list. Rachael was able to review Rose's chart and learned that she was 27 years old, 35 weeks pregnant, and had steadily rising blood pressure and urine protein.

When Rachael arrived, she greeted Rose, who was clearly worried. Rachael and the nurse midwife did not like what they saw on the monitors and arranged a web-based consult with the obstetrician and the neonatologists. After reviewing the data, the obstetrician and neonatologists decide the safest method of delivery is a C-section. The team decides to make a medication change that will buy some time and hopefully improve the outcome for the mother and baby. Once the order is entered in the EHR, the pharmacy receives an electronic alert, and prepares and delivers the medication.

In the monitoring room, Rachael hangs the IV with the new medication and prepares Rose for a C-section delivery. The patient is wheeled to the OR. The baby is delivered and other than moderate prematurity, Michael is healthy and will go home within a week or ten days. Easy access to information, web-based consultation, and electronic ordering made all the difference for Rose, Michael and the rest of the Turner family.

THE PHYSICIAN

Sam Roth has been an obstetrician for 15 years and joined West Coast OB/GYN Associates three years ago, just as the practice and the hospital were embarking on a large information technology initiative. While the implementation was slow and painful, today Dr. Roth does not know how he did his job without the IT systems. The system afforded his practice the kind of data necessary to be efficient and effective in the delivery of obstetric care.

In his practice, Dr. Roth works with two other physicians, two nurse midwives, an RN and two medical assistants. This week he is assigned to overflow coverage. He just received an alert to attend an electronic consult in one hour. He is relieved that he can attend from home using his laptop, since he was in attendance at a delivery until 2:30 am. Before the new technology, he would have to make the 45 minute drive to the hospital after only a few hours of sleep.

The labor and delivery nurse, the nurse midwife, Dr. Roth, and the neonatologists consult on Rose Turner. The team decides on a medication change suggested by the built-in decision support from the EHR, which allows Dr. Roth enough time to make the trip to the hospital without putting himself or the patient in danger.

Once at the hospital, Dr. Roth confers with the rest of the team in person, greets Rose, and reassures her that delivering Michael early is the safest alternative for her and the baby. In the operating room, Dr. Roth is guided by high quality ultrasound images on large plasma screens mounted on the walls. The baby is delivered without incident. Dr. Roth enters the post partum orders in the computer from a station just outside the OR.

Now that Rose is stable, he can check the computer for the status of the patient he delivered yesterday, and if everything is normal, enter her discharge orders. He will also check on the lab and ultrasound results he ordered last week on the patient he saw in the office. After he reviews the results, he can approve, post the test results to the web portal for patients, and the patient will automatically receive an email that her data has been updated. Finally, after checking to make sure Rose and her new family are stable, Dr. Roth can return home for some much needed rest. He will be able to check on her progress and the progress of the baby from home.

What Do You Think?

1. How was the experience of Rose and her baby enhanced by technology in place at this hospital?
2. What are the potential challenges of this sort of system?
3. What is the greatest advantage for the patient using a hospital system with fully integrated, state-of-the-art information technology? For the staff? For the physician?

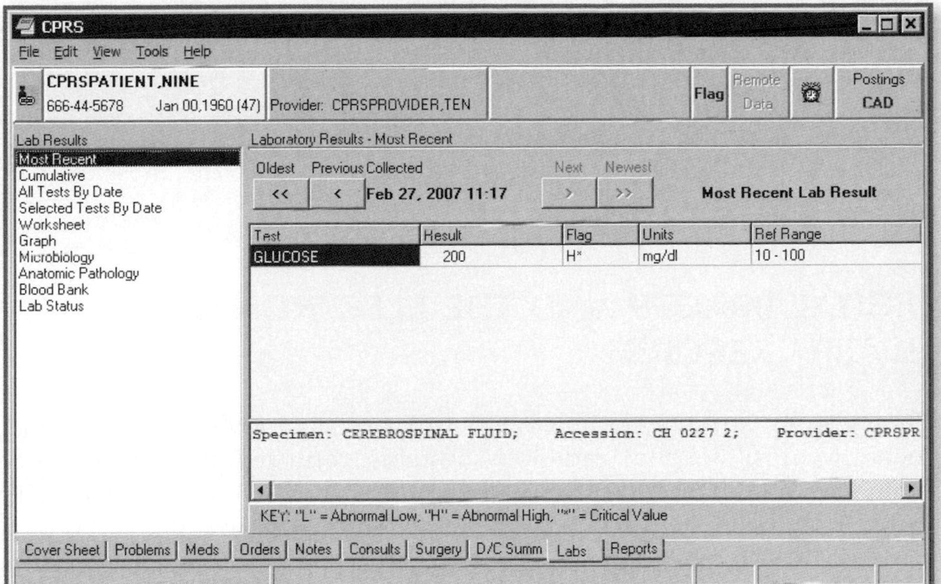

Figure 4-9

Laboratory test results in an inpatient EHR.

comes to the emergency room complaining of chest pains. She recently had a same-day procedure done at the hospital to clear a small blockage in an artery. The emergency room doctor orders an ECG and has blood drawn to check cardiac markers. A call is made requesting a consulting cardiologist in the emergency room. Within minutes, the physician and the cardiologist are able to view the test results on a computer in the ER. Since the hospital also has a picture archiving and communication system, the doctors can compare the current ECG with the patient's most recent ECG and make critical decisions about the patient's condition.

The results reporting function in an electronic health record program allows providers to receive and review laboratory and imaging test results from within the EHR. Whenever laboratory, radiology, or other tests are performed in the hospital, the ordering clinician is notified when results are available; the test results are automatically sent to the patient's EHR (see Figure 4-9). The provider accesses the patient's EHR and clicks on a laboratory or imaging icon that contains the results of the test along with relevant reports and images. At a glance, it is easy to see which results are new as well as which are normal and abnormal. Results that are critical are identified so that they can be easily recognized. The clinician is also able to view current and past results, making it easy to spot and track trends over time.

In a digital environment, the process of results reporting follows these steps:

1. Physician orders the test through the electronic health record.
2. The department conducting the test receives the order via its computer system and schedules the patient for the test.
3. Once the test is complete, the ordering physician receives an alert via computer. Special alerts are sent when the test results are

outside the normal range; critical alerts are sent when a test indicates that the patient is in danger and requires immediate intervention.

4. Once the physician reads the alert and reviews the test results, the testing department is automatically notified that the message has been received.

DIGITAL IMAGES AND THE ELECTRONIC HEALTH RECORD

Photographic images are an essential part of the medical record. Until recently, most hospital radiology systems captured images on film, including angiography, computed tomography (CT) scans, magnetic resonance imaging (MRI), ultrasound, and X-ray procedures. Today, more and more hospitals are using digital imaging to replace film. In digital imaging systems, images are created without using film and are captured and stored in a computerized picture archiving and communication system (PACS) (see Figure 4-10).

PACS is a computerized system for capturing, transmitting, archiving, and displaying medical images. Images stored in the system can be viewed via a network computer or through a computer with an Internet connection. The Department of Defense developed the first PACS system to make it possible for physicians away from the battlefield to view images of soldiers' injuries and consult with medics on the front lines.

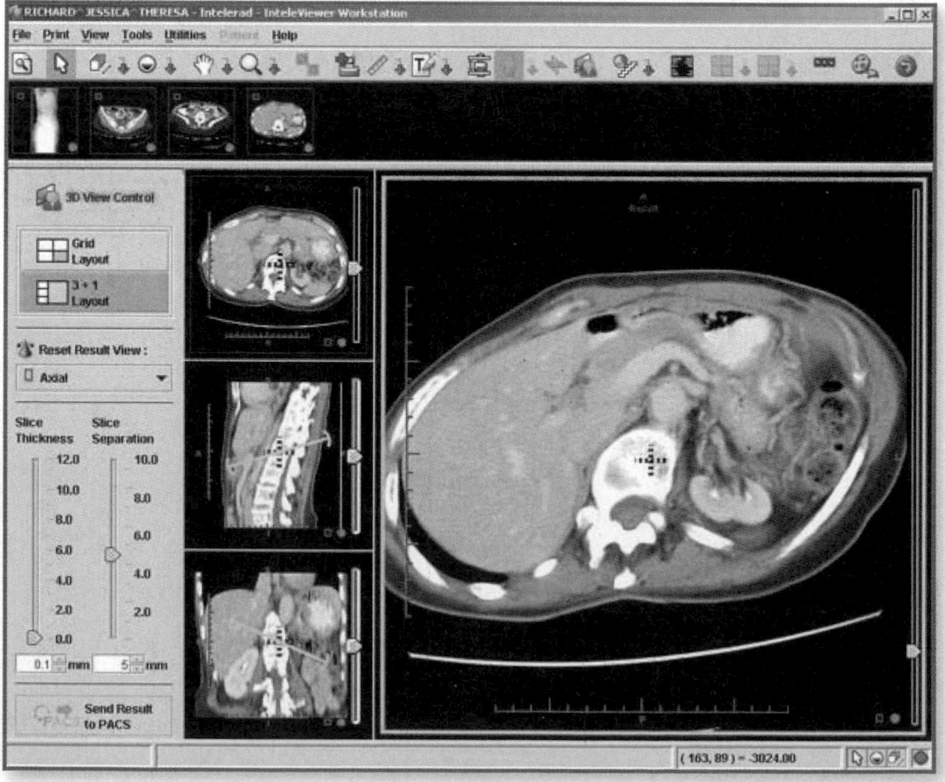

Figure 4-10

An image viewed in a picture archiving and communication system (PACS).

A PACS is able to transfer data to the patient's EHR, which makes it an efficient method of distributing test results. As soon as the technologist completes the procedure, the image is sent to PACS, where it is reviewed by a radiologist. Once the radiologist finishes the report, the information is available to the patient's physician. The physician can view the report and the images from any computer that has access to the EHR. If the EHR system is web-based, physicians are able to view images from anyplace that has an Internet connection—the hospital, the office, home, or elsewhere.

Integrating PACS with an EHR provides clinicians with rapid access to images. Current images can be compared with previous images to discover whether changes have occurred. For example, a physician may want to compare a woman's current mammogram with the one taken at an earlier time to determine whether a cyst has changed in size.

Since PACS provides access to images via a computer network or via a website, it takes little time to get the opinions of other clinicians. For example, a physician may want an orthopedic surgeon to look at an MRI to determine whether a patient requires knee surgery. Since the clinician can be in any location that has computer access, it is possible for the two doctors to collaborate no matter where they are located. In the end, patients benefit since they will most likely be diagnosed and treated more quickly than if everything had to be done with film and paper files.

Implementation of a PACS also eliminates the problem of lost films and saves time, since staff members no longer spend time looking for missing films. A PACS can reduce the need for duplicate testing, resulting in lower costs and less patient inconvenience.

ADVANTAGES OF ELECTRONIC RESULTS REPORTING

Electronic results reporting within an EHR offers a number of advantages over traditional paper-based reporting systems, including:

- *Faster turnaround time:* There is minimal delay between the time the test is finished and the availability of results. Results can be accessed from any computer with network access.
- *Faster diagnosis and treatment:* Once clinicians are alerted that results are available, they can review the results and consider how that information affects the possible diagnosis. By making results available in less time, clinicians may be able to make a diagnosis more quickly and begin providing appropriate care.
- *Efficient consultations:* More than one physician can view the images at the same time, even if the physicians are not in the same location. For example, a cardiologist and a surgeon both view a patient's angiogram and echocardiogram while speaking on the telephone. In the past, results would have to be sent from one physician to another, often requiring several days for a coordinated assessment to be completed.

- *Faster medication administration:* The laboratory test results for hospitalized patients are available more quickly, which makes it possible for patients to receive their medication sooner. Without an electronic reporting system, nurses would have to wait for a paper report to arrive, usually via a fax machine at the nurse's station. If a report did not arrive, nurses had to call the hospital laboratory and inquire about the patient's results. All this took time, and the end results were delay in administering the medication to the patient and time spent tracking down results instead of caring for patients.
- *Fewer duplicate tests:* Since there is a computerized record of every test ordered during a patient's hospital stay, providers will see that a test has already been preformed before unknowingly ordering a duplicate test.
- *Enhanced analysis:* Results from lab tests such as glucose levels or cholesterol levels can be viewed in graphical format, making it easier to spot trends in results over time.
- *Easier retrieval:* Since images and results are stored on a computer, they are easy to locate and review when necessary. In addition, the reports stored in a computer can be searched for keywords, a process that would be time-consuming with paper records. This is much more efficient than filling out a request form, submitting it to the records department, and waiting for the chart to arrive.

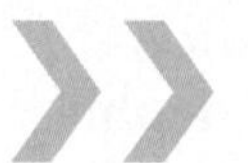

CHAPTER REVIEW

CHAPTER SUMMARY

1. In an inpatient hospital environment, an EHR serves as a single point of access for clinical information about a patient. By integrating data from other hospital systems, such as pharmacy, laboratory, and radiology, the EHR provides caregivers with a complete and up-to-date picture of the patient's condition and status. The primary function of an inpatient EHR is to assist in managing the transactions involved in a patient's care, such as ordering diagnostic tests, viewing lab results, and administering medications, with the goal of improving quality and increasing patient safety.
2. The primary benefits of hospital EHRs include (a) access to complete, up-to-date information about patients, including progress notes, results of laboratory tests and imaging studies, medication administration, and responses to treatment; (b) decreased turnaround time for medication delivery and completion of diagnostic tests; (c) increased efficiency by standardizing work processes and by integrating information from different departments; and (d) access to decision-support tools that help physicians make diagnosis and treatment decisions that provide patients with the safest, most effective care.
3. Clinical documentation is used in an inpatient setting for many purposes, including (a) to assist in patient care planning and continuity of care; (b) to provide evidence of the course of the patient's care and treatment during the hospital stay; (c) to facilitate communication among members of the patient care team; (d) to serve as a legal record to protect the interests of the patient, the hospital, and the clinician; (e) to supply data for research purposes; (f) to supply data for utilization review and quality improvement analysis and reporting; and (g) to provide information that enables coders to determine the appropriate diagnosis and procedure codes to substantiate patient billing.
4. Computerized physician order entry (CPOE) eliminates errors that occur as a result of illegible handwriting by enabling physicians to enter patient orders using a computer. Electronic ordering is more efficient and also eliminates the possibility of losing or misplacing an order. Orders can be entered from any computer that has access to the hospital system. CPOE systems also contain decision-support tools that (a) provide alerts that warn against the possibility of drug interaction, allergy, overdose, and other problems; (b) provide accurate, up-to-date information on new medications, procedures, research, and so on; and (c) reduce costs by improving efficiency, eliminating duplicate tests, and reducing the number of lawsuits due to medication errors.

5. Decision-support tools allow physicians to select medications, diagnostic tests, and treatments that result in improved quality of care and patient outcomes. Such tools can be used to select the best treatment based on evidence-based guidelines; to reduce variation in care by incorporating standard order sets; to alert the physician to possible drug interactions, improper dosages, and allergy conflicts during the ordering process; and to provide computerized access to up-to-date clinical research.
6. When a physician orders a medication using CPOE, the order is automatically entered in the electronic medication administration records (eMAR). From that point on, the medication order and its administration are tracked by computer using barcode technology. The medication itself is labeled with a barcode by the pharmacy, and the patient has a wristband with a barcode. The nurse uses a handheld device to scan the label on the medication and on the patient's wristband as part of the process of checking the five rights of medication administration.
7. Electronic results reporting in an EHR has several advantages over traditional paper-based reporting systems, including faster turnaround time for results, which makes it possible for the physician to diagnose and treat the patient more efficiently. Consultations are more convenient, since clinicians can view the results from any computer with access to the EHR. Patients are given medications more quickly, since the orders are sent and received in less time. Electronic reporting also results in fewer duplicate tests, since the test is recorded in the EHR. Electronic results can be viewed in graphical format, which makes it easy to spot trends. Images and reports stored on a computer can be easily retrieved from any computer that has access to the EHR.

CHECK YOUR UNDERSTANDING

Part 1. Write *T* or *F* in the blank to indicate whether you think the statement is true or false.

____ **1.** The most important feature of CPOE systems is the reduced turnaround time for medication orders.

____ **2.** Electronic health records in a hospital setting are one of several clinical information systems.

____ **3.** Recent studies indicate that medication errors continue to be a serious problem.

____ **4.** Electronic health records that incorporate CPOE and decision-support reduce errors by providing built-in error checking of orders.

____ **5.** A picture archiving and communication system (PACS) is a computerized system for reporting the results of laboratory tests.

____ **6.** Medication errors occur primarily during the prescribing and administering stages of medication management.

_____ **7.** Clinical documentation is an important component of a hospital's efforts to meet quality standards set by payers.

_____ **8.** A hospital can incorporate evidence-based guidelines into clinical practice through the use of order sets.

_____ **9.** Even in a hospital that uses CPOE, physicians are still required to handwrite prescriptions for medications.

_____ **10.** Decision-support tools can be used for diagnosis as well as for selecting the best medication for a patient.

Part 2. In the space provided, write a definition of the term.

11. adverse drug event (ADE)

____

____

12. computerized physician order entry (CPOE)

____

____

13. electronic medication administration records (e-MARs)

____

____

14. five rights

____

____

15. medication administration record (MAR)

____

____

16. medication reconciliation

____

____

17. order sets

____

____

18. transition points

THINKING ABOUT THE ISSUES

Part 3. In the space provided, write a brief paragraph describing your thoughts on the following issues.

19. It is generally agreed that implementing an electronic health record system in a hospital is more difficult than implementing one in a physician's office. Why do you think this is true?

20. Hospitals are counting on information technology to play a role in reducing medical errors and improving the quality of care provided to patients. Some researchers do not believe that technology can fix some problems, and also believe that it can introduce problems of its own. Based on your own experiences with computers in school, at work, or at home, what problems do you think computers might introduce in a hospital setting?

Personal Health Records

CHAPTER OUTLINE

The Need for Personal Health Records
- *Consumer Responsibility*
- *The Rise of Consumer-Driven Health Plans*
- *Consumer Health Information on the Internet*

The Role of Personal Health Records in Managing Health

Defining Personal Health Records
- *Personal Health Record Content*

Types of Personal Health Record Applications
- *Computer-Based Stand-Alone*
- *Internet-Based, Tethered*
- *Internet-Based, Untethered*
- *Internet-Based, Networked and Interoperable*

Benefits of Networked Personal Health Records
- *Access to Evidence Based Health Information*
- *Assessment of Risk*
- *Enhanced Communication with Providers*
- *Empowerment of Patients*
- *Increased Patient Safety*
- *Improved Quality of Care*
- *Improved Emergency Care*
- *Potential Cost Savings*

Barriers to the Implementation of Personal Health Records
- *Interoperability*
- *Consumer Awareness*
- *Privacy and Security*

LEARNING OUTCOMES

After completing this chapter, you will be able to define key terms and:

1. Explain why consumers are being encouraged to take a more active role in their health care.
2. List five tools that personal health records offer that enable individuals to manage their health care.
3. Explain the differences among the four types of personal health records.
4. Explain the major advantage that a networked personal health record has over the other types of personal health records.
5. Describe the three major barriers to the implementation of networked personal health records.

KEY TERMS

consumer-driven health plans (CDHPs)
networked personal health record
patient portal
personal health record (PHR)
tethered
untethered

Why This Chapter Is Important to You

The information in this chapter will enable you to:

- Understand why personal health records are becoming important to individuals in managing their own health care.
- Understand the ways in which personal health records are more than repositories for health records.
- Understand the advantages and disadvantages of the four major categories of personal health records.
- Understand the barriers to the implementation of personal health records.

During the last several years, consumers have been encouraged to take a more active role in their health care. The rationale is that individuals have the most to gain—and lose—when it comes to making key medical decisions. Traditionally, patients relied solely on their physicians for answers to health questions, and physicians made most of the treatment decisions. Today, many patients and providers make joint decisions. An individual faced with a diagnosis is likely to have done some of his or her own research before agreeing to a plan of treatment, including:

- Asking relatives about diseases that run in the family
- Looking back over past test results stored in a file cabinet
- Contacting another provider for a second opinion
- Searching the Internet for the latest information on the disease

To participate in the decision-making process, individuals need information—about their family history, their own medical history, and the latest medical knowledge about their condition. The difficulty is that people do not have easy access to this information. It is stored in multiple locations and scattered among providers and facilities, such as primary care providers, specialists, surgeons, hospitals, pharmacies, and health plans. Patients seeking comprehensive, up-to-date medical records have to contact the different offices and request copies. Even then, answering questions such as "when did I have my last tetanus shot?" or "when was the dose of my medication increased?" requires searching through the many printouts.

The Need for Personal Health Records

As individuals become more active in managing their health care, there is a growing recognition of the need to maintain up-to-date records of essential personal health information. While physicians store records of patient encounters in electronic health records (EHRs), patients save information about their health in personal health records (PHRs) (see Table 5-1). A **personal health record (PHR)** is an electronic version of a comprehensive record of a person's lifelong health that is collected and maintained by the patient (see Figure 5-1). It can be shared with providers if the patient chooses to do so. When stored and maintained on a secure Internet website, it is the most efficient way to manage personal health care information.

personal health record (PHR) electronic version of person's life-long, comprehensive health record.

CONSUMER RESPONSIBILITY

The development of PHRs is not just a result of individuals' greater role in managing their own health care. It has come at a time when employers, the government, and insurance plans are all asking

TABLE 5-1 **Differences Between PHRs and EHRs**

Personal health records are different from electronic health records in a number of areas:
EHR files are owned and managed by providers or facilities; PHR files are owned and updated by the individual.
EHRs are legal documents that must be created and maintained according to state and federal laws; PHRs are not legal records.
EHR access is controlled by the provider with the patient's authorization; PHR access is controlled by the patient.
An EHR contains information about treatment by a single provider; a PHR contains information about treatment by multiple providers.
EHR data are entered by a provider or the medical staff; PHR data are entered by the patient.
An EHR is used by a medical office or facility; a PHR is used by an individual patient.

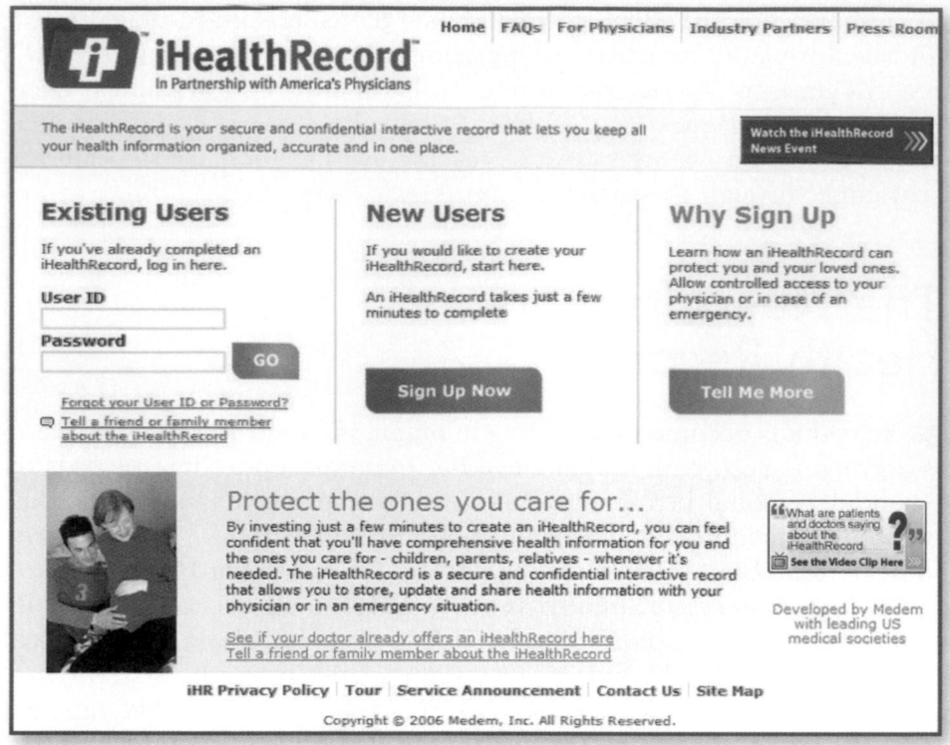

Home
FAQs
For Physicians
Industry Partners
Press Room
iHealthRecord
In Partnership with America's Physicians
The iHealthRecord is your secure and confidential interactive record that lets you keep all your health information organized, accurate and in one place.
Watch the iHealthRecord News Event
Existing Users
If you've already completed an iHealthRecord, log in here.
User ID
Password
GO
Forgot your User ID or Password?
Tell a friend or family member about the iHealthRecord
New Users
If you would like to create your iHealthRecord, start here.
An iHealthRecord takes just a few minutes to complete
Sign Up Now
Why Sign Up
Learn how an iHealthRecord can protect you and your loved ones. Allow controlled access to your physician or in case of an emergency.
Tell Me More
Protect the ones you care for...
By investing just a few minutes to create an iHealthRecord, you can feel confident that you'll have comprehensive health information for you and the ones you care for - children, parents, relatives - whenever it's needed. The iHealthRecord is a secure and confidential interactive record that allows you to store, update and share health information with your physician or in an emergency situation.
See if your doctor already offers an iHealthRecord here
Tell a friend or family member about the iHealthRecord
What are patients and doctors saying about the iHealthRecord
See the Video Clip Here
Developed by Medem with leading US medical societies
iHR Privacy Policy
Tour
Service Announcement
Contact Us
Site Map
Copyright © 2006 Medem, Inc. All Rights Reserved.

Figure 5-1
Sign-up page for the iHealthRecord personal health record.

individuals to take more responsibility for their health care in the form of higher insurance premiums and higher out-of-pocket expenses.

THE RISE OF CONSUMER-DRIVEN HEALTH PLANS

consumer-driven health plans (CDHPs) health plans with high deductibles, low premiums, and tax-free savings accounts.

Employers are turning to consumer-driven health plans to lower the cost of providing health insurance to their employees. **Consumer-driven health plans (CDHPs)** combine high deductibles, low premiums, and tax-free savings accounts that are used to cover out-of-pocket expenses. Since the plans have high deductibles (the average is around $2,000) and may require coinsurance of as much as 30 percent, annual out-of-pocket costs can exceed $5,000 for an individual and $10,000 for a family.

With no insurance benefits until the deductible is met and even then less than 100 percent coverage, individuals are faced with decisions about how much of their money to spend on routine medical care. They are asking questions such as:

Do I really need this test?

Is there a less expensive medication that I can take?

Will my condition go away on its own, or do I need to see a doctor?

When insurance plans covered most routine visits, consumers often did not question the necessity of a visit. Proponents of CDHPs believe that individuals who are spending their own money will be more selective by going to the doctor less often and choosing treatments that are cost-efficient as well as medically effective.

CONSUMER HEALTH INFORMATION ON THE INTERNET

Consumers faced with decisions about seeking medical care educate themselves about their conditions, just as they would educate themselves when buying a big-ticket item such as a car. Before going to the local auto dealership, they read about the car's features, gas mileage, reliability, and safety. Armed with that information, they use the Internet to learn what others are paying for the same vehicle. Only then do they go to the dealership to purchase the car. The concept is similar in consumer-directed health care. For example, an individual considering nonemergency major surgery researches the procedure, looks into the quality of local surgeons and hospitals, and compares costs before making a decision. Fortunately, PHRs provide a number of tools that can help consumers make educated decisions.

The Role of Personal Health Records in Managing Health

Personal health records are more than just places to store health information; they offer a number of tools intended to help individuals manage their health and wellness. PHRs allow individuals to:

- View personal health information
- Send e-mail messages to providers
- Provide health care information to selected individuals
- Receive, review, and graph test results
- Schedule appointments
- Track compliance with recommended screening guidelines
- Obtain information about diseases and treatments
- Renew prescriptions
- Access self-assessment tools (for example, how great is my risk for developing Type 2 diabetes)
- Set up alerts and reminders regarding appointments, tests, and so on
- Track insurance claims, deductibles, and health savings accounts online
- Check medical records for errors
- Record data from home care devices such as glucose monitors
- Record symptoms, observations, and responses to medications or allergies (see Figure 5-2 on page 142)

To understand the importance of PHRs in managing health, consider the following examples.

Examples In an emergency, it can be difficult to remember critical information. Persons taken to the emergency room may be unable to recall all relevant health information because of their medical condition or because they are afraid or confused. Patients who are unconscious when they arrive have no ability to communicate information about medications, allergies, and other factors that might affect treatment. A PHR is always available where there is Internet access. If the hospital has been granted access to the patient's PHR ahead of time, staff members would be able to view up-to-date health information even if the person was unconscious.

In a natural disaster, residents may have to leave their homes and their local health care facilities. This happened to many of the people who fled the Gulf Coast during Hurricane Katrina. People who had filed medical documents in a desk or file cabinet lost all their records. Many providers also lost all medical records; only a few had electronic health records with off-site backup. If the individuals who were evacuated had PHRs, they could access their health records wherever they were located.

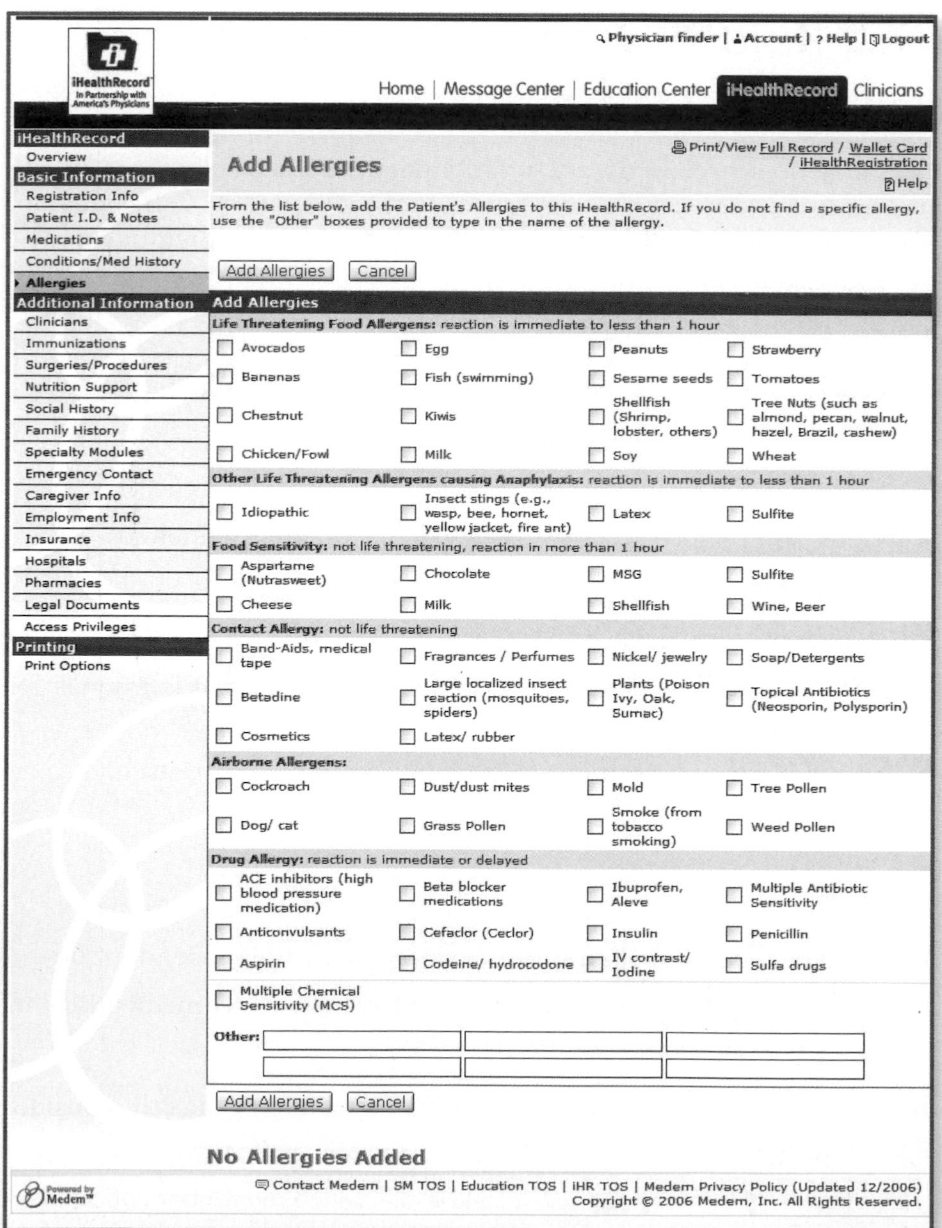

Figure 5-2

A screen for entering allergy information in a PHR.

Many people forget to schedule important preventive health screenings. Screening tests and procedures are recommended at different times for patients who are predisposed to a disease. For example, a patient with a family history of colon cancer (cancer or polyps in a first-degree relative younger than sixty or in two first-degree relatives of any age) should begin screening earlier than an individual without this risk factor. A PHR can take family history and other risk factors into account and can provide a customized health screening schedule.

When a patient visits a doctor for the first time, filling out all the forms can be time-consuming. The patient may make errors or lack important information. With a PHR in place, the individual can grant the new provider access to selected sections of the PHR. This information can be used to populate corresponding sections of the provider's EHR.

A person traveling away from home may need to request a prescription refill. While it would be possible to find out the pharmacy's telephone number without a PHR, trying to obtain a refill without a prescription number and lacking contact information for the pharmacy that originally filled the prescription would be difficult and time-consuming. A PHR contains a complete list of medications as well as pharmacy contact information (see Figure 5-3).

Many people with chronic conditions are regularly treated by more than one physician. Keeping track of all the appointments, visit details, and care plans can be overwhelming. A PHR sends appointment requests to providers, tracks scheduled appointments, and sends reminders to the patient via e-mail. It also maintains records of visits with each provider.

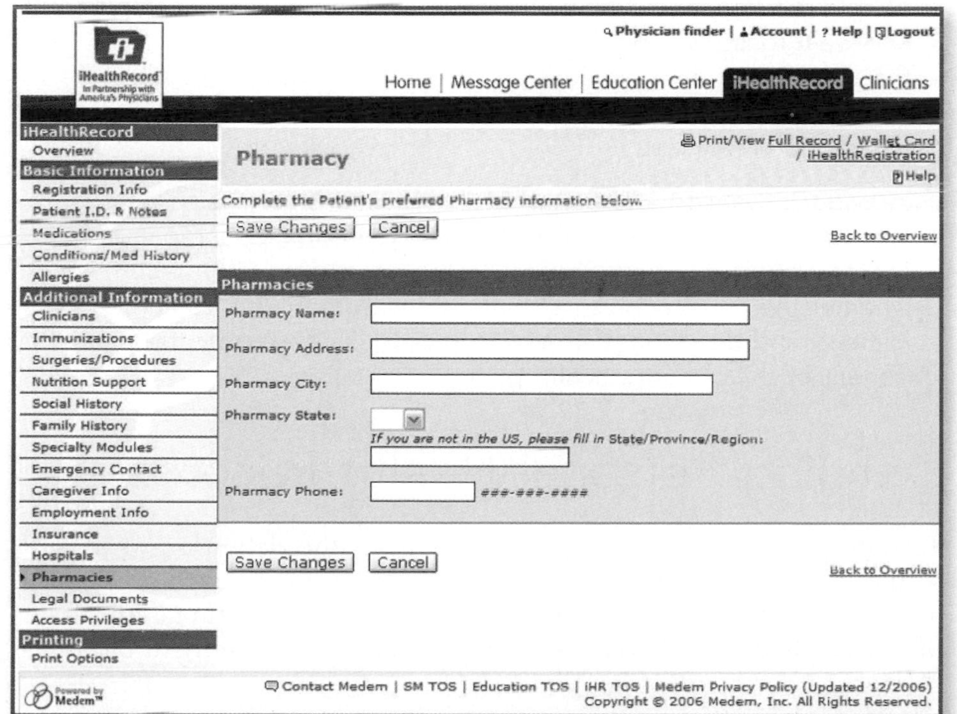

Figure 5-3

A screen for recording pharmacy information in a PHR.

Figure 5-4

A screen for inserting immunization information in a PHR.

Physician finder | Account | ? Help | Logout

iHealthRecord In Partnership with America's Physicians

Home | Message Center | Education Center | iHealthRecord | Clinicians

iHealthRecord
- Overview

Basic Information
- Registration Info
- Patient I.D. & Notes
- Medications
- Conditions/Med History
- Allergies

Additional Information
- Clinicians
- Immunizations
- Surgeries/Procedures
- Nutrition Support
- Social History
- Family History
- Specialty Modules
- Emergency Contact
- Caregiver Info
- Employment Info
- Insurance
- Hospitals
- Pharmacies
- Legal Documents
- Access Privileges

Printing
- Print Options

Add Immunizations

Print/View Full Record / Wallet Card / iHealthRegistration

Help

From the list below, add the Patient's Immunizations to this iHealthRecord. If you do not find a specific immunization, use the "Other" boxes provided to type in the name of the immunization.

[Add Immunizations] [Cancel]

Add Immunizations

List of Immunizations:

☐ Anthrax	☐ Immune Serum Globulin	☐ Pertussis/Whooping Cough	☐ Rubella
☐ Chickenpox (Varicella or VZV)	☐ Influenza	☐ Plague	☐ Smallpox
☐ Cholera	☐ Japanese Encephalitis	☐ Pneumococcal conjugate vaccine (PCV7 or PCV)	☐ Tetanus
☐ Diphtheria	☐ Lyme Disease	☐ Pneumococcal polysaccharide vaccine (PPV23 or PPV)	☐ Tuberculosis (BCG)
☐ Haemophilus influenzae type b (Hib)	☐ Measles	☐ Polio (IPV)	☐ Typhoid
☐ Hepatitis A	☐ Meningococcal Vaccine	☐ Rabies	☐ Yellow Fever
☐ Hepatitis B (Hep B)	☐ Mumps		

Combination Vaccines:

☐ Diphtheria/Tetanus/Pertussis (DTaP)	☐ Measles/Mumps/Rubella (MMR)	☐ Tetanus and Diphtheria booster (Td)

Other:

[Add Immunizations] [Cancel]

No Immunizations Added

Powered by Medem

Contact Medem | SM TOS | Education TOS | iHR TOS | Medem Privacy Policy (Updated 12/2006)

Parents like to keep track of their children's health, including pediatrician visits, immunizations, dates of diseases such as chickenpox, height and weight readings, and school physicals (see Figure 5-4). A PHR keeps all this information in one secure location.

People are concerned about diseases that are present in their family and want to know what they can do to reduce their risks of developing the diseases. A PHR provides access to risk assessment tools, to a list of preventive measures, and to the latest guidelines for common diseases and conditions.

Individuals want to know the best medications for their illnesses, the side effects of the drugs, and whether the insurance company will pay for them. A PHR provides access to the latest drug information, checks whether the medication would interact with the patient's current medications, and determines whether the drug is covered by the pharmacy benefit of the patient's health plan.

Defining Personal Health Records

To date, there is no universal agreement on the definition of a PHR. Without a common definition, the range of products that are labeled as PHRs is very broad. In an attempt to narrow this range and focus on critical features to provide a definition, several prominent organizations have come up with definitions.

The Markle Foundation Connecting for Health Initiative Group developed a list of seven characteristics of a PHR:

1. Each person controls his or her own PHR.
2. PHRs contain information from one's entire lifetime.
3. PHRs contain information from health care providers.
4. PHRs are accessible from any place at any time.
5. PHRs are private and secure.
6. PHRs are transparent. Individuals can see who entered each piece of data, where it was transferred from, and who has viewed it.
7. PHRs permit easy exchange of information across health care systems (*Connecting Americans to Their Healthcare—Final Report of the Working Group on Policies for Electronic Information Sharing Between Doctors and Patients*, July 2004, www.connectingforhealth.org./resources/wg_eis_final_report_0704.pdf).

The American Health Information Management Association (AHIMA) defines a PHR as:

> an electronic, universally available, lifelong resource of health information needed by individuals to make health decisions. Individuals own and manage the information in the PHR, which comes from healthcare providers and the individual. The PHR is maintained in a secure and private environment, with the individual determining rights of access. The PHR is separate from and does not replace the legal record of any provider. ("The Role of the Personal Health Record in the EHR," *Journal of AHIMA* 76, 7 2005: 64A–D.)

The Healthcare Information and Management Systems Society (HIMSS) focuses on electronic personal health records, which they refer to as ePHRs. HIMSS defines an ePHR as:

> An electronic Personal Health Record ("ePHR") is a universally accessible, layperson comprehensible, lifelong tool for managing relevant health information, promoting health maintenance and assisting with chronic disease management via an interactive, common data set of electronic health information and e-health tools. The ePHR is owned, managed, and shared by the individual or his or her legal proxy(s) and must be secure to protect the privacy and confidentiality of the health information it contains. It is not a legal record unless so defined and is subject to various legal limitations. (www.himss.org/content/files/PHRDefinition071707.pdf.)

In these three definitions, a PHR shares several common attributes:

- It is owned and managed by the individual.
- It is universally accessible.
- It is a lifelong tool.
- It is secure and private.
- The individual decides who can have access to the information.

Many organizations that call their products personal health records (PHRs) do not conform to these definitions. At this time, there are more than seventy-five PHR products available on the Internet, and more are being developed. Among the groups that offer PHRs are employers, health plans, physician practices, Internet companies, non-profit organizations, and hospitals.

PERSONAL HEALTH RECORD CONTENT

Regardless of who provides the product, PHRs generally contain personal information and health information.

Personal Information

- Demographic information (name, address, and so on; see Figure 5-5)
- Emergency contacts (see Figure 5-6)
- Insurance information
- List of health care providers, including contact information
- List of individuals granted access to PHR (see Figure 5-7)
- Spiritual/religious affiliation
- Living wills, advance directives, or medical power of attorney (see Figure 5-8)

Figure 5-5

Screen for recording identifying demographic information.

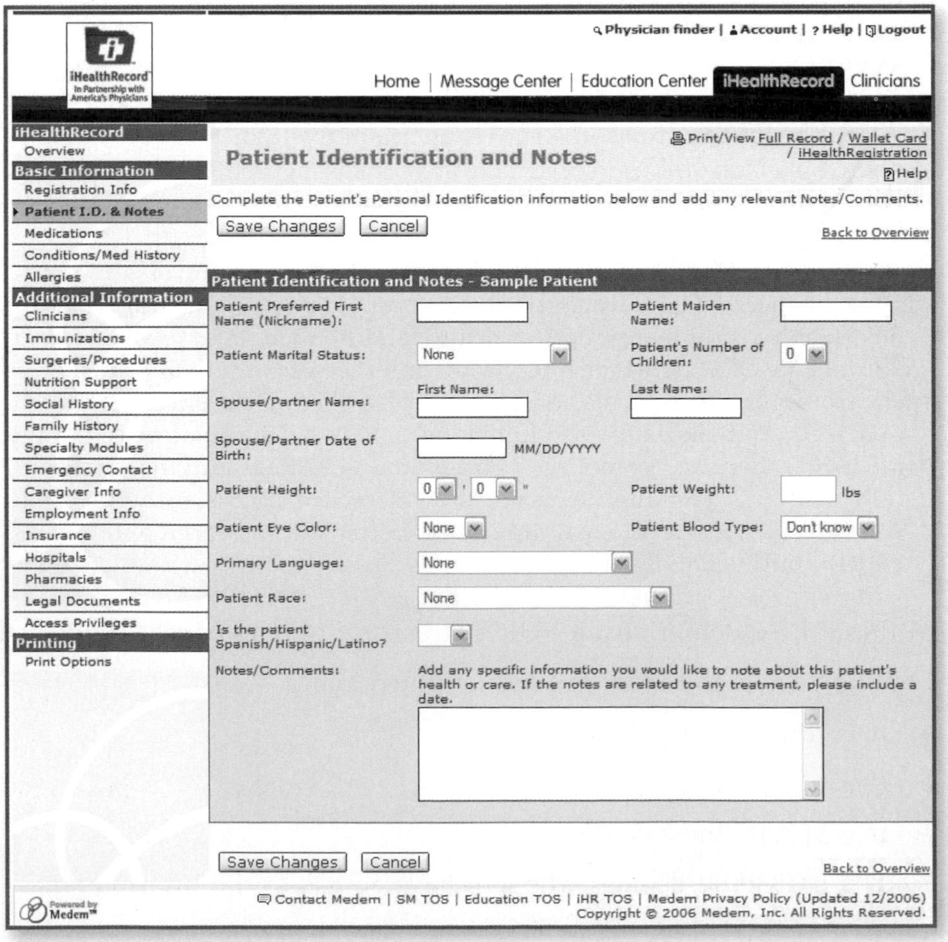

Physician finder | Account | ? Help | Logout

iHealthRecord In Partnership with America's Physicians

Home | Message Center | Education Center | iHealthRecord | Clinicians

iHealthRecord
Overview
Basic Information
Registration Info
Patient I.D. & Notes
Medications
Conditions/Med History
Allergies
Additional Information
Clinicians
Immunizations
Surgeries/Procedures
Nutrition Support
Social History
Family History
Specialty Modules
Emergency Contact
Caregiver Info
Employment Info
Insurance
Hospitals
Pharmacies
Legal Documents
Access Privileges
Printing
Print Options

Print/View Full Record / Wallet Card / iHealthRegistration

Help

Patient Identification and Notes

Complete the Patient's Personal Identification information below and add any relevant Notes/Comments.

Save Changes | Cancel

Back to Overview

Patient Identification and Notes - Sample Patient

Patient Preferred First Name (Nickname):
Patient Maiden Name:
Patient Marital Status: None
Patient's Number of Children: 0
Spouse/Partner Name: First Name: Last Name:
Spouse/Partner Date of Birth: MM/DD/YYYY
Patient Height: 0 ' 0 "
Patient Weight: lbs
Patient Eye Color: None
Patient Blood Type: Don't know
Primary Language: None
Patient Race: None
Is the patient Spanish/Hispanic/Latino?
Notes/Comments: Add any specific information you would like to note about this patient's health or care. If the notes are related to any treatment, please include a date.

Save Changes | Cancel

Back to Overview

Powered by Medem

Contact Medem | SM TOS | Education TOS | IHR TOS | Medem Privacy Policy (Updated 12/2006)
Copyright © 2006 Medem, Inc. All Rights Reserved.

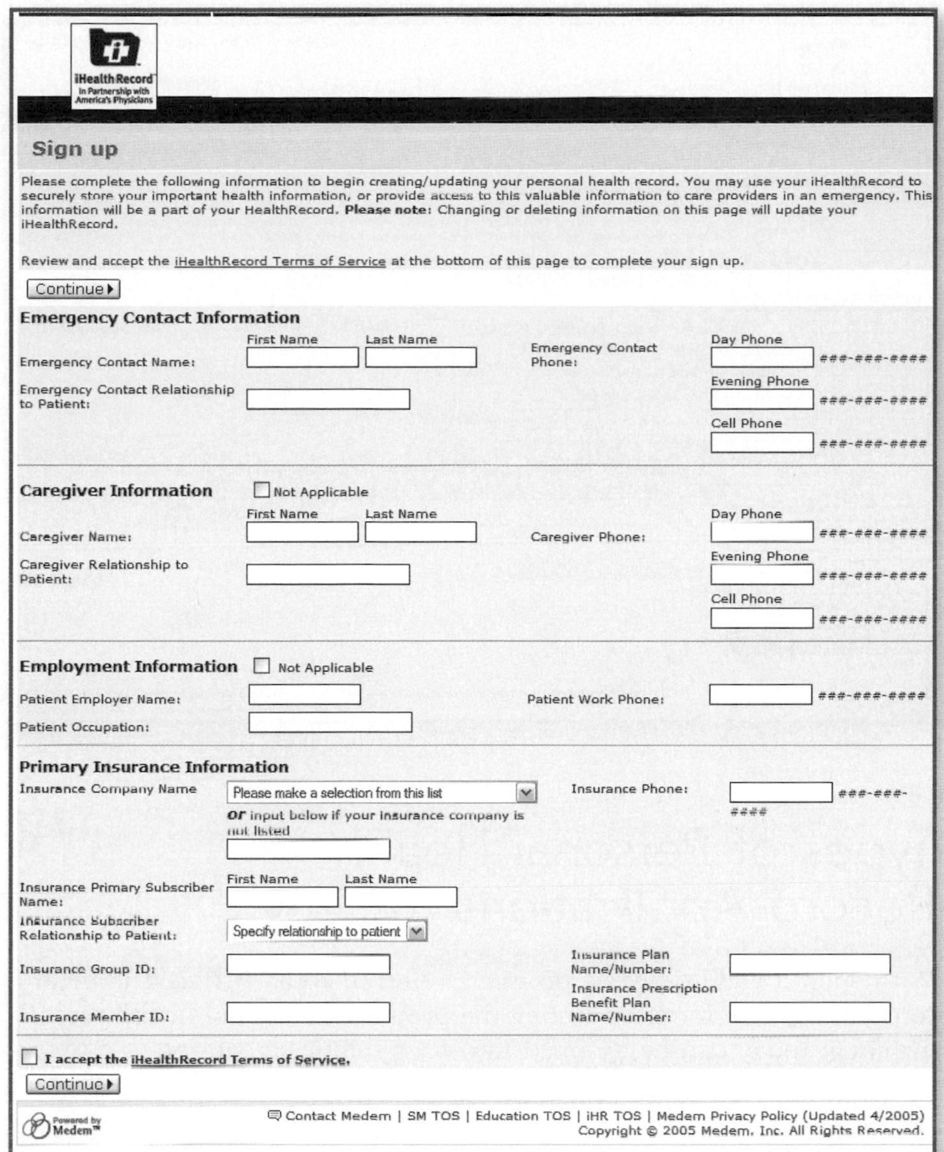

iHealthRecord
In Partnership with America's Physicians

Sign up

Please complete the following information to begin creating/updating your personal health record. You may use your iHealthRecord to securely store your important health information, or provide access to this valuable information to care providers in an emergency. This information will be a part of your HealthRecord. **Please note:** Changing or deleting information on this page will update your iHealthRecord.

Review and accept the iHealthRecord Terms of Service at the bottom of this page to complete your sign up.

Continue ▸

Emergency Contact Information

Emergency Contact Name: First Name ___ Last Name ___

Emergency Contact Relationship to Patient: ___

Emergency Contact Phone: Day Phone ___ ###-###-#### Evening Phone ___ ###-###-#### Cell Phone ___ ###-###-####

Caregiver Information ☐ Not Applicable

Caregiver Name: First Name ___ Last Name ___

Caregiver Relationship to Patient: ___

Caregiver Phone: Day Phone ___ ###-###-#### Evening Phone ___ ###-###-#### Cell Phone ___ ###-###-####

Employment Information ☐ Not Applicable

Patient Employer Name: ___

Patient Occupation: ___

Patient Work Phone: ___ ###-###-####

Primary Insurance Information

Insurance Company Name: Please make a selection from this list
or input below if your insurance company is not listed ___

Insurance Phone: ___ ###-###-####

Insurance Primary Subscriber Name: First Name ___ Last Name ___

Insurance Subscriber Relationship to Patient: Specify relationship to patient

Insurance Group ID: ___

Insurance Plan Name/Number: ___

Insurance Member ID: ___

Insurance Prescription Benefit Plan Name/Number: ___

☐ **I accept the iHealthRecord Terms of Service.**

Continue ▸

Powered by Medem™

Contact Medem | SM TOS | Education TOS | iHR TOS | Medem Privacy Policy (Updated 4/2005)
Copyright © 2005 Medem, Inc. All Rights Reserved.

Figure 5-6
Screen for entering emergency contact, caregiver, employment, and insurance information.

Health Information

- List of current and previous health problems (see Figure 5-9 on page 150)
- Medications (see Figure 5-10 on page 150)
- Allergies
- Preventive screenings
- Immunizations
- Laboratory and test results
- List of hospitalizations and surgeries (see Figure 5-11 on page 151)
- Eye and dental care information
- E-mail, letters, and telephone calls with providers, insurance plan representatives, hospital representatives, and others

Figure 5-7

Screen for granting or denying access privileges to the PHR.

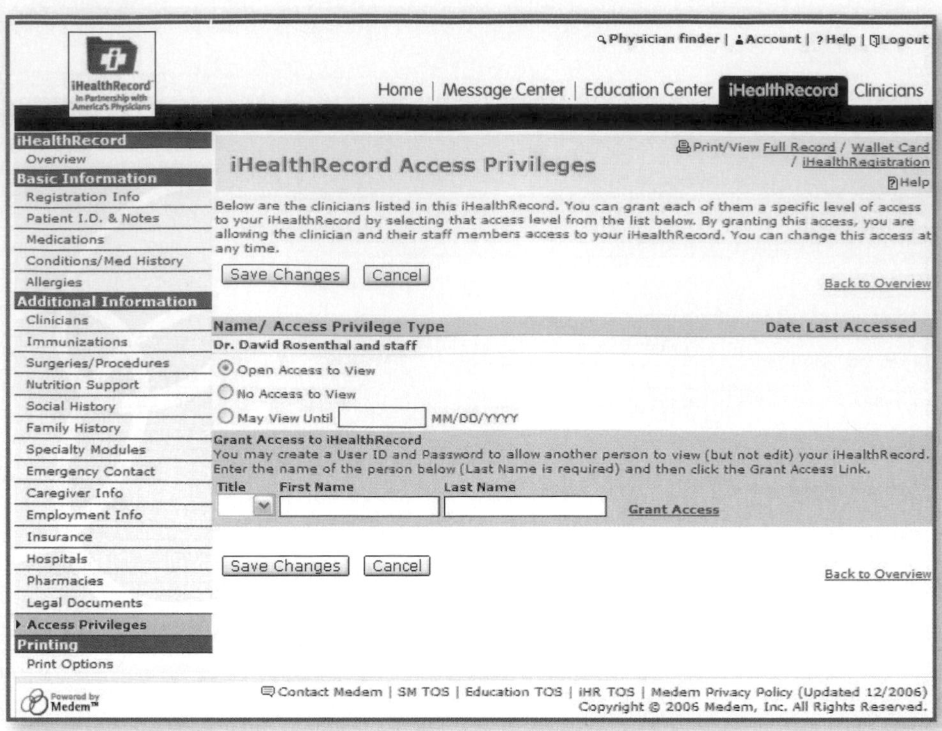

Types of Personal Health Record Applications

With such a wide range of products referred to as PHRs, it is helpful to note major differences among the products. Personal health records available today can be grouped into four major categories:

1. Computer-based, stand-alone
2. Internet-based, tethered
3. Internet-based, untethered
4. Internet-based, networked and interoperable

While these categories are useful for grouping purposes, it should be noted that they are not mutually exclusive.

COMPUTER-BASED STAND-ALONE

In a computer-based stand-alone PHR, individuals enter their own health information in a software program that resides on their home computer. Consumers first either purchase or download the PHR software program and install it on their computer. Information is entered by keying it in manually and/or by scanning documents or images such as lab reports and hospital discharge instructions.

This type of PHR is not designed to send or receive information with other health information systems. It is known as a stand-alone or

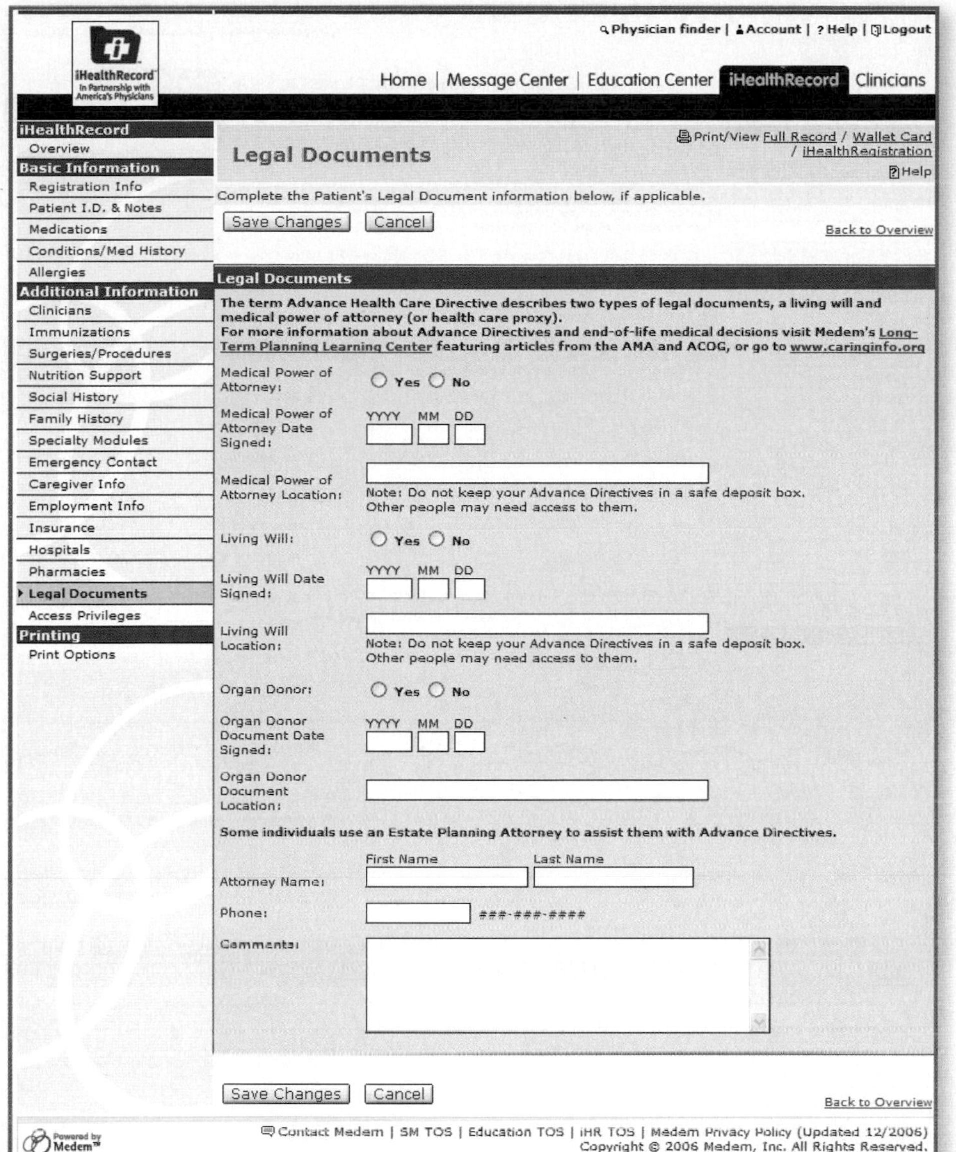

Figure 5-8

Screen for specifying which legal documents are included in the PHR.

untethered PHR, which means that it is not connected to any other computer system. The only way information gets into an untethered PHR is if it is entered by the patient or by someone to whom the patient has granted permission.

untethered information system not connected to another information system.

This type of PHR is portable; information can be copied to a portable storage device, such as a memory card or a CD, and taken to a doctor or hospital visit. Once at the office, the information can be uploaded to a computer and accessed by a patient's physician. However, this requires the physician to have software that is compatible with the program that the patient is using. If the programs are not compatible, the physician will not be able to access the data on the portable device. However, it is still possible to print pages ahead of time and bring them to the office

Figure 5-9

Partial list of past and present medical conditions.

Physician finder | Account | ? Help | Logout

iHealthRecord In Partnership with America's Physicians

Home | Message Center | Education Center | iHealthRecord | Clinicians

iHealthRecord
Overview
Basic Information
Registration Info
Patient I.D. & Notes
Medications
Conditions/Med History
Allergies
Additional Information
Clinicians
Immunizations
Surgeries/Procedures
Nutrition Support
Social History
Family History
Specialty Modules
Emergency Contact
Caregiver Info
Employment Info
Insurance
Hospitals
Pharmacies
Legal Documents
Access Privileges
Printing
Print Options

Add Conditions and Patient's Medical History

Print/View Full Record / Wallet Card / iHealthRegistration
Help

From the list below, add the Patient's Conditions/Diagnoses to this iHealthRecord. You can select current and past Conditions and Diagnoses. You do not need to list Allergies here. For Allergies, please use the Allergies section of the iHealthRecord.

If you do not find a specific condition or diagnosis, use the "Other" boxes provided to type in the name of the condition/diagnosis.

Add Conditions/Med Hx | Cancel

Add Conditions and Patient's Medical History

List of Common Conditions / Medical History Diagnoses:

Alzheimer's Disease	Pneumonia	Sexual Dysfunction	Gonorrhea
Dizziness	Pulmonary Embolism	Urinary Tract Infections	Herpes
Epilepsy	Upper Respiratory Infection	Hemorrhoids	Infertility
Fainting	Angina	Rectal Bleeding	Pelvic Inflammatory Disease
Meningitis	Atherosclerosis	Arthritis	Scabies
Migraine Headache	Congestive Heart Failure	Bursitis	Syphilis
Multiple Sclerosis	Coronary Artery Disease	Carpal Tunnel Syndrome	Chickenpox
Parkinson's Disease	Heart Condition / Heart Disease	Chronic Pain	Lyme disease
Periods of Unconsciousness	High Blood Cholesterol	Fibromyalgia	Measles
Seizures / Seizure Disorder	High Blood Pressure	Gout	Mononucleosis
Stroke	High Lipids	Limb Pain	Mumps

Figure 5-10

Screen for adding medications to the PHR.

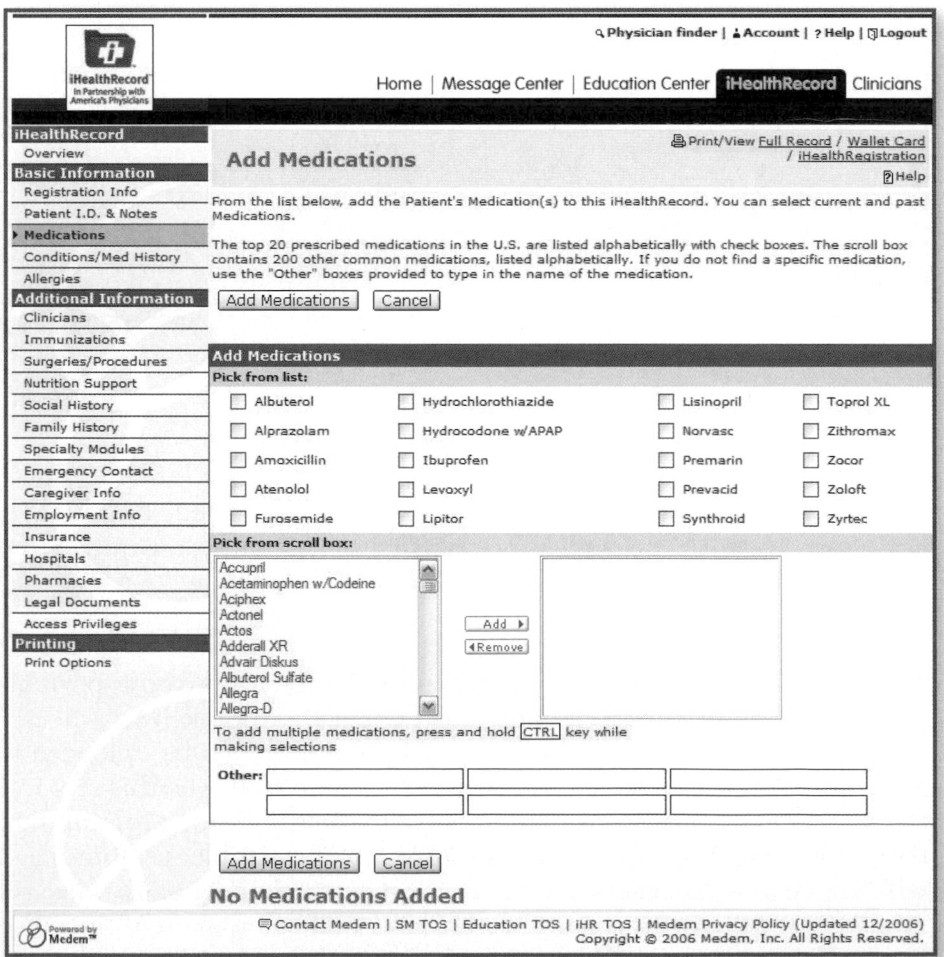

Physician finder | Account | ? Help | Logout

iHealthRecord In Partnership with America's Physicians

Home | Message Center | Education Center | iHealthRecord | Clinicians

iHealthRecord
Overview
Basic Information
Registration Info
Patient I.D. & Notes
Medications
Conditions/Med History
Allergies
Additional Information
Clinicians
Immunizations
Surgeries/Procedures
Nutrition Support
Social History
Family History
Specialty Modules
Emergency Contact
Caregiver Info
Employment Info
Insurance
Hospitals
Pharmacies
Legal Documents
Access Privileges
Printing
Print Options

Print/View Full Record / Wallet Card / iHealthRegistration

Add Surgeries and Procedures

Help

From the list below, add the Patient's Surgeries/Procedures to this iHealthRecord. You can add both current and past Surgeries and Procedures. Surgeries/Procedures are listed alphabetically. If you do not find a specific surgery or procedure, use the "Other" boxes provided to type in the name of the surgery/procedure.

[Add Surgeries/Procedures] [Cancel]

Add Surgeries and Procedures

Pick from list:

Abdominal Surgery	Circumcision	Hemorrhoid Surgery	Pacemaker
Abortion	Colonoscopy	Hernia Repair	PET scan
Angiogram	Colorectal Resection	Hip Replacement	Prostatectomy
Angioplasty	Colposcopy	Hysterectomy	Pulmonary Artery Catheter placement
Ankle / Leg Fracture Repair	Coronary Artery Bypass Grafting (CABG)	In vitro Fertilization (IVF)	Radial Keratotomy (RK)
Appendectomy	Cosmetic Surgery	Joint Aspiration	Radiation Treatment
Arterial Line Placement	Craniotomy	Knee Replacement	Radiograph
Artificial Insemination	CT Scan	Knee Surgery	Shoulder Surgery
Aspiration of Breast Cyst	Cystoscopy	Laminectomy	Sigmoidoscopy
Back Surgery	Dialysis	Laparoscopy	Spinal Tap /Lumbar Puncture
Bladder Repair	Dilation & Curettage (D&C)	Laparotomy	Splenectomy
Blood Transfusion	Electrocardiogram (EKG, ECG)	LASIK	Stress Test
Bone Scan	Episiotomy	LEEP	Thyroidectomy
Cardiac Catheterization	Fusions (e.g., Lumbar)	Lumpectomy	Tonsillectomy
Carpal Tunnel Surgery	Gall Bladder Removal (Cholecystectomy)	Mammogram	Tracheostomy
Cataract Surgery	Gastroscopy	Mastectomy	Transurethral Prostate Surgery
Cesarean Section	Glaucoma Surgery	MRI	Tubal Ligation (Female Sterilization)
Chemotherapy	Heart Bypass Surgery	Myelogram	Ultrasound
Chest Tube Placement	Heart Valve Replacement	Oophorectomy	Vasectomy (Male Sterilization)

Other:

[Add Surgeries/Procedures] [Cancel]

No Surgeries or Procedures Added

Powered by Medem™

Contact Medem | SM TOS | Education TOS | iHR TOS | Medem Privacy Policy (Updated 12/2006)
Copyright © 2006 Medem, Inc. All Rights Reserved.

Figure 5-11
Screen for indicating which surgeries and procedures have been performed.

visit. Figure 5-12 on page 154 shows an example of a PHR that can be completed online and downloaded to a user's computer or storage device.

Advantages

On the positive side, the computer-based stand-alone PHR is totally owned and controlled by the patient. The information is more secure than it would be in a PHR that exchanged data with other information systems, since it does not send and receive information over a network.

Disadvantages

This lack of data exchange also has a downside, since the patient must enter all the information and manually update the record on a regular basis. The program is unable to receive data from other sources, such as a physician office. Since no one else has access to the record, the only way information becomes part of this type of PHR is if the patient enters it, which requires a commitment on the part of the patient to keep

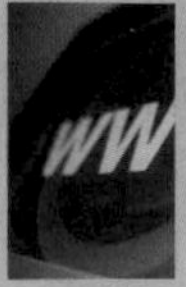

Online Discovery

iHealthRecord is an Internet-based PHR that is offered by the iHealth Alliance, a not-for-profit organization. The website allows individuals to create and store personal health records at no charge. In this exercise, you will have the option of starting your own PHR or following the steps below to explore the iHealthRecord website. Open a web browser and go to www.ihealthrecord.org.

If you are interested in starting your own PHR, click the Sign Up Now button on the website. Follow the directions provided on the screen to register and begin entering your information.

If you would rather look at the website without creating your own PHR, Click the Tell Me More button.

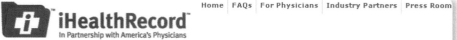

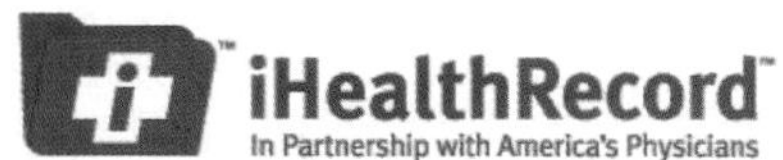

Home | FAQs | For Physicians | Industry Partners | Press Room

The secure and confidential, interactive record for your health information.

What is an iHealth Record?

The iHealth Record is a secure and confidential, interactive personal record of your medical history. You can create, manage and share (with your authorized physicians) your personal health information.

The iHealthRecord is:

1. **Easy**
2. **Efficient**
3. **Accurate**
4. **Accessible**
5. **Secure**

The privacy and security of your iHealth Record is governed by the iHealth Alliance - committed to bringing an iHealth Record to every American.
Tell me more

About the iHealthRecord

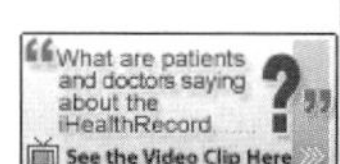

By investing just a few minutes to create an iHealthRecord, you can feel confident that you'll have comprehensive health information for you and the ones you care for (your spouse, children, parents or other loved ones) whenever you may need it. The iHealthRecord is a secure and confidential interactive record that allows you to store, update and share health information with your physician or in an emergency situation.

- The iHealthRecord is simple and quick. It's easy to create, update and access your iHealthRecord online.
- You can store all of your health information in one place. By keeping all of your :health information in one place, you can ensure accurate, comprehensive information can be provided to physicians and other healthcare providers when needed.
- Confidence in the privacy and security of your information.. The privacy of your iHealthRecord will be overseen by the iHealth Alliance, a not-for-profit advisory board whose mission is to protect the interests of physicians and patients.
- You control access. You can share your health information with whomever you choose, including physicians and family members, whenever needed because you control access to your iHealthRecord.
- Carry important information with you. You can print a wallet card to carry important health information with you at all times.
- Participate in education programs. Based on your condition and medication information, you will begin receiving education programs from trusted health authorities including the Food and Drug Administration (FDA), the Centers for Disease Control (CDC), the American Heart Association (AHA), and the nation's leading medical societies.
- Available through physicians. The iHealthRecord is already widely available today on 100,000 physician web sites. Check to see if your doctor offers the iHealthRecord.

iHR Privacy Policy | Tour | Service Announcement | Contact Us | Site Map

Copyright © 2007 Medem, Inc. All Rights Reserved.

Read the information on the page, and then scroll to the bottom of the page and click on the word Tour.

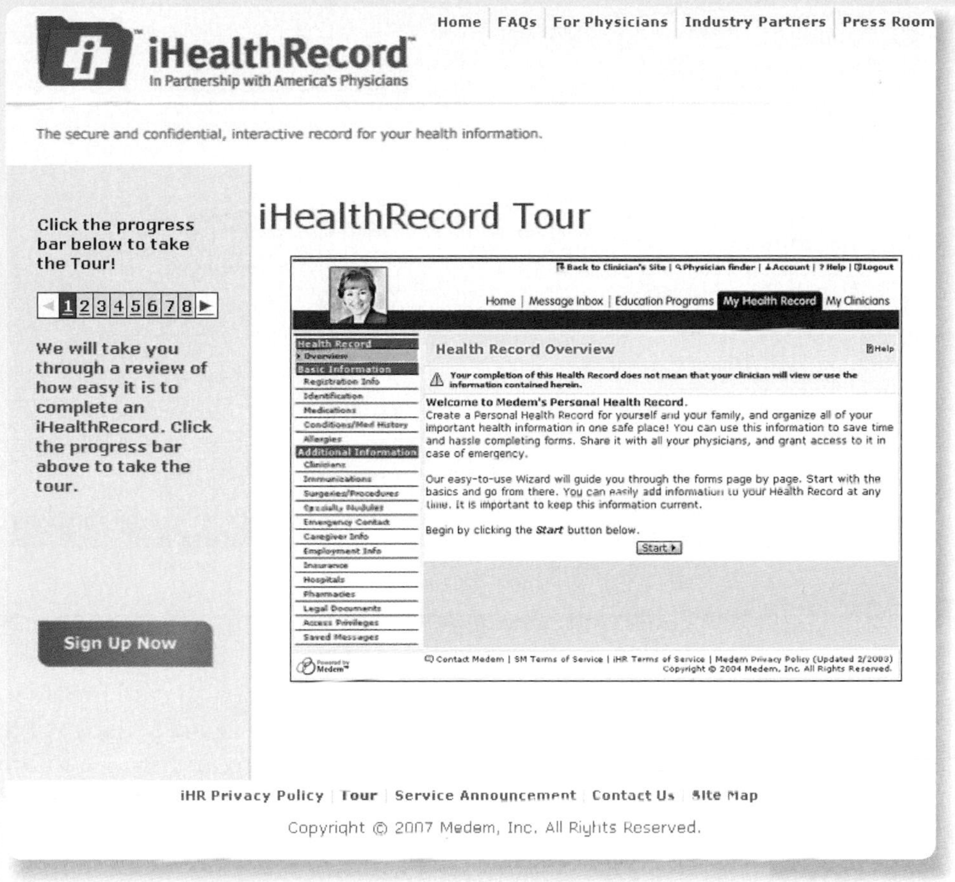

Using the progress bar on the left side of the page, view the iHealthRecord tour.

Thinking About It

1. What are some of the obstacles to creating your own PHR?

   ____

2. Can the iHealthRecord exchange information with health care providers?

   ____

3. What do you think is the greatest advantage of storing personal health information on a site such as this one? Do you see any disadvantages?

   ____

When you are finished viewing the website and answering the questions, close your web browser.

Figure 5-12

A computer-based stand-alone PHR offered by the federal government.

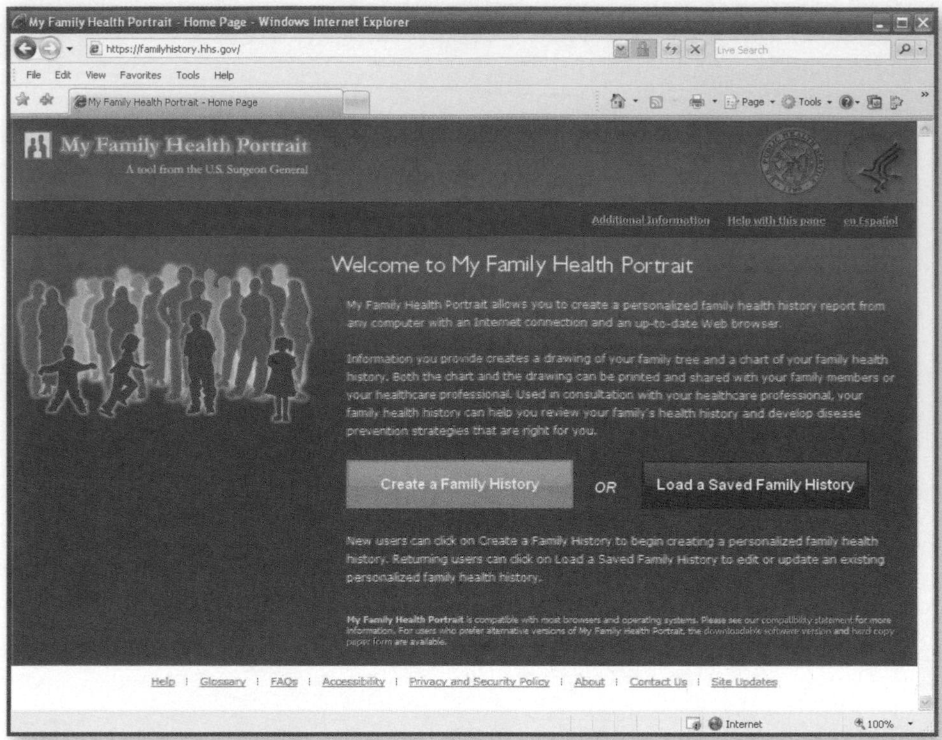

information up-to-date. After each encounter with a health care provider, the record must be manually updated. The patient is also responsible for remembering to copy the data to a portable device and take it to the health care facility. Not all doctors will use the information provided.

INTERNET-BASED, TETHERED

The term *personal health record* is also used to refer to health records that are stored and maintained on websites owned by outside organizations rather than by patients. Some physician practices, insurance companies, employers, and hospitals offer what is known as tethered PHRs. The word **tethered** refers to the fact that the PHR is attached to the health information system of a particular organization. Rather than bringing together information from all the patient's providers, this type of record provides information from one provider's database. In most cases, the patient can only view the information; no information can be added or removed.

tethered information system attached to another information system.

Physician Office-Based

For example, a physician office may allow patients to access a portion of their electronic health records via the Internet. Some physician EHRs contain a linked application referred to as a **patient portal,** a website that allows patients to interact with a particular provider or facility (see Figure 5-13). Common activities that can be accomplished via a portal include sending and receiving e-mail messages to and from the provider's office, requesting appointments, viewing medical history and test results, requesting prescription refills, accessing patient education materials, and receiving automated alerts and reminders when preventive screenings or tests are due. While some providers' sites actually allow patients to create

patient portal website that allows patients to interact with provider or facility.

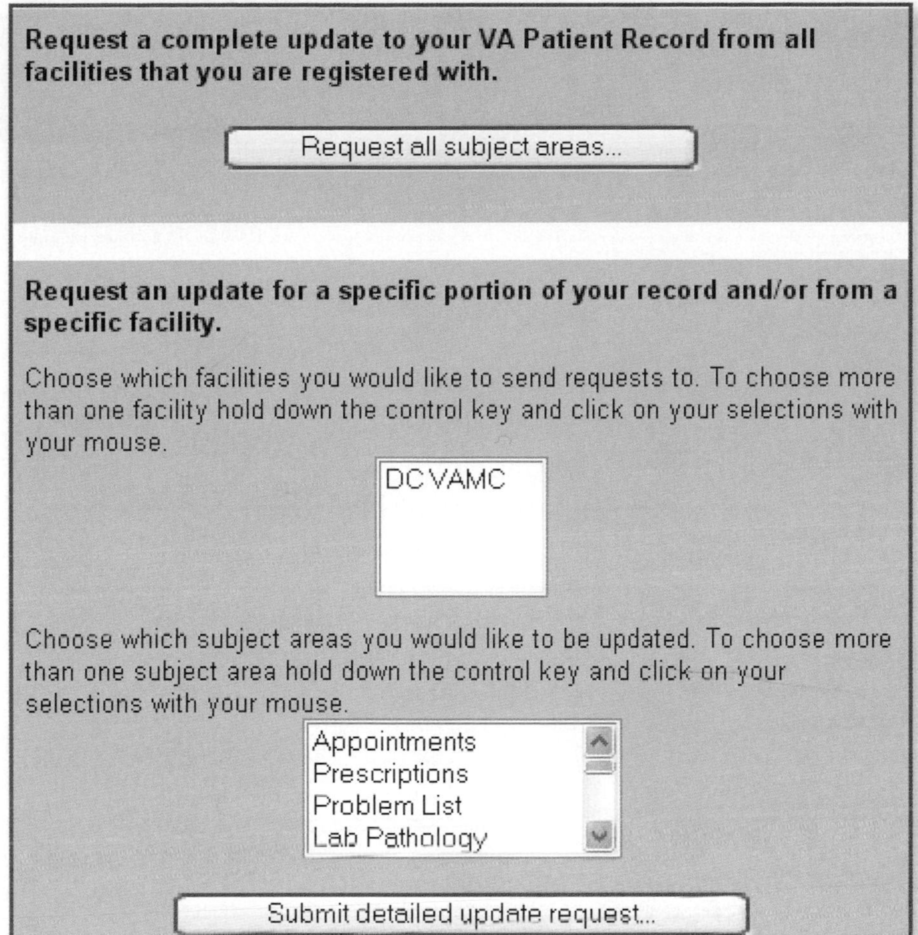

Figure 5-13
A tethered PHR can be updated by the provider or facility that offers the PHR.

their own PHRs, most just permit the patient to view information in the EHR, which is owned and maintained by the provider.

Insurance Plan-Based

Some health plans offer subscribers an opportunity to create and maintain PHRs on their websites (see Figure 5-14). In addition to information the individual enters, the PHR provides access to information maintained by the company, including insurance claims, lists of participating providers, benefit coverage information, and so on. Health insurers are encouraging subscribers to take a more active role in managing their health. Many insurers provide information on their websites to educate individuals about medical conditions and the costs and benefits of various treatments. Discounts are offered on programs designed to improve an individual's health, such as weight loss, exercise, and smoking cessation programs. The insurance carriers hope that education and incentives will motivate individuals to make choices that will improve their quality of life and that will result in reduced costs to the company. While the patient actually enters some of the information in this type of program, the file is still owned by the insurer, not by the individual.

In this example, the PHR is integrated with another application, whether it is a physician office EHR or a claim database at a health plan. Some of these programs do little more than allow patients access

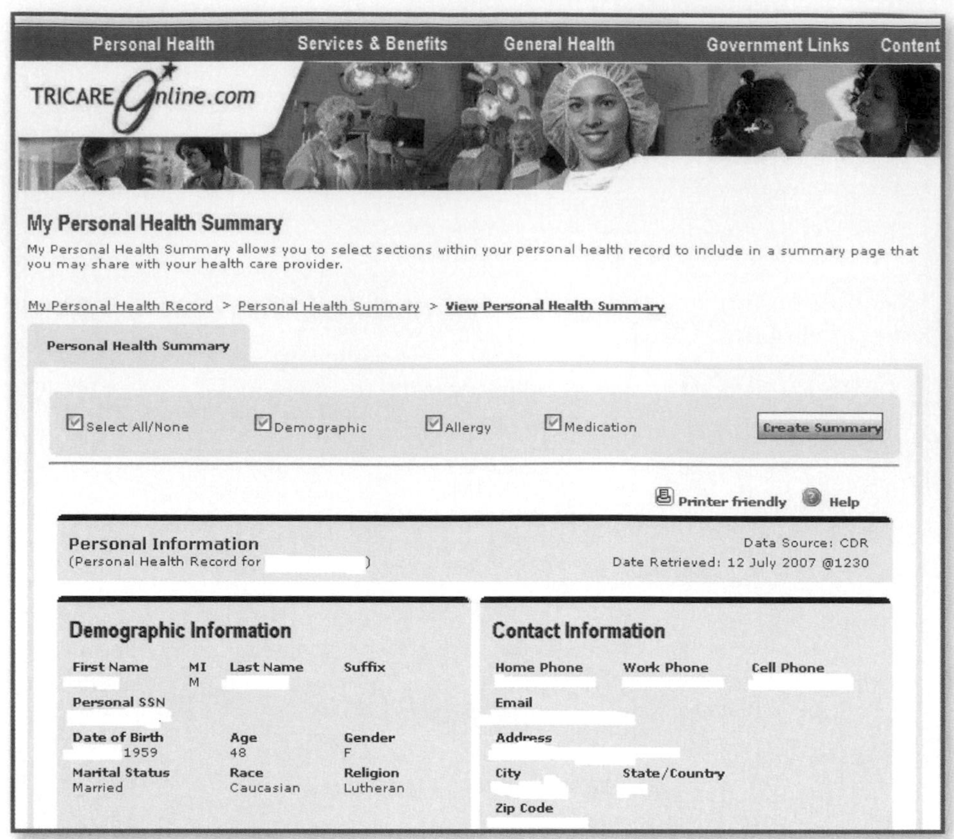

Figure 5-14

A PHR offered by Tricare, the federal health care program for members of the uniformed services, their families, and survivors.

to information that already exists on the provider's computer. In all these instances, the individual has no independent access to the information without going through the website of the outside entity. This group owns the software program and grants access to the individual.

Although often referred to as PHRs, these patient portals are actually not true PHRs, since the files are owned and maintained by the provider, not by the patients. In addition, the majority of the data is entered by the provider or a staff member, not by the patient. In a true PHR, the individual owns and maintains the data and determines who has access to the information in the PHR.

Advantages

Tethered PHRs do not require regular updating by the individual, since much of the information is entered by the staff of the organization that hosts the PHR. Because of this, the information may be more up-to-date.

Disadvantages

A tethered PHR does not include information from multiple providers and facilities. It is stored and maintained by a single organization, and it is primarily designed to address the organization's needs rather than the needs of the patient. It does not, then, provide a comprehensive picture of the patient's past and present medical condition. Since most tethered PHRs do not make it possible for patients to extract data and send the information to other providers or facilities, patients' health information is still scattered among various groups, such as physicians, labs, and outpatient clinics.

INTERNET-BASED, UNTETHERED

In an Internet-based, untethered PHR, consumers access a PHR software application using a web browser and enter health-related information, which is stored by the application provider. An untethered PHR does not rely on another database for content; such as a provider's EHR or an insurance plan's claim database. The individual creates all the content, owns the information, and controls access to the file. For example, individuals can grant permission for doctors and family members to access selected information in the record. Because the information is accessible via the Internet, it is available whenever it is needed, which is particularly important in emergencies.

Patients access the application from a web browser, create user IDs and passwords, and then enter and store their health information. The data are stored in a secure, private database. The individual can view and update the information at any time. Some PHR applications are free, while others charge a fee.

Employer-Based

A number of large employers are providing web-based PHRs to their employees. Individuals can enter and store information about their past and current health and can access educational materials and self-help tools to use to improve their health. Individuals may also be able to take self-assessment tests that provide information on risk status for common diseases such as heart conditions and diabetes. In 2006, a number of large companies formed an organization known as Dossia (see Figure 5-15). In 2008, Dossia will begin offering PHRs to employees of the member companies.

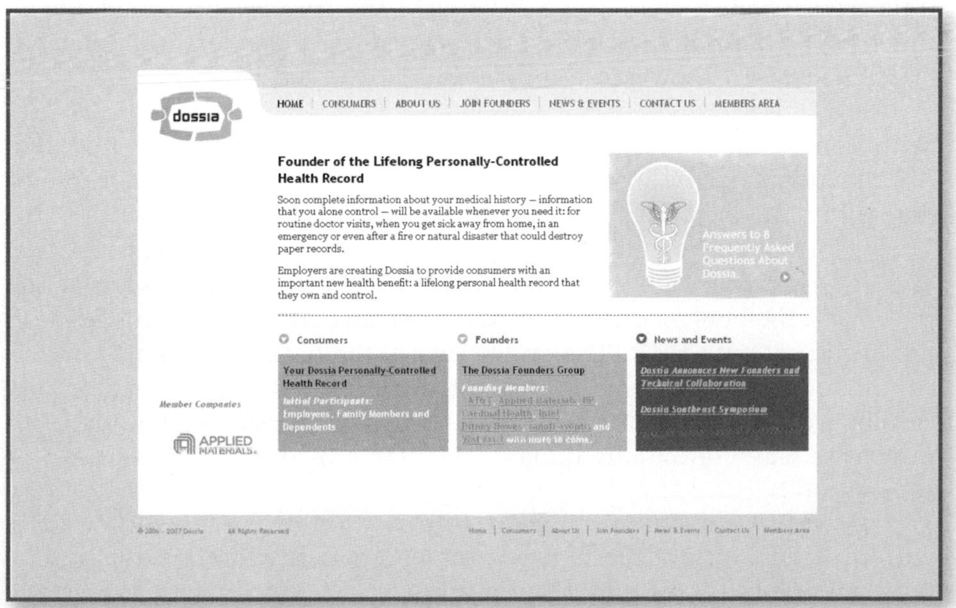

Figure 5-15

The web site of Dossia, a non-profit organization formed by a number of large corporations, to provide PHRs to employees (www.dossia.org).

Advantages

Since the content is entered by individuals, this type of PHR includes data from all providers who are treating the patient. It is not limited to the records on file at one provider's office. In addition, the PHR can be viewed at any time from any location. A patient who is in a provider's office for the first time can access the PHR data from an office computer and share relevant medical information with the provider.

Disadvantages

As with the stand-alone PHR model, this model relies on the individual to enter health information, and the consumer is responsible for keeping the PHR up-to-date.

INTERNET-BASED, NETWORKED AND INTEROPERABLE

All the models just described have one major limitation—they do not support the exchange of information to and from the computer systems of all the providers and facilities that are involved in the patient's health care.

The health records of an individual reside in a number of different software applications located at each of the health care sites. The primary care provider maintains patient records in one EHR program, while the dermatologist uses a different EHR application. The laboratory that performs the tests uses a laboratory information system. Similarly, the hospital, pharmacy, and insurance company all use different systems. To maintain an up-to-date PHR, individuals must collect information from the different sources and manually update the record. Not everyone has the time or inclination to do this. For a PHR to be useful, it must be easy for ordinary people to use, and maintaining it should not require a major commitment of time. Recognizing the problem, key organizations are now recommending what are called networked PHRs. A **networked personal health record** allows the transfer of information to and from multiple sources, including the systems of the patient's providers and of other health care organizations such as insurance carriers and pharmacies. Figure 5-16 shows an example of a networked PHR.

networked personal health record PHR that transfers information to and from multiple health information systems.

With a networked PHR in place, information is continually updated. After an office visit with a physician, relevant portions of the information entered in the doctor's EHR are automatically sent to the patient's PHR. This information includes the diagnosis, treatment plan, prescriptions, and any follow-up care. After the patient fills a new prescription at the pharmacy, the new medication is automatically added to the medication list in the patient's PHR. The system alerts the patient if the new medication interacts with any current medication. Any laboratory or test results are sent to the PHR from the ordering physician. The patient's insurance plan continually updates the status of insurance claims.

The individual can choose to share information in the networked PHR with providers or facilities. For example, a patient who is being admitted to a hospital can allow the admitting office to access necessary

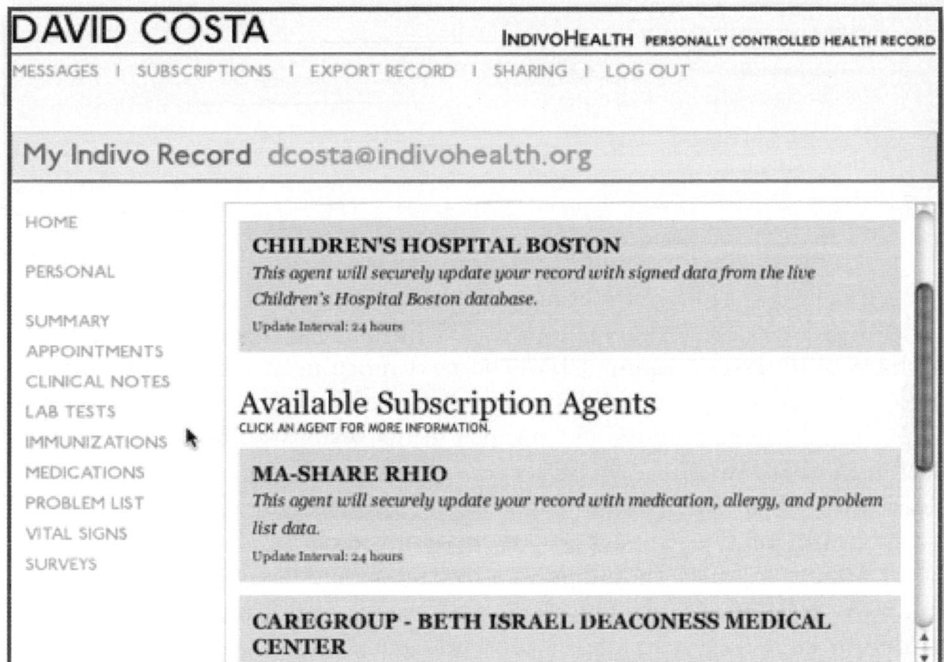

Figure 5-16
An Internet-based PHR that allows patients to share information with providers and facilities.

information in the PHR, such as a list of medications, information about the patient's allergies and current condition, and insurance information. A patient can also allow a primary care provider to view information from office visits with specialists.

Advantages

With a networked PHR, the patient has a complete, up-to-date electronic personal health record. It can be accessed at any time from any location with an Internet connection. Both patients and their providers benefit from having access to complete, current information. The patient is in control of the flow of information—deciding which incoming information is accepted and which outside systems are allowed access. Information from other health information systems is automatically updated, so the patient is not required to manually maintain all the information.

Disadvantages

Consumers will not want to use a PHR that does not ensure complete privacy and security. The exchange of health information across multiple computer networks is of concern to many people. Another problem with the idea of a networked PHR is the lack of the necessary infrastructure to exchange data among health information systems. In late 2007, the organization that developed a functional model for EHRs (EHR-S-FM) created a similar model for PHRs. The Health Level Seven (HL7) model for the functionality of a PHR is known as PHR-S. The EHR-S-FM model was used by the Certification Commission for Healthcare Information Technology (CCHIT) to develop certification guidelines for EHR software programs. Eventually, PHR applications may be certified in a similar manner to EHR programs.

Case Study

"THE LIST"

Ellis Johnston had more than his share of illnesses. Ten years ago he suffered a heart attack and since then he has been on a beta blocker, a blood thinner, and a cholesterol-lowering medication. A year later, he developed a gastrointestinal bleed and had to be rushed to the emergency room, as a result of the aspirin he was taking after this heart attack. A year later, he had a cough that would not go away. After a chest x-ray showed nothing, his doctor suggested a CT scan. He knew Ellis had been a cigarette smoker for over 40 years, until he quit when he had his heart attack. The CT scan found a nodule in a lobe of his left lung. Surgery was performed, and the nodule turned out to be malignant. As a precaution, Ellis underwent 16 weeks of chemotherapy. This year, Ellis developed Type II diabetes. His endocrinologist prescribed glucophage to try to keep his blood sugar under control.

Ellis retired last year and now he and his wife Mamie are fulfilling their retirement dream to spend the summer months in Ohio near their children and grandchildren, and the winter months in Florida. They were leaving in five days. As they were raking leaves and mowing the lawn one last time, Ellis accidentally scraped his leg on the shed door as he put the lawnmower away. It was more of a scrape than a cut, but since Ellis is on blood thinners, it bled quite a bit. The next morning it was oozing slightly, but Ellis was not concerned. He had seen plenty of cuts and scrapes in his seventy-some years.

That afternoon, Ellis and Mamie went to the local walk-in clinic for their annual flu shots. Ellis showed his leg to the nurse at the clinic, and she told him he should go to a nearby wound center to have it looked at. The doctor at the wound center examined the scrape closely, and suspected that the wound was infected. Ellis mentioned that he was a diabetic, and that they were leaving for Florida in two days. The doctor looked concerned as he cleaned and bandaged the wound. He had taken a culture and would send it out to see if Ellis had developed a staph infection. As he handed him a prescription for the antibiotic Bactrim, he suggested that Ellis visit a wound center in Florida as soon as he arrived. Mamie called a friend in Florida and asked her to look up "wound center" in the phonebook. After calling several places, she finally found one who could see Ellis the day after they would arrive.

Five days later, Ellis went to the wound center near his home in Florida. In the waiting room, he is asked to complete a form listing all the medications

The HL7 Personal Health Record System Functional Model

The newly developed PHR-S FM identifies the features and functions that could be included in a networked PHR. It also links functions in the PHR to functions in the EHR, creating a road map for exchanging data between providers and patients. While other functions may be added in the future, thus far the model consists of three sections: Personal Health, Supportive, and Information Infrastructure (see Table 5-2).

Personal Health Functions The personal health functions enable individuals to capture, view, and manage records of their health care over time. This includes demographic information, clinical data about past and present medical conditions, wellness and preventive care, self-help

he is taking, including the dose amounts. He asks his wife to complete that part of the form for him. In her purse, she carries what they call "the list"—a set of 3 × 5 cards that list all his medications, dates of surgeries, and the names and phone numbers of all his doctors. She has done this ever since he had his heart attack. She used to update it regularly, but with all the chores required to get ready to leave for the winter, Mamie realized she had done so for quite awhile. Realizing that some of Ellis's medications had changed, she turned and asked him if he could remember the newer medications.

Ellis tried to remember, but he was worried about his leg. He knows the implications of infections for diabetes sufferers. What was the name of his new diabetes medication? What was the name of the medication they had given him at the wound center in Ohio? By the time he was ushered into the examining room, the medical assistant noted that he seemed anxious. The doctor asked Ellis whether the culture taken in Ohio had come back positive. Ellis said that since they had been traveling, he had not been in contact with the wound center. The doctor decided it was easier to take another culture than to track down a phone number for the wound center in Ohio.

A few days later, the doctor phoned Ellis to say that he had a staph infection, and would need follow-up care. Eventually, the wound healed, and Ellis was back to his old self.

Yesterday, Ellis and Mamie went to an information session on the Medicare Prescription Drug Plan. The facilitator mentioned the importance of creating a personal health record, and listed several web sites with additional information.

The next day, Mamie went online and read more about PHRs. She was on the computer regularly, sending emails to her children and grandchildren. Convinced of the benefits, she took the list of Ellis's medications, surgeries, past problems, and contact information for all his doctors and began to enter it into an online PHR.

What Do You Think?

1. What risks is Ellis taking by not having an up-to-date personal health record?
2. Would you consider Mamie's list a paper-based personal health record? Why or why not?
3. Once Mamie finishes creating the online personal health record, what additional steps must she take to realize the benefits?

tools for managing care, decision support, and managing encounters with providers. The PHR would be able to:

- Provide information about the owner, such as demographic information and administrative statements such as advanced directives, consents, and authorizations
- Enable the owner to enter, import, and maintain clinical information, such as:
    - Problems
    - Medications
    - Allergies
    - Past medical history

TABLE 5-2 The Major Functional Areas in the HL7 PHR-S Model

Personal Health	PH.1	Account Holder Profile
	PH.2	Manage Historical Clinical Data and Current Data State
	PH.3	Wellness, Preventive Medicine, and Self-Care
	PH.4	Manage Health Education
	PH.5	Account Holder Decision Support
	PH.6	Manage Encounters with Providers
Supportive	S.1	Provider Management
	S.2	Financial Management
	S.3	Administrative Management
	S.4	Other Resource Management
Information Infrastructure	IN.1	Health Record Information Management
	IN.2	Standards-Based Interoperability
	IN.3	Security
	IN.4	Auditable Records

- Surgical history
- Immunizations
- Family history
- Genetic data
- Social history
- Physical examinations
- Diagnostic studies

- Assist the owner in taking steps necessary to maintain health and/or manage current health conditions
- Provide tools to assist the owner in managing health care information, such as details regarding insurance plans, providers and their contact information, and appointments already scheduled or that need to be scheduled
- Allow the owner to enter observations about his or her own health, such as symptoms, reactions to medications, and readings from home care monitors
- Provide the ability to communicate with public health agencies to monitor and control threats to public health
- Provide clinical decision support, such as diagnosis aids, drug interaction databases, and clinical guidelines for treating diseases
- Provide access to educational materials
- Manage information associated with provider encounters, such as office visits, emergency room visits, hospitalizations, e-mail, and telephone calls

Supportive Functions The supportive functions of the PHR-S model include administrative and financial information related to individuals' medical care. The supportive functions also provide information required by financial and administrative systems to process claims and share data with public health systems, researchers, and systems designed to measure and improve the quality of care provided. Some of these functions provide the support necessary to:

- Allow the owner to search for a provider in a geographic area or one who participates in a specific health plan, as well as provide access to current provider contact information
- Manage financial data concerning health plan coverage and utilization of services
- Enable the PHR to exchange information with EHRs and other health care information systems

Information Infrastructure Functions The information infrastructure section of the model enables the PHR to function effectively and efficiently. The functions ensure that the information is stored and exchanged in a secure manner and that individuals' privacy is maintained. The functions also make certain that the system is easy for ordinary people to use. Some of the capabilities include being able to:

- Ensure that information in the PHR is accurately represented through the use of common data sets
- Provide the appearance of an automated, seamless exchange of information through standards-based solutions
- Manage the permissions granted by the owner for access to information and prevent data from being lost, stolen, or viewed by unauthorized parties

It is important to note that while the PHR-S functional model contains many of the functions of currently available PHRs, it is not intended to list all functions or to restrict a PHR to the listed functions. The development of the PHR-S model is important because it outlines the functions of a PHR and specifies the relationship of data in the PHR to data in the EHR.

Benefits of Networked Personal Health Records

A personal health record has many benefits. The primary benefit is that it provides the individual with a complete, up-to-date record of health information in a single location, available wherever there is an Internet connection. By placing ownership and control in the hands of the individual, the PHR encourages individuals to more actively participate in their own health care.

ACCESS TO EVIDENCE-BASED HEALTH INFORMATION

While physicians are able to access evidence-based health information about medical conditions, individuals have not had the same opportunity.

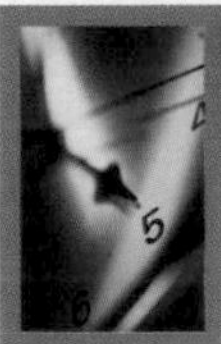

Making It Real

PHRs: A Sticky Subject

A number of companies are developing technologies that make it possible to access personal health records radio-frequency identification (RFID) chips. The chips do not contain the actual personal health record, but contain a link to a secure online database where the patient's personal health record is stored. When the chip is read by a portable RFID reader, the identifying information on the chip is entered in a secure online database that contains the patient's personal health record. The identifying information does not contain any personal information—it is just a code that is assigned to that patient's record. While there is conflicting information on whether chips implanted under the skin are safe, the chips can also be enclosed in thin, adhesive skin patches. The major advantage of an RFID chip application is that is always with the patient, since it is located on the body.

If hospitals acquire the RFID readers, the allergy and medication lists of patients would be available in seconds, reducing the likelihood of adverse drug events in the emergency room. The PHR would also provide demographic information, insurance information, and emergency contact information. This method of storing personal health information would be especially beneficial to patients who speak a different language or who are unconscious or unable to communicate when they arrive in the emergency room.

PHRs provide access to the latest medical information through the Internet, which helps people make medical decisions in partnership with their providers.

ASSESSMENT OF RISK

Personal health records educate patients about diseases that are present in their families, as well as diseases that they may be at risk for due to age, weight, social habits, and the like. Personal health records also provide tools for evaluating risk factors and identifying steps that can be taken to prevent diseases from developing.

ENHANCED COMMUNICATION WITH PROVIDERS

Personal health records provide consumers with the ability to send e-mail messages to their providers (see Figure 5-17). Messaging allow patients to communicate their health situations and concerns to their physicians at their convenience. E-mail may be more efficient than leaving messages with front desk staff or answering services. This form of messaging updates the provider on the patient's condition and improves communication between patients and clinicians.

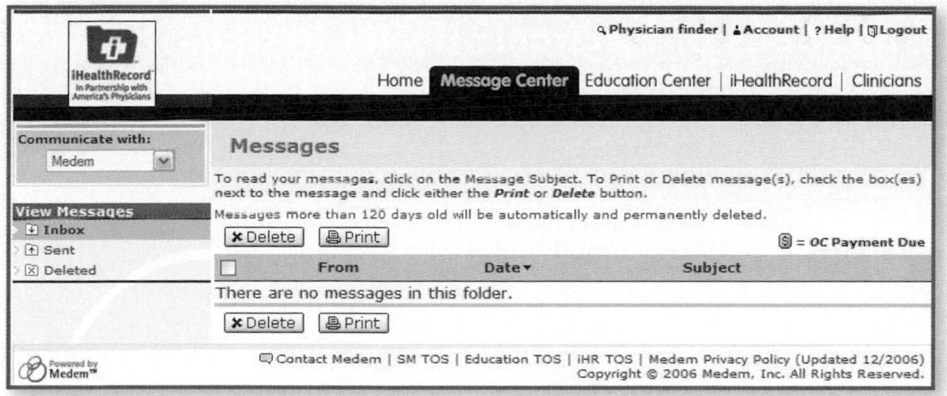

Figure 5-17

Screen in a PHR where electronic messages are sent and received.

EMPOWERMENT OF PATIENTS

In many diseases, the behavior of the patient outside the physician office is more important to overall health than is the brief time spent in the office. Personal health records make it easier for patients to monitor their health, record their observations, and follow care plan recommendations. In addition, patients are responsible for maintaining the records and ensuring that information is accurate and up-to-date, which makes them more involved in their health care.

INCREASED PATIENT SAFETY

More than anyone, patients know whether information in their health record is correct. The use of PHRs makes it possible to reduce errors in medical records, since patients are more likely to recognize incorrect information. Also, similar to the features in an electronic health record, a PHR provides automated alerts. This feature informs patients of medication interactions, overdue tests, and out-of-range test results.

IMPROVED QUALITY OF CARE

By providing a physician with a complete, up-to-date picture of a patient's health, the PHR makes the doctor better able to provide quality care. If a patient grants permission, a doctor may view information in the PHR. Patients have the ability to limit the information a provider may see—providing access to one section while restricting access to another.

IMPROVED EMERGENCY CARE

Since PHRs can be accessed in any location with an Internet connection at any time, patient health information is available to paramedics and emergency room personnel (if the patient has granted permission for access). This can save critical time in an emergency and can also prevent problems such as allergic reactions to medications.

The ABCs of Electronic Health Records

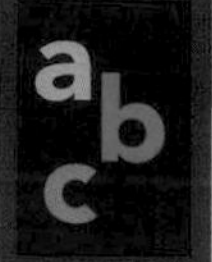

CDHP—Consumer-Directed Health Plan

A type of health plan that combines a high deductible with low premiums and a tax-free savings account used for out-of-pocket health costs.

HIPAA—The Health Insurance Portability and Accountability Act of 1996

Federal legislation, part of which is designed to protect the privacy and security of personal health information.

HL7—Health Level Seven

An organization that develops health care standards.

PHR—Personal Health Record

An electronic version of a person's lifelong, comprehensive health record that is collected and maintained by the patient and can be shared with providers if the patient chooses.

ePHR—Electronic Personal Health Record

Another term used to refer to a personal health record that is created and saved on a computer.

PHR-S FM—Personal Health Record System Functional Model

A model of the features of personal health records developed by the HL7 organization.

POTENTIAL COST SAVINGS

Using information available through a PHR, consumers may select lower-cost medications or treatments. Costs are also reduced by the elimination of duplicate testing, since the patient has easy access to a list of completed tests.

Barriers to the Implementation of Personal Health Records

The features that make PHRs appealing are the same features that make them difficult to implement. Standing in the way of implementation are the lack of interoperability, the lack of consumer awareness, and privacy and security concerns.

INTEROPERABILITY

While an individual is the source of much of the information in a PHR, the products that have the greatest value are able to exchange data electronically with physician practices, laboratories, hospitals, and other health care providers. At present, there is no simple way of enabling PHR programs to send data to and receive data from other health care information systems. As discussed in Chapter 2, for health information systems to be interoperable, they must share common standards for data sets such as diagnoses and procedures, laboratory information, and medication.

Likewise, PHRs and the systems with which they exchange data need to use the same standards. The PHR-S functional model created by HL7 identifies links between information in a PHR and information in an EHR. For example, the data field for the patient's date of birth in a PHR contains the same information as that field in the EHR. While progress is being made, there is much still to be done before PHRs work seamlessly with other health information systems.

CONSUMER AWARENESS

A 2007 survey sponsored by Aetna and the Financial Planning Association found that almost two-thirds of people surveyed "do not know or are unsure" about the concept of personal health records ("Nearly Two-Thirds of Americans Are Not Familiar with Personal Health Records, a Resource Available to Millions of Consumers," Aetna Press Release, July 17, 2007). In a 2006 Markle Foundation study (*Connecting Americans to Their Health Care: A Common Framework for Networked Personal Health Information,* The Markle Foundation, December 2006), most people felt that PHRs would improve the quality of health care. Two-thirds said they were interested in having their own PHRs. They felt that having PHRs would give them more control of their health care. However, the findings also indicated that 80 percent of consumers were "very concerned" about the possibility of identity theft and fraud involving their health information. If PHRs are going to be in widespread use, consumers need to be educated about what they are and the benefits they offer.

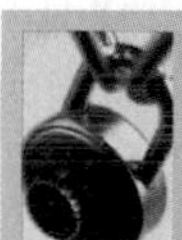

Privacy and Security Alert

The Same or Different?

The type of personal health records advocated by groups such as AHIMA and the Markle Foundation are capable of sharing data with other health information systems over the Internet. However, several studies have found that consumers are hesitant to put their personal health records online because of privacy and security concerns.

While PHRs are a relatively new product and there is little consumer awareness of them, most people already consent to have sensitive financial information stored and sent via the Internet. The most prominent example is online banking, which offers account management, funds transfer, bill paying, and a number of other features. Although some people are not comfortable with online banking, most have realized that the benefits outweigh the risks, and Internet banking has became commonplace. It remains to be seen whether the acceptance and use of personal health records will follow a course similar to that of online banking.

PRIVACY AND SECURITY

Almost every week, there is another story in the media about consumers' electronic medical information being lost or stolen. While most people support the idea of an electronic network for the exchange of health information, they are also concerned that their personal health information will not be safe. They wonder how they can be sure their information is safe and how they can find out who has accessed their information.

If people do not feel that effective security and confidentiality safeguards are in place, they are unlikely to sign up for PHRs. Individuals need to be able to trust the organization that offers the PHR as well as the providers of the other health information systems, such as physicians, insurance plans, and pharmacies.

The Health Insurance Portability and Accountability Act (HIPAA) passed by the federal government in 1996 goes a long way toward protecting individuals' private health information. However, due to the widespread use of computer networks to send and receive confidential health information, some experts are suggesting that the legislation be reevaluated and perhaps updated to reflect the current environment. For example, some sponsors of PHRs on the Internet do not fit the definition of covered entities under the current HIPAA legislation, so they are not required to inform consumers of their privacy policies.

Until consumers feel confident about the security of their online health information, they are unlikely to want PHRs that allow data to be exchanged with other health care providers. The privacy and security issue is a major obstacle to PHR adoption, and it must be addressed before consumers can realize the many benefits of PHRs. The privacy and security of health information as it applies to EHRs and PHRs is the topic of the next chapter.

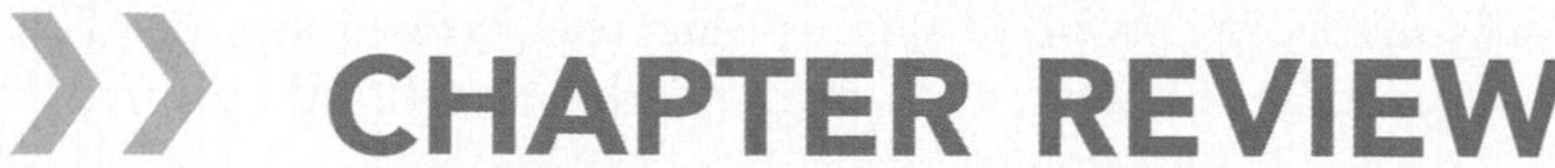

CHAPTER REVIEW

CHAPTER SUMMARY

1. As consumers become active partners in their health care, there is recognition of the need to maintain an up-to-date record of essential personal health information.
2. Personal health records are more than locations to store health information; they offer a number of tools to help individuals manage health and wellness. For example, individuals can send e-mail messages to providers, receive and review test results, renew prescriptions, and track insurance claims.
3. Personal health records can be grouped into four categories:
   - A computer-based stand-alone personal health record does not share information with other health information systems. It offers the most security, since there is no electronic exchange of data.
   - An Internet-based tethered personal health record is aligned with a single outside organization and allows individuals to view information in that organization's system.
   - Internet-based untethered records are not limited to records stored on a single external website. Consumers are responsible for keeping the records up-to-date.
   - Networked personal health records are able to send and receive data from other health information systems, such as the provider's electronic health record and a pharmacy information system. Some information is entered by the patient, and some is received electronically from these external systems.
4. Networked personal health records have a number of advantages over the other types. Information is continually updated, and relevant portions of information are sent to and from a provider's electronic health record system. When a patient fills a new prescription at a pharmacy, the new medication is automatically added to the medication list in the patient's personal health record. Laboratory test results and updates on the status of insurance claims are also available. Most importantly, the patient is in control of the flow of information, deciding when to grant access to others.
5. The three major barriers to the implementation of personal health records are:
   - *Lack of interoperability:* At present, it is difficult to exchange data with other health information systems due to the lack of common standards.
   - *Lack of consumer awareness:* Most people are not aware that computerized personal health records exist. If personal health

records are going to be in widespread use, consumers need to be educated about what they are and the benefits they offer.

- *Privacy and security concerns:* The biggest barrier to implementation is the security and confidentiality of the data. Until consumers feel confident that their online health information is safe and secure, they are unlikely to want personal health records that exchange data over the Internet.

CHECK YOUR UNDERSTANDING

Part 1. Write *T* or *F* in the blank to indicate whether you think the statement is true or false.

____ **1.** Individuals are being encouraged to become more active partners in their health care.

____ **2.** Consumer-driven health plans (CDHPs) reduce the deductible and out-of-pocket expenses for individuals.

____ **3.** While there is no universal definition of a personal health record, all definitions agree that a PHR is owned and managed by the individual.

____ **4.** A computer-based stand-alone personal health record sends and receives information from a patient's provider.

____ **5.** An Internet-based tethered personal health record that is linked to a single outside database does not meet the definition of a true personal health record.

____ **6.** An Internet-based untethered personal health record is also known as a patient portal.

____ **7.** A networked personal health record supports the exchange of information with the computer systems of providers and other health information systems.

____ **8.** A major problem with networked personal health records is the lack of necessary infrastructure to exchange data among systems.

____ **9.** In addition to providing a complete, up-to-date record of health information in a single location, personal health records also provide access to the latest evidence-based health information.

____ **10.** The objections of insurance companies are a major barrier to the implementation of personal health records.

Part 2. In the space provided, write a definition of the term.

11. consumer-driven health plans (CDHPs)

____

____

12. networked personal health record

____

____

13. personal health record (PHR)

14. patient portal

15. tethered

16. untethered

THINKING ABOUT THE ISSUES

Part 3. In the space provided, write a brief paragraph describing your thoughts on the following issues.

17. Despite the benefits of personal health records, few consumers have created them. What could be the reasons for this?

18. Since information in a networked personal health record is sent over the Internet, some people may not include sensitive information such as HIV status, alcohol or drug dependency, or mental health treatment. What are the risks to the patient's health of not including this information?

19. If a physician uses information in a patient's personal health record to make a diagnosis, and if that diagnosis is later found to be incorrect, do you think the doctor should be held liable for the incorrect diagnosis?

6 The Privacy and Security of Electronic Health Information

CHAPTER OUTLINE

The Health Insurance Portability and Accountability Act of 1996 (HIPAA)
- *Title I and Title II of HIPAA*
- *Administrative Simplification Standards*

The HIPAA Privacy Rule
- *Covered Entities*
- *Business Associates*

Protected Health Information (PHI)
- *Minimum Necessary Standard*
- *Designated Record Set*
- *Disclosure of Personal Health Information (PHI)*
- *Release of Information for Purposes Other Than TPO*
- *Notice of Privacy Practices (NPP)*
- *Rights of Individuals*
- *HIPAA Enforcement*

Threats to the Security of Electronic Information
- *The Actions of Individuals*
- *Environmental Hazards*
- *Computer Hardware, Software, or Network Problems*

The HIPAA Security Rule
- *Administrative Safeguards*
- *Physical Safeguards*
- *Technical Safeguards*

Privacy and Security Risks of Electronic Health Information Exchange
- *Clinical Data Available in Electronic Form*
- *Portable Computers and Storage Devices*
- *Problems Not Adequately Addressed by Existing Privacy Laws*

The Importance of Public Trust
- *Public Attitudes Toward the Electronic Use of Health Information*

LEARNING OUTCOMES

After completing this chapter, you will be able to define key terms and:

1. Describe the purpose of the Administrative Simplification provisions of the Health Insurance Portability and Accountability Act (HIPAA).
2. Discuss how the HIPAA Privacy Rule protects patient health information.
3. Describe when protected health information can be released without patients' authorization.
4. List three categories of threats to the security of electronic information.
5. Describe the safeguards outlined in the HIPAA Security Rule.

6. Discuss the ways that increased use of information technology places protected health information at greater risks.
7. Explain why the existing HIPAA laws may not be adequate in today's health care environment.
8. Explain why public trust is key to the development of electronic health records and a nationwide health information network.

KEY TERMS

administrative safeguards
Administrative Simplification
antivirus software
audit trails
authentication
authorization
availability
business associates
clearinghouses
confidentiality
covered entities (CEs)
de-identified health information
designated record set (DRS)
disclosure
electronic protected health information (ePHI)
encryption
firewall
health information exchange
health plan
HIPAA Privacy Rule
HIPAA Security Rule
integrity
intrusion detection system (IDS)
minimum necessary standard
Notice of Privacy Practices (NPP)
passwords
physical safeguards
protected health information (PHI)
providers
role-based authorization
technical safeguards
treatment, payment, and operations (TPO)

Why This Chapter Is Important to You

The information in this chapter will enable you to:

- Understand the importance of the HIPAA Privacy Rule to the protection of personal health information.
- Understand when protected health information (PHI) can be released with a patient's consent and when an authorization must be obtained.
- Understand how the increasing use of computers and networks such as the Internet places health information at risk.
- Understand the types of safeguards included in the HIPAA Security Rule.
- Understand how the health care environment has changed since the HIPAA legislation was enacted and why existing privacy and security laws may no longer be adequate.

The problems with the current paper-based health record system have been well documented. One of the most serious issues is the fragmentation of health records. Patients today use several providers to meet their health care needs, and each physician maintains a separate medical record on a patient. Unless the patient volunteers information, providers do not know whether the patient is being treated by another physician, let alone what medications might have been prescribed. Important medical decisions may be made without a complete picture of the patient's health. This is not a situation in which patients are provided with the safest, most effective care.

At the same time, by its very nature, the fragmented paper-based system possesses built-in security measures. Paper medical records stored in a physician office are more difficult for unauthorized persons to access. The only people who have access to the records are the health care professionals working in the office. If computers are used, it is for administrative functions such as scheduling and billing, rather than for clinical information. The paper records are confined to a single location, and even if someone were to break in to the office, the number of bulky paper files they could carry would be limited.

On the other hand, one lost laptop or one computer hacker who gains access to a network can put thousands of health records at risk. While paper records restrict the ability to exchange information with other health care professionals, privacy and confidentiality may be easier to maintain. However, to realize the many benefits that electronic health records have to offer, information must be computerized and exchanged among providers and facilities.

The challenge facing the health care field today is protecting electronic health information exchanged over computer networks with many access points and convincing the public to trust the electronic system, just as they have trusted their physicians with personal health information. Consumer attitudes and behaviors are influenced by reports in the media of stolen credit card numbers, Internet fraud, and identity theft. Because of the size and scope of today's computer networks, a breach puts thousands of people's records at risk.

Examples The records of 365,000 patients were stolen when a car belonging to an employee of Providence Health System in Portland, Oregon, was broken in to. Backup tapes the employee had been asked to store were in the car, and the data were not encrypted. As a result, Providence was fined $95,000 under Oregon state laws, and a civil lawsuit was filed.

A CD containing the protected health information of 75,000 members of Empire Blue Cross and Blue Shield in New York went missing for over a month. A subcontractor had sent the disk to Magellan Behavioral Health via United Parcel Service. Before shipping the CD, the subcontractor had removed the coding and passwords that protected the information.

In May 2006, a laptop computer with the Social Security numbers of more than 26 million veterans was stolen from the home of a Department of Veterans Affairs employee. The device was eventually recovered.

The Health Insurance Portability and Accountability Act of 1996 (HIPAA)

HIPAA, the Health Insurance Portability and Accountability Act of 1996, is the most significant legislation affecting the health care field since the Medicare and Medicaid programs were introduced in 1965. The legislation was designed to:

- Ensure the portability of insurance coverage as employees moved from job to job
- Increase accountability and decrease fraud and abuse in health care
- Improve the efficiency of health care transactions and mandate standards for health information
- Ensure the security and privacy of health information

More than a decade later, HIPAA continues to have a major impact on organizations and professionals in the health care field. Health care organizations need to understand what information is covered under the law, how it is being used, and when it can be disclosed. Professionals working in health care must be familiar with the legal requirements as they apply to patient health records.

TITLE I AND TITLE II OF HIPAA

The legislation consists of two parts, or "titles." Title I, health insurance reform, is the section of the law that allows individuals to continue health insurance coverage when they change jobs. Title II, known as the Administrative Simplification standards (see Figure 6-1 on page 176), is the section of HIPAA that is important to the discussions in this chapter.

ADMINISTRATIVE SIMPLIFICATION STANDARDS

In the 1990s, health care industry leaders, the Department of Health and Human Services (HHS), and the U.S. Congress became increasingly concerned about rising health care costs. A significant share of each health care dollar was going toward administrative costs, such as checking patient eligibility for benefits, filing insurance claims, and requesting authorization for services. At the same time, it was estimated that more than four hundred different formats existed for processing claims. Many in Congress believed that establishing national standards for electronic health information, and the greater use of technology in transaction processing, would lead to gains in efficiency and significant cost savings.

The **Administrative Simplification** provisions, in addition to mandating formats for the transfer of electronic health care data, provided patients with rights with regard to their health records and required putting privacy and security mechanisms in place to ensure that their personal health information was kept confidential. Some of the provisions that HHS was required to establish included:

Administrative Simplification HIPAA Title II on the uniform transfer of electronic health care data and privacy protection.

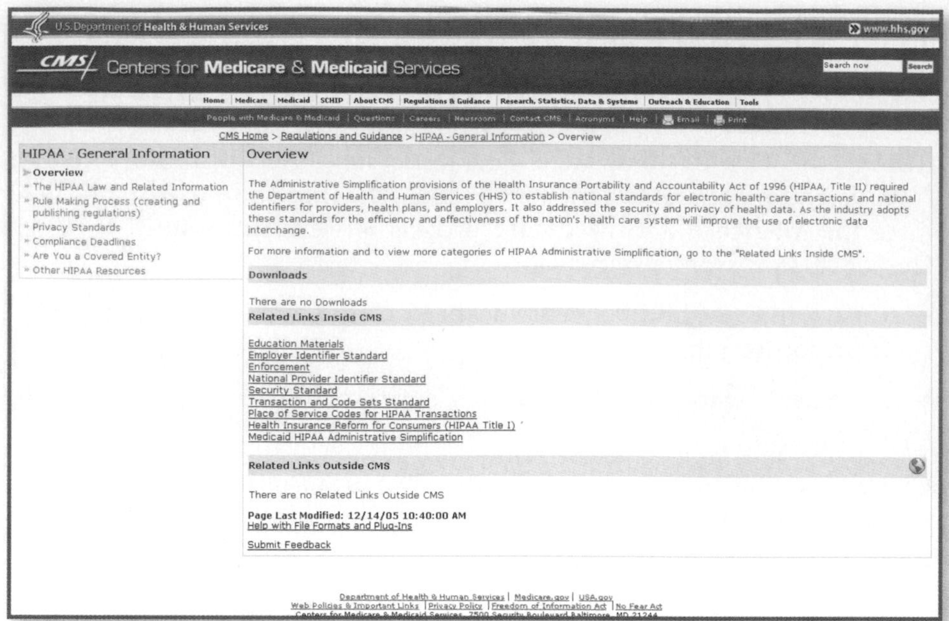

Figure 6-1 The website for the Administrative Simplification section of HIPAA (www.cms.hhs.gov/hipaageninfo).

- National standards for electronic health care transactions
- National identifiers for providers, health plans, and employers
- Rules to protect the privacy and security of health information, known as the Privacy Rule and the Security Rule

The range and scope of Title II of HIPAA are more extensive than the information discussed in this chapter. This chapter presents an overview of the Privacy Rule and the Security Rule, and then introduces the challenges electronic health records present to information security and confidentiality.

The HIPAA Privacy Rule

HIPAA Security Rule protects the confidentiality, integrity, and availability of electronic health information.

The HIPAA Standards for Privacy of Individually Identifiable Health Information rule, known as the **HIPAA Privacy Rule,** was enacted on April 14, 2003. It provides protection for individually identifiable health information and grants certain rights to individuals in regard to their medical records. Before that, an individual's medical records had no federal protection. They were protected by state privacy laws—if they existed; not all states had privacy laws for the protection of health information.

COVERED ENTITIES

HIPAA was created in part to improve the efficiency of financial and administrative health care transactions. As such, its regulations do not apply to every health care organization or professional. HIPAA applies only to health care professionals and organizations that provide health care in the normal course of business and that electronically transmit information that is protected under HIPAA. Those who meet these conditions are referred to as **covered entities (CEs).** The Privacy Rule says that covered entities must:

covered entities (CEs) professionals and organizations that normally provide health care and electronically transmit PHI.

- Have privacy policies and procedures that are appropriate for their health care services
- Notify patients about their privacy rights and how their information can be used or disclosed
- Train employees so that they understand the privacy practices
- Appoint a privacy official responsible for seeing that the privacy policies and procedures are implemented
- Safeguard patients' records

Under HIPAA, health plans, providers, and clearinghouses are considered covered entities.

Health Plans

A **health plan** is defined by HIPAA as an insurance plan that provides or pays for medical care. Health plans include government and private-payer plans. Certain health care benefits are exempt from the HIPAA standards even when provided by health plans:

health plan insurance plan that provides or pays for medical care.

- Workers' compensation
- Coverage for on-site medical clinics
- Accident or disability income insurance
- General and automotive liability insurance
- Automobile medical payment insurance

Providers

Health care **providers** are people or organizations that furnish, bill, or are paid for health care in the normal course of business, including physicians, nurses, hospitals, home health agencies, outpatient clinics, laboratories, pharmacies, dentists, long-term care facilities, and others. Providers who do not send claims electronically (either themselves or through third parties) are not subject to HIPAA rules, but may be required to follow state privacy laws.

providers people or organizations that furnish, bill, or are paid for health care in the normal course of business.

Clearinghouses

Health care **clearinghouses** are companies that process health information and execute electronic transactions, such as the submission of insurance claims, on behalf of providers.

clearinghouses companies that process health information and execute electronic transactions.

Covered entities must comply with a number of requirements, including:

- Possessing a set of privacy practices that are appropriate for their health care services
- Notifying patients about their privacy rights and how their information can be used or disclosed

- Training employees so that they understand the privacy practices
- Appointing a member of the staff to be the privacy official responsible for seeing that the privacy practices are implemented
- Keeping patients' records safe and secure

BUSINESS ASSOCIATES

business associate entity that works under a contract for a covered entity and is therefore subject to the CE's HIPAA policies and procedures.

On a regular basis, covered entities interact with a number of other individuals and organizations to accomplish business tasks. For example, a physician office uses legal services, information technology products and services, transcription services, and collection agencies, among others. Since these businesses are not considered covered entities, they are not directly required to comply with the law. However, in the course of doing business, covered entities disclose personal health information to these groups. To ensure that confidential health information is protected once it is exchanged with a non-CE, HIPAA requires CEs to enter into contracts with **business associates.** The contracts must state that a business associate that provides services to a CE must perform its work in a manner that abides by the HIPAA Privacy Rule. The CE may be held responsible for the actions of its business associates if it

The ABCs of Electronic Health Records: HIPAA Privacy and Security

CE—Covered Entity

Health care professionals and organizations that provide health care in the normal course of business and that electronically transmit information that is protected under HIPAA.

DRS—Designated Record Set

Any item, collection, or grouping of information that includes protected health information and is maintained by a covered entity.

ePHI—Electronic Protected Health Information

Protected health information that is created, received, maintained, or transmitted in electronic form.

NPP—Notice of Privacy Practices

Document that describes practices regarding the use and disclosure of protected health information.

PHI—Protected Health Information

Individually identifiable health information that is transmitted or maintained by electronic media or transmitted or maintained in any other form or medium.

TPO—Treatment, Payment, and Operations

Conditions under which protected health information can be released without consent from the patient.

knew of a pattern of activity that was in violation of the contract and it failed to take reasonable steps to fix the problem.

Protected Health Information (PHI)

Covered entities must follow HIPAA regulations for the protection of health information. However, not all of a patient's information is subject to the law. The HIPAA Privacy Rule covers the use and disclosure of patients' **protected health information (PHI).** PHI is defined as individually identifiable health information that is transmitted or maintained by electronic media, such as over the Internet, or is transmitted or maintained in any other form or medium. Table 6-1 lists the information that meets the definition of PHI.

protected health information (PHI) individually identifiable health information transmitted or maintained by electronic media.

The Privacy Rule applies to PHI in any form, whether it is communicated verbally, written or printed on paper, or maintained in an electronic format.

TABLE 6-1 **Information Considered Protected Health Information (PHI)**

Name
Address (including street address, city, county, ZIP code)
Names of relatives and employers
Birth date
Telephone numbers
Fax number
E-mail address
Social Security number
Medical record number
Health plan beneficiary number
Account number
Certificate or license number
Serial number of any vehicle or other device
Website address
Fingerprints or voiceprints
Photographic images

MINIMUM NECESSARY STANDARD

minimum necessary standard safeguards to protect PHI from being accidentally released.

When using or disclosing protected health information, a covered entity must try to limit the information to the minimum amount of PHI necessary for the intended purpose. The **minimum necessary standard** means using reasonable safeguards to protect PHI from being accidentally released—to those who do not need access to the information—during an appropriate use or disclosure.

The minimum necessary standard does not apply to uses and disclosures for treatment purposes or to uses and disclosures that an individual has authorized, among other limited exceptions.

DESIGNATED RECORD SET

For purposes of the HIPAA Privacy Rule, *record* means any item, collection, or grouping of information that includes PHI and is maintained by a covered entity. The HIPAA term for a group of records is **designated record set (DRS).**

designated record set (DRS) information that includes PHI and is maintained by a covered entity.

The exact contents of the DRS depend on the role of the organization or provider. For example, the DRS for a physician includes medical and billing records but not appointment schedules, requests for lab tests, or birth and death records. For a health plan, the designated record set includes information about enrollment, payment, claim decisions, and medical management systems of the plan.

DISCLOSURE OF PERSONAL HEALTH INFORMATION (PHI)

HIPAA contains detailed requirements for the use or disclosure of protected health information. Covered entities may use and disclose PHI only as permitted by HIPAA or by a more protective state rule if one applies.

treatment, payment, and operations (TPO) conditions under which PHI can be released without patient consent.

disclosure release of PHI to an outside provider or organization.

Under the HIPAA privacy standards, covered entities may use and disclose PHI for **treatment, payment, and operations (TPO)** purposes without special permission from a patient. In this context, the term *use* refers to activities within the entity that holds the information. **Disclosure** refers to the release of PHI to an outside provider or organization.

Treatment, payment, and operations are defined as follows:

- *Treatment:* This purpose primarily consists of discussion of the patient's case with other providers. For example, a physician may document the role of each member of the health care team in providing care. Each team member then records actions and observations so that the ordering physician knows how the patient is responding to treatment.

- *Payment:* Providers usually submit claims to health plans on behalf of patients, which involves exchanging demographic and diagnostic information. Payment activities include determining insurance eligibility and coverage as well as billing and collections.
- *Operations:* This purpose includes activities such as tracking and measuring adherence to quality standards, accreditation (such as by the Joint Commission), staff training, and business planning.

RELEASE OF INFORMATION FOR PURPOSES OTHER THAN TPO

Medical office personnel receive many requests for information about patients from a range of sources, such as insurance companies, lawyers, and employers. Each request must be evaluated, taking the HIPAA regulations protecting PHI into account. The decision must be made about whether the information can legally be released. In some cases, this is relatively easy to determine; in others, it is not so clear. The basic HIPAA guideline states that covered entities must have patients' authorization to use or disclose information that is not for TPO purposes. For example, TPO is not involved when a town's personnel office requests the records of an individual who has applied for a position as a police officer.

Special permission, called **authorization,** must be obtained for uses and disclosures other than for TPO. This type of permission is known as *general authorization*. Information about alcohol and drug abuse, sexually transmitted diseases (STDs), human immunodeficiency virus (HIV), and behavioral and mental health services may not be released without a *specific authorization* from the patient. The authorization document must be easy to understand and must include the following:

authorization permission to use and disclose information for uses other than TPO.

- A description of the information to be used or disclosed
- The name or other specific identification of the persons authorized to use or disclose the information
- The name of the persons or group to whom the covered entity may make the use or disclosure
- A description of each purpose of the requested use or disclosure
- An expiration date
- The signature of the individual (or authorized representative) and the date

In addition, the rule states that a valid authorization must include statements:

- Of the individual's right to revoke the authorization in writing
- About whether the covered entity is able to base treatment, payment, enrollment, or eligibility for benefits on the authorization
- That information used or disclosed after the authorization may be disclosed again by the recipient and may no longer be protected by the rule

Covered entities must document these disclosures and, if requested, provide that information to the patient. Disclosures made in connection with TPO, or after an authorization has been obtained, do not need to be documented this way. Figure 6-2 contains a sample authorization form for the release of information.

Figure 6-2

A sample authorization form.

Sample Authorization to Use or Disclose Health Information

Patient Name: ____________________

Health Record Number: ____________________

Date of Birth: ____________________

1. I authorize the use or disclosure of the above named individual's health information as described below.

2. The following individual(s) or organization(s) are authorized to make the disclosure: ____________________

3. The type of information to be used or disclosed is as follows (check the appropriate boxes and include other information where indicated)

❑ problem list
❑ medication list
❑ list of allergies
❑ immunization records
❑ most recent history
❑ most recent discharge summary
❑ lab results (please describe the dates or types of lab tests you would like disclosed): ____________________
❑ x-ray and imaging reports (please describe the dates or types of x-rays or images you would like disclosed): ____________________
❑ consultation reports from (please supply doctors' names): ____________________
❑ entire record
❑ other (please describe): ____________________

4. I understand that the information in my health record may include information relating to sexually transmitted disease, acquired immunodeficiency syndrome (AIDS), or human immunodeficiency virus (HIV). It may also include information about behavioral or mental health services, and treatment for alcohol and drug abuse.

5. The information identified above may be used by or disclosed to the following individuals or organization(s):

Name: ____________________

Address: ____________________

Name: ____________________

Address: ____________________

6. This information for which I'm authorizing disclosure will be used for the following purpose:

❑ my personal records
❑ sharing with other health care providers as needed/other (please describe): ____________________

7. I understand that I have a right to revoke this authorization at any time. I understand that if I revoke this authorization, I must do so in writing and present my written revocation to the health information management department. I understand that the revocation will not apply to information that has already been released in response to this authorization. I understand that the revocation will not apply to my insurance company when the law provides my insurer with the right to contest a claim under my policy.

8. This authorization will expire (insert date or event): ____________________

If I fail to specify an expiration date or event, this authorization will expire six months from the date on which it was signed.

9. I understand that once the above information is disclosed, it may be redisclosed by the recipient and the information may not be protected by federal privacy laws or regulations.

10. I understand authorizing the use or disclosure of the information identified above is voluntary. I need not sign this form to ensure health care treatment.

Signature of patient or legal representative: ____________________ Date: ____________

If signed by legal representative, relationship to patient

Signature of witness: ____________________ Date: ____________

Distribution of copies: Original to provider; copy to patient; copy to accompany use or disclosure

Note: This sample form was developed by the American Health Information Management Association for discussion purposes. It should not be used without review by the issuing organization's legal counsel to ensure compliance with other federal and state laws and regulations.

Source: ***AHIMA*** *Practice Brief: Requried Content for Authorizations to Disclose*

Exceptions to Disclosure Standards

These rules for use and disclosure do not apply to the release of PHI in certain circumstances, including such public interest purposes as public health, law enforcement, research, workers' compensation cases, and national security situations. Even though the rules do not apply, there may be other conditions that must be met before PHI can be released. For example, if the patient's PHI is required as evidence by a court of law, the provider may release it without the patient's approval if a judicial order is received.

There use and disclosure rules also do not apply to de-identified health information. **De-identified health information** is information that neither identifies nor provides a reasonable basis for identifying an individual. The identifiers that must be removed are listed in Table 6-2.

de-identified health information information that neither identifies nor provides a basis to identify an individual.

NOTICE OF PRIVACY PRACTICES (NPP)

Under the HIPAA Privacy Rule, covered entities must list their privacy policies and procedures in a **Notice of Privacy Practices (NPP).** This

Notice of Privacy Practices (NPP) document describing practices regarding use and disclosure of PHI.

TABLE 6-2 Information That Must Be Removed for De-identification

1. Names
2. All geographic subdivisions smaller than a state, including street address, city, county, precinct, ZIP code, and their equivalent geographical codes, except for the initial three digits of a ZIP code if, according to the current publicly available data from the Bureau of the Census:
   a. The geographic unit formed by combining all ZIP codes with the same three initial digits contains more than 20,000 people
   b. The initial three digits of a ZIP code for all such geographic units containing 20,000 or fewer people are changed to 000
3. All elements of dates (except year) for dates directly related to an individual, including birth date, admission date, discharge date, date of death; and all ages over eighty-nine, and all elements of dates (including year) indicative of such age, except that such ages and elements may be aggregated into a single category of age ninety or older
4. Telephone numbers
5. Facsimile numbers
6. Electronic mail addresses
7. Social Security numbers
8. Medical record numbers
9. Health plan beneficiary numbers
10. Account numbers
11. Certificate/license numbers
12. Vehicle identifiers and serial numbers, including license plate numbers
13. Device identifiers and serial numbers
14. Web universal resource locators (URLs)
15. Internet protocol (IP) addresses numbers
16. Biometric identifiers, including fingerprints and voiceprints
17. Full-face photographic images and any comparable images
18. Any other unique identifying number, characteristic, or code, unless otherwise permitted by the Privacy Rule for re-identification

document describes the CE's practices regarding the use and disclosure of PHI. It also establishes privacy complaint procedures, explains that disclosure is limited to the minimum necessary information, and discusses how consent for other types of information release is obtained. Patients must be given a copy of the NPP at the time of their first encounter, and at least once every three years thereafter. In a physician office, the NPP is usually a paper form that is handed to the patient; in the case of a provider conducting business electronically, the information is delivered as an electronic file. A sample NPP is displayed in Figure 6-3.

For compliance purposes, CEs keep track of when patients receive the Notice of Privacy Practices form. The office must make a good-faith effort to obtain a patient's acknowledgment of having received and read the NPP. This is accomplished through a form known as the Acknowledgment of Receipt of Notice of Privacy Practices. This form states that the patient has read the privacy practices and understands how the provider intends to protect the patient's rights to privacy under HIPAA. Again, this form can be paper, or it can be electronic. A sample is illustrated in Figure 6-4 on page 186.

RIGHTS OF INDIVIDUALS

The HIPAA Privacy Rule also provides significant rights to patients, including the right to:

- Receive a written notice of information practices
- Ask to access, inspect, and obtain a copy of their PHI
- Request an accounting of disclosures
- Request amendment of records
- Request restrictions on uses and disclosures of their PHI
- Receive accommodation of reasonable alternate communications requests
- File a complaint about a violation with the organization or with the Office for Civil Rights (OCR) in the Department of Health and Human Services

HIPAA ENFORCEMENT

One of Americans' civil rights is the right to privacy. The Office for Civil Rights (OCR) in the U.S. Department of Health and Human Services is charged with investigating complaints that HIPAA privacy regulations have been violated. Anyone who believes that a health care provider, health plan, or other entity covered by the privacy rule has violated can file a complaint with OCR. Complaints to OCR must be in writing and sent either on paper or electronically, and must be filed within 180 days of when the individual knew or should have known that the act had occurred. Figure 6-5 on page 186 shows a portion of OCR's factsheet on filing a complaint.

Notice of Privacy Practices for the Original Medicare Plan

THIS NOTICE DESCRIBES HOW MEDICAL INFORMATION ABOUT YOU MAY BE USED AND DISCLOSED AND HOW YOU CAN GET ACCESS TO THIS INFORMATION. PLEASE REVIEW IT CAREFULLY.

By law, Medicare is required to protect the privacy of your personal medical information. Medicare is also required to give you this notice to tell you how Medicare may use and give out ("disclose") your personal medical information held by Medicare.

Medicare **must** use and give out your personal medical information to provide information:

- To you or someone who has the legal right to act for you (your personal representative),
- To the Secretary of the Department of Health and Human Services, if necessary, to make sure your privacy is protected, and
- Where required by law.

Medicare **has the right** to use and give out your personal medical information to pay for your health care and to operate the Medicare program. For example:

- Medicare Carriers use your personal medical information to pay or deny your claims, to collect your premiums, to share your benefit payment with your other insurer(s), or to prepare your Medicare Summary Notice.
- Medicare may use your personal medical information to make sure you and other Medicare beneficiaries get quality health care, to provide customer services to you, to resolve any complaints you have, or to contact you about research studies.

Medicare **may** use or give out your personal medical information for the following purposes under limited circumstances:

- To State and other Federal agencies that have the legal right to receive Medicare data (such as to make sure Medicare is making proper payments and to assist Federal/State Medicaid programs),
- For public health activities (such as reporting disease outbreaks),
- For government health care oversight activities (such as fraud and abuse investigations),
- For judicial and administrative proceedings (such as in response to a court order),
- For law enforcement purposes (such as providing limited information to locate a missing person),
- For research studies that meet all privacy law requirements (such as research related to the prevention of disease or disability),
- To avoid a serious and imminent threat to health or safety,
- To contact you about new or changed benefits under Medicare, and
- To create a collection of information that can no longer be traced back to you.

By law, Medicare must have your written permission (an "authorization") to use or give out your personal medical information for any purpose that isn't set out in this notice. You may take back ("revoke") your written permission at any time, except if Medicare has already acted based on your permission.

By law, you have the right to:

- See and get a copy of your personal medical information held by Medicare.
- Have your personal medical information amended if you believe that it is wrong or if information is missing, and Medicare agrees. If Medicare disagrees, you may have a statement of your disagreement added to your personal medical information.
- Get a listing of those getting your personal medical information from Medicare. The listing won't cover your personal medical information that was given to you or your personal representative, that was given out to pay for your health care or for Medicare operations, or that was given out for law enforcement purposes.
- Ask Medicare to communicate with you in a different manner or at a different place (for example, by sending materials to a P.O. Box instead of your home address).
- Ask Medicare to limit how your personal medical information is used and given out to pay your claims and run the Medicare program. Please note that Medicare may not be able to agree to your request.
- Get a separate paper copy of this notice.

Look at our **Medicare Privacy Practices (HIPAA) FAQs** for more information on:

- Exercising your rights set out in this notice.
- Filing a complaint, if you believe the Original Medicare Plan has violated these privacy rights. Filing a complaint won't affect your benefits under Medicare.

You can also call 1-800-MEDICARE (1-800-633-4227) to get this information. Ask to speak to a Customer Service Representative about Medicare's privacy notice. TTY users should call 1-877-486-2048.

You may file a complaint with the Secretary of the Department of Health and Human Services. Visit www.hhs.gov/ocr/hipaa or contact the Office for Civil Rights at 1-866-627-7748. TTY users should call 1-800-537-7697.

By law, Medicare is required to follow the terms in this privacy notice. Medicare has the right to change the way your personal medical information is used and given out. If Medicare makes any changes to the way your personal medical information is used and given out, you will get a new notice by mail within 60 days of the change.

The Notice of Privacy Practices for the Original Medicare Plan became effective April 14, 2003.

Figure 6-3

A Notice of Privacy Practices for a Medicare program

Source: www.medicare.gov/privacypractices.asp

Acknowledgment of Receipt of Notice of Privacy Practices

I understand that the providers of ABC Clinic may share my health information for treatment, billing, and health-care operations. I have been given a copy of the organization's notice of privacy practices that describes how my health information is used and shared. I understand that ABC Clinic has the right to change this notice at any time. I may obtain a current copy by contacting the practice's office or by visiting the website at www.xxx.com.

My signature below constitutes my acknowledgment that I have been provided with a copy of the notice of privacy practices.

Signature of Patient or Legal Representative   Date __________

____

If signed by legal representative, relationship to patient: ____________________________

Figure 6-4

A sample Acknowledgment of Receipt of Notice of Privacy Practices

Figure 6-5

A portion of the factsheet available from the Office for Civil Rights (OCR) that describes procedures for filing a complaint

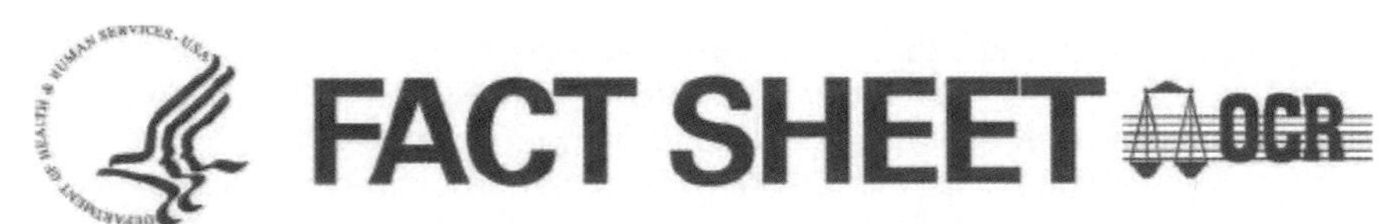

U.S. Department of Health and Human Services • Office for Civil Rights

HOW TO FILE A HEALTH INFORMATION PRIVACY COMPLAINT WITH THE OFFICE FOR CIVIL RIGHTS

If you believe that a person, agency or organization covered under the HIPAA Privacy Rule ("a covered entity") violated your (or someone else's) health information privacy rights or committed another violation of the Privacy Rule, you may file a complaint with the Office for Civil Rights (OCR). OCR has authority to receive and investigate complaints against covered entities related to the Privacy Rule. A covered entity is a health plan, health care clearinghouse, and any health care provider who conducts certain health care transactions electronically. For more information about the Privacy Rule, please look at our responses to Frequently Asked Questions (FAQs) and our Privacy Guidance. (See the web link near the bottom of this form.)

Complaints to the Office for Civil Rights must: (1) Be filed in writing, either on paper or electronically; (2) name the entity that is the subject of the complaint and describe the acts or omissions believed to be in violation of the applicable requirements of the Privacy Rule; and (3) be filed within 180 days of when you knew that the act or omission complained of occurred. OCR may extend the 180-day period if you can show "good cause." Any alleged violation must have occurred on or after April 14, 2003 (on or after April 14, 2004 for small health plans), for OCR to have authority to investigate.

Anyone can file written complaints with OCR by mail, fax, or email. If you need help filing a complaint or have a question about the complaint form, please call this OCR toll free number: 1-800-368-1019. OCR has ten regional offices, and each regional office covers certain states. You should send your complaint to the appropriate OCR Regional Office, based on the region where the alleged violation took place. Use the OCR Regions list at the end of this Fact Sheet, or you can look at the regional office map to help you determine where to send your complaint. Complaints should be sent to the attention off the appropriate OCR Regional Manager.

You can submit your complaint in any written format. We recommend that you use the OCR Health Information Privacy Complaint Form which can be found on our web site or at an OCR Regional office. If you prefer, you may submit a written complaint in your own format. Be sure to include the following information in your *written* complaint:

Your name, full address, home and work telephone numbers, email address.

If you are filing a complaint on someone's behalf, also provide the name of the person on whose behalf you are filing.

Name, full address and phone of the person, agency or organization you believe violated your (or someone else's) health information privacy rights or committed another violation of the Privacy Rule.

Briefly describe what happened. How, why, and when do believe your (or someone else's) health information privacy rights were violated, or the Privacy Rule otherwise was violated?

Threats to the Security of Electronic Information

As health information migrates from paper systems to computer systems and electronic networks, the threats to protected health information multiply. Instead of limiting access to office personnel, electronic networks provide hundreds or even thousands of access points. The threats to information security come from a number of sources, including individuals, the environment, and computer hardware, software, and networks.

THE ACTIONS OF INDIVIDUALS

People pose a significant threat to the security of data stored on computers. The actions of individuals, both intentional and unintentional, can undermine data security. For example, when former president Clinton was hospitalized for open heart surgery in 2004, many people tried to "hack" into his electronic records, including hospital employees (New York Times, December 3, 2006). The basic types of threats from individuals are:

- Employees who make unintentional mistakes, such as accidentally deleting a file or entering information inaccurately
- Employees who abuse their security privileges, as in the case of an employee who sees a former spouse come in for an appointment and accesses his or her record without a legitimate need to do so
- Outsiders who try to damage or steal information, otherwise known as computer hackers
- Employees who hold grudges or make threats, as in the case of someone who feels he or she was wrongfully passed over for a promotion and threatens to post portions of patient records on the Internet

ENVIRONMENTAL HAZARDS

Electronic information is also at risk from environmental hazards, such as fires, floods, and earthquakes as well as utility failures such as electrical power outages. For this reason, medical practices create regular backups of computerized information and store backup files at remote physical locations to minimize the likelihood of data loss in a large-scale disaster. In the event of a major disaster, data from the remote site can easily be recovered.

The experiences of doctors and hospitals during and after Hurricane Katrina points out the value of storing copies of data at a remote location. Medical groups that had off-site backups at a distant location were able to restore their records once the crisis subsided. In many cases, those that did not have off-site backup or that stored backup material in a nearby location lost all health records.

COMPUTER HARDWARE, SOFTWARE, OR NETWORK PROBLEMS

Some security threats come directly from problems with computer systems and software, such as insufficient security in the hardware or software, programming errors, changes to existing software including upgrades, and the addition of new users to the system.

The HIPAA Security Rule

HIPAA Privacy Rule provides protection for individually identifiable health information.

In 2005, the **HIPAA Security Rule** was enacted to protect the confidentiality, integrity, and availability of electronic health information. The Security Rule applies to health care professionals and organizations that meet the definition of a covered entity, just as the HIPAA Privacy Rule does. However, while the Privacy Rule applies to all forms of protected health information, whether electronic, paper, or oral, the Security Rule covers only **electronic protected health information (ePHI)**—protected health information that is created, received, maintained, or transmitted in electronic form. The regulations cover physical devices such as computers, USB flash drives, CDs, and magnetic tapes as well as computer networks and information sent or received over the Internet.

electronic protected health information (ePHI) PHI created, received, maintained, or transmitted in electronic form.

The goals of the HIPAA security standards are to ensure:

confidentiality sharing of electronic PHI among authorized individuals or organizations only.

integrity authenticity, completeness, and reliability of electronic PHI.

availability accessibility of systems for delivering, storing, and processing electronic protected health information.

- The **confidentiality** of ePHI. The information is shared only among authorized individuals or organizations.
- The **integrity** of ePHI. The information is not changed in any way during storage or transmission, is authentic and complete, and can be relied on to be sufficiently accurate for its purpose.
- The **availability** of ePHI. The systems responsible for delivering, storing, and processing data are accessible, when needed, by those who need them under both routine and emergency circumstances.

The HIPAA security standards do not state specific actions that CEs must take to protect ePHI. The rule is intentionally flexible, recognizing that security policies and procedures vary according to the size of the organization and the nature of the work performed. For example, the policies and procedures required in a two-physician practice are different from those needed in a large city hospital. Each CE must determine which security measures and specific technologies are reasonable and appropriate for implementation in its organization.

The security standards are divided into three categories: administrative, physical, and technical.

ADMINISTRATIVE SAFEGUARDS

administrative safeguards policies and procedures designed to protect electronic health information.

Administrative safeguards are administrative policies and procedures designed to protect electronic health information. The management of security is assigned to one individual, who conducts a risk assessment of the current level of data security. Once that assessment is complete, security policies and procedures are developed or modified to meet current needs. Security training is provided to educate staff members on the policies and to raise awareness of security and privacy issues.

PHYSICAL SAFEGUARDS

Physical safeguards are mechanisms to protect electronic systems, equipment, and data from threats, environmental hazards, and unauthorized intrusion. These include devices that limit physical access to facilities housing protected information, such as reinforced doors, locks, and identification badge readers.

physical safeguards mechanisms to protect electronic systems, equipment, and data.

TECHNICAL SAFEGUARDS

Technical safeguards are the automated processes used to protect data and control access to data. They include firewalls, intrusion detection systems, access control, and antivirus software.

technical safeguards automated processes to protect and control access to data.

Firewalls

A **firewall** examines traffic entering and leaving a computer network, determining (according to defined rules) whether to allow it to continue toward its destination. Packet filtering is a process in which a firewall examines each piece of information traveling into or out of the network. A firewall acts as a gatekeeper, deciding who has legitimate access to a network and what data should be allowed in and out. Firewalls can log attempted intrusions and report them to appropriate security personnel.

firewall examines traffic entering and leaving a computer network.

Intrusion Detection Systems

An **intrusion detection system (IDS)** provides constant surveillance of the network. Unlike firewalls, an IDS monitors and analyzes packet data streams, searching for unauthorized activity. If such an activity is suspected, the suspicious user's access to the network is immediately terminated.

intrusion detection system (IDS) provides surveillance of a computer network.

Access Control

User authentication procedures are necessary to confirm the claimed identity of all users who access the data. In this context, **authentication** is a confirmation of the identity of a user—that the user is the person he or she claims to be. In contrast, authorization is the process of determining whether an identified individual has been granted access rights to information. Authorization procedures are necessary to ensure that only appropriate users view the information.

authentication confirmation of the identity of a computer user.

Passwords, a very basic user authentication system, are specific codes that are required for gaining access to information on a computer or network. The code is known by the user, but is not known to others. Passwords are used in most health care organizations, since they are easy to implement. Used successfully, a password utilization program can keep unauthorized users from successfully logging onto a system

passwords codes for gaining access to information on a computer or network.

or network. Password logging programs can track all successful and failed log-in attempts, which can be useful in detecting possible break-in attempts.

Much more sophisticated systems are being used to identify individuals who gain entry to the information, including biometric methods. These techniques use a person's physical characteristics such as fingerprints, facial features, or retinal patterns to confirm identity. Biometric devices use some measurable feature of an individual to authenticate their identity. Because they are based on unique physical characteristics, they cannot be forged, stolen, or duplicated.

role-based authorization limits access to patient information based on the user's organizational role.

Role-based authorization limits access to patient information based on the user's role in an organization. Once access rights have been assigned, each user is given a key to the designated databases. A user must enter an ID and a key to see files to which he or she has been granted access rights. Role-based authorization meets the HIPAA standard of releasing only the minimum amount of information necessary to provide care. In a medical office, for example, a billing specialist needs access to different parts of a health record than does a medical assistant. Technology permits the system to prevent users from viewing or modifying any part of the record that is not directly related to their jobs.

encryption process of converting data into an unreadable format.

Encryption is the process of converting data into an unreadable format before it is distributed. To read a message, the recipient must have a key that deciphers the information. For example, encryption can protect the privacy of restricted data that are stored on a laptop computer even if the computer is stolen. Similarly, it can protect data that are transmitted over a network even if that network is accessed by an unauthorized third party. These techniques also make it possible to determine whether the information has been altered in any way.

audit trails records of who has accessed a computer or network and the operations preformed.

Audit trails are records that show who has accessed a computer or network and what operations were preformed. At a minimum, an audit trail should contain the following information:

- Type of event
- Date and time of occurrence
- User ID associated with the event
- Program, command, or method used to initiate the event
- Patient and data elements that were changed

The log is reviewed on a regular basis to detect irregularities. If an error or a suspicious entry has been made, the program lists the name of the person and the date the information was entered.

Antivirus Software

antivirus software software that scans for viruses and attempts to remove them.

Antivirus software scans a system for known viruses. After detection, antivirus software attempts to remove the virus from the system and, in some cases, fix any problems the virus created. Antivirus tools, however, cannot detect and eliminate all viruses. New viruses are

Making It Real

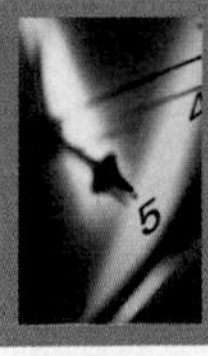

Protecting Celebrities' Records

Twenty-seven Palisades Medical Center workers were suspended without pay for a month after being accused of accessing actor George Clooney's electronic health record while was being treated at the hospital for injuries sustained in a motorcycle accident. While hospital officials found no evidence that the employees leaked Clooney's information to the public, they disciplined the employees for violating the HIPAA privacy rule.

It is believed that the unauthorized logins were discovered through the hospital's own internal auditing system. Electronic health record systems keep an audit trail of everyone who accesses the system. If the hospital was still using a paper record-keeping system, there might not be such an easy way to find out who accessed the person's record.

While the hospital did detect the unauthorized use, it seemingly did not have measures in place to protect the file from being looked at in the first place. Some hospitals take additional steps to protect the medical records of well-known patients, such as requiring a special code to access the records.

continually being developed, and antivirus software must be regularly updated to maintain its effectiveness.

Privacy and Security Risks of Electronic Health Information Exchange

Despite these and other security measures, electronic health information remains at risk. A study by the eHealth Vulnerability Reporting Program (eHVRP) designed to assess the degree of risk associated with current electronic health information systems found serious security flaws in them. Largely due to weaknesses in the EHR software, investigators were able to gain access to a program and to view personal health data. The fifteen-month study, reported on in the fall of 2007, uncovered a number of security loopholes in commercial EHR systems, including in ambulatory (physician offices, outpatient clinics) systems certified by the Certification Commission for Healthcare Information Technology (CCHIT). As part of the report, eHVRP recommended additional security measures (www.ehvrp.org/report.html). The eHVRP is made up of representatives of health care industry organizations as well as of the technology and security industries.

The increased use of information technology in health care to cut costs, improve patient safety, and provide the best possible care places large amounts of protected health information at greater risk. Reasons for this include the following:

- A greater volume of confidential clinical patient information is available in electronic form, while the proliferation of health information networks provides many points of access to patient information, increasing the possibility of unauthorized access.
- The increase in the use of portable computing and storage devices means that health information can be moved from place to place with ease. This increases the possibility of data being lost or devices being stolen.
- Personal health information is increasingly in the hands of groups not covered under current HIPAA privacy laws. In addition, information in networks that cross state lines is sometimes subject to conflicting privacy laws.

CLINICAL DATA AVAILABLE IN ELECTRONIC FORM

More personal health information is being created, accessed, and maintained on computers than ever before. In an electronic health record system, personal health information is entered and stored in a computer database. The database then connects to other databases in health information networks, making it possible to share health information with authorized providers, hospitals, pharmacies, laboratories, and others. The larger the network, the greater the risk, so while a nationwide health information network brings the most benefits, it also presents the greatest privacy and security challenges.

PORTABLE COMPUTERS AND STORAGE DEVICES

In the past, personal health information did not commonly leave a physician office or hospital facility. Desktop computers, bulky paper files, and large backup tapes made it difficult to move data from one place to another. In large part, the locks on office doors were safeguards against intruders.

Today, as the examples in this chapter have illustrated, data are portable and leave medical offices and hospital buildings regularly. The widespread use of portable hardware and small storage devices makes it more difficult to control access to a person's health information.

Many health care professionals use laptops, personal digital assistants (PDAs), and smart cell phones to access and store data. Laptops are popular because they can be moved from one location to another, such as from a physician's desk to an examining room. It is not uncommon for employees to take laptops to and from work, since doing so enables them to access files wherever they are. One of the benefits of electronic health records is being able to access data when and where it is needed, but this cannot be done without portable computer hardware.

Case Study

Just after midnight, Bill Ahern, a nineteen year-old college student, was wheeled in to the emergency room at South Shore Hospital (SSH). He and two friends had been watching a baseball game on the large-screen televisions at a restaurant/bar just a few miles from campus. While driving back, Bill lost control of the car, and swerved off the shoulder of the road and into a tree.

The driver of a car going in the opposite direction stopped to see if everyone was alright. The passengers in the backseat were shaken up, but not seriously injured. Bill had not been wearing his seatbelt, which was customary for him when driving a short distance. He had lacerations on his face and arms and was unconscious. The driver of the other car called 911, and police and an ambulance were dispatched to the scene.

Bill was transported to South Shore, where Dr. Virind R. Gupta, the attending physician, quickly began to assess Bill's injuries. At Dr. Gupta's direction, a technician took a vial of blood for analysis.

At the nurses' station in the hall, the police officer investigating the accident was talking to the head trauma nurse, and requested that a blood-alcohol test be conducted. Since it was a single car accident with no obvious cause, he suspected the men might have been drinking.

In the meantime, one of the passengers in the car had called Bill's parents, who lived within an hour's drive of the hospital. When Bill's parents heard the news, they headed for the hospital. As they drove, they wondered whether Bill was going to be alright, and how this could have happened. They felt that Bill had changed in the past few months. In his freshman year, Bill stopped home almost once a week for a home cooked meal and to do his laundry. But this year had been different. They hadn't seen Bill since he left in September, and when they called, he always seemed to be on his way out to do something, and had no time to talk.

Bill was still unconscious when his parents arrived. They wanted to talk to Dr. Gupta about Bill's condition, and to find out what had happened, but Dr. Gupta was busy with another patient. They left Bill's room to look for someone to ask. Bill's father saw a computer at a station outside Bill's room. He walked over and glanced at the information on the screen. A nurse walking by excused herself, and then pressed a key that caused the screen to change and display login and password prompts.

Still trying to find out what was happening, they asked the nurse about Bill's condition. Was he going to be alright? How did the accident happen? Had any tests been done? Had he been drinking? Did they test him for alcohol or drugs? Did they need insurance information? (Bill was still covered by his parents' health insurance, as well as their automobile insurance.) They asked the nurse to give them a printout of his record from the computer.

What Do You Think?

1. Does the nurse need Bill's permission to answer his parent's questions? Does it matter that he is still covered by his parent's health insurance policy?
2. Does the hospital need his permission to release the results of the blood alcohol test to the police?
3. Did the hospital take adequate measures to protect patients' electronic health information? Why or why not?

USB flash drives and other removable storage devices are smaller and less expensive than they were just a year ago. They function like hard drives, and people require little in the way of instruction before they can use the devices to store data. Small storage devices, including CDs and DVDs, easily fit in a briefcase.

PROBLEMS NOT ADEQUATELY ADDRESSED BY EXISTING PRIVACY LAWS

HIPAA is not a universal law; that is, it does not apply to every person or organization. It was designed to provide protection for personal health information that was exchanged by certain groups and individuals in certain electronic transactions. Since HIPAA was enacted (1996) and the Privacy Rule (2003) and Security Rule (2005) went into effect, the field of health information technology has changed dramatically. Table 6-3 lists some differences between today's health care environment and that of 1996. Increasingly, an individual's personal health information is accessed, maintained, and exchanged by groups that may not be covered under current HIPAA privacy laws:

- New computer networks permit doctors, hospitals, pharmacies, health plans, and others to electronically exchange health information. Many have been developed by groups that may not fit the HIPAA definition of a covered entity.
- A wide variety of entities now offer personal health records directly to individuals. The information in these PHRs may not be protected, since the organization that provides the service may not fit the definition of a covered entity or a business associate.
- Providers and health care facilities use overseas companies for administrative, financial, and clinical tasks, making oversight and enforcement of privacy laws more difficult.
- Many states have privacy laws that are more protective that the federal HIPAA Privacy Rule. In these states, personal health information is safeguarded by the stricter state legislation. With the rapid rise in the number of electronic data networks that span state lines, it is unclear which states' law would apply if a privacy breach occurred.

Private Sector Electronic Networks

While the federal government continues its work on developing a strategy for the creation of a national health information network (NHIN), businesses and organizations in the private sector (meaning

TABLE 6-3 Changes in the Health Record Environment

	1996	2008
Medical records format	Mostly paper	Mixture of paper and electronic
Privacy and security concerns	Physical, limited to office	Online as well as physical
Computer use	Financial and administrative purposes	Clinical, financial, and administrative
Access to data	Limited to single physical location	Available through any Internet connection
Data entered by	Physician and staff	Physician, staff, and patient

nongovernmental) have created new models of health information networks for sharing information. For example, health information exchanges (HIEs) have been created at the state, regional, and community levels. A **health information exchange** enables health care information to be exchanged electronically across organizations and retain its meaning. A regional health information organization (RHIO) is a type of HIE in which a group of health care entities in a geographic area exchange health information over an electronic network for the purpose of improving the delivery of health care. Participants may include health care providers, clinics, hospitals, laboratories, pharmacies, health plans, mental health agencies, and local health departments. While some of these providers, such as health care providers and health plans, are subject to HIPAA privacy laws, the overall organization is not. It is estimated that health information exchanges exist in more than 150 communities.

health information exchange state, regional, or community network that enables electronic exchange of health care information.

Personal Health Records (PHRs)

Many different organizations, including employers, health plans, and providers, offer personal health records (PHRs) to individuals, as discussed in Chapter 5. Companies including Wal-Mart, Intel, BP, Pitney Bowes, and Allied Materials have joined together to provide personal health record systems for their 2.5 million employees. Commercial software vendors are offering PHRs to individuals at no charge or for a fee. These companies do not meet the HIPAA definition of provider, health plan, or health care clearinghouse. They also do not file any electronic health care transactions. As a result, many of the PHRs offered today are not covered by the Privacy Rule, leaving protected health information subject to release without a patient's consent or authorization. Some states are working on laws that protect an individual's health information in these instances, but it will take time for state legislatures to enact legislation.

Overseas Business Associates

Overseas companies in India and other countries are providing services to the health care providers and organizations in the United States, including coding, transcription processing, and claim management. Some of these tasks cannot be completed without access to protected health information. Some developing companies lack security systems that protect sensitive health data. Also, offshore vendors are not covered entities under HIPAA, so they do not have to comply with HIPAA security and privacy legislation. If HIPAA applies at all, it is only indirectly through a business associate agreement they signed with the U.S. covered entity. Even then, if a violation occurs, it is up to the U.S. company to resolve, since the Department of Health and Human Services cannot impose penalties against business associates.

Multistate Exchange of Data with Different Laws

It is now commonplace for health information to speed across state lines via a computer network, such as the Internet. Many health care providers, health plans, pharmacies, laboratories, and hospitals already exchange data electronically. As health information exchange expands

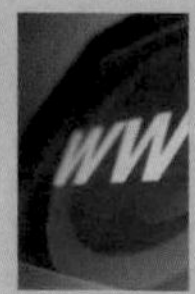

Chapter 6 Online Discovery

The shootings at Virginia Tech that took place on April 16, 2007, raised questions about the use and disclosure of students' health records, mental health records in particular. On June 13, 2007, the Report to the President on Issues Raised by the Virginia Tech Tragedy was released. The report was made available to the public on a government website.

Open a web browser, and go to www.hhs.gov/vtreport.html.

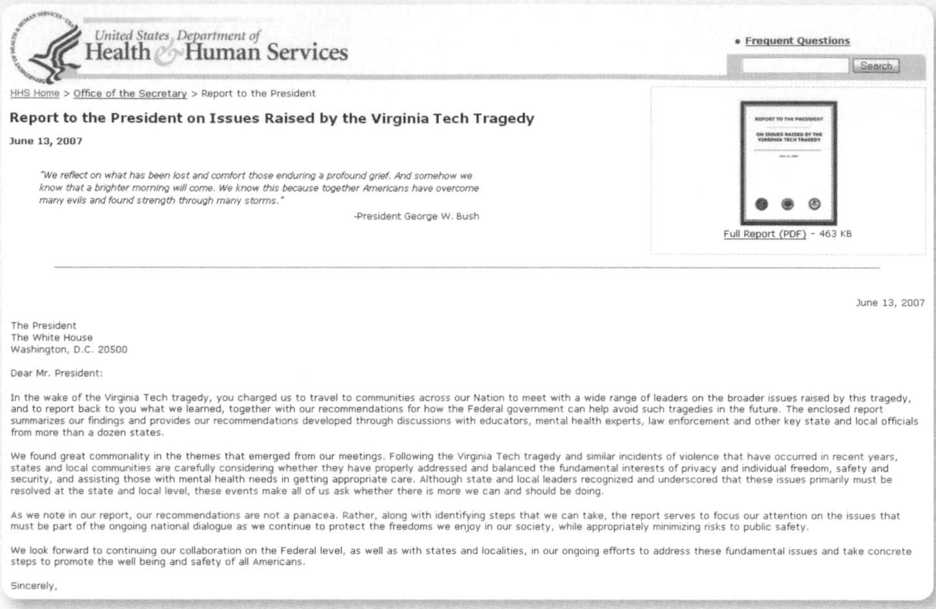

United States Department of Health & Human Services

• Frequent Questions

Search

HHS Home > Office of the Secretary > Report to the President

Report to the President on Issues Raised by the Virginia Tech Tragedy

June 13, 2007

"We reflect on what has been lost and comfort those enduring a profound grief. And somehow we know that a brighter morning will come. We know this because together Americans have overcome many evils and found strength through many storms."

-President George W. Bush

Full Report (PDF) - 463 KB

June 13, 2007

The President
The White House
Washington, D.C. 20500

Dear Mr. President:

In the wake of the Virginia Tech tragedy, you charged us to travel to communities across our Nation to meet with a wide range of leaders on the broader issues raised by this tragedy, and to report back to you what we learned, together with our recommendations for how the Federal government can help avoid such tragedies in the future. The enclosed report summarizes our findings and provides our recommendations developed through discussions with educators, mental health experts, law enforcement and other key state and local officials from more than a dozen states.

We found great commonality in the themes that emerged from our meetings. Following the Virginia Tech tragedy and similar incidents of violence that have occurred in recent years, states and local communities are carefully considering whether they have properly addressed and balanced the fundamental interests of privacy and individual freedom, safety and security, and assisting those with mental health needs in getting appropriate care. Although state and local leaders recognized and underscored that these issues primarily must be resolved at the state and local level, these events make all of us ask whether there is more we can and should be doing.

As we note in our report, our recommendations are not a panacea. Rather, along with identifying steps that we can take, the report serves to focus our attention on the issues that must be part of the ongoing national dialogue as we continue to protect the freedoms we enjoy in our society, while appropriately minimizing risks to public safety.

We look forward to continuing our collaboration on the Federal level, as well as with states and localities, in our ongoing efforts to address these fundamental issues and take concrete steps to promote the well being and safety of all Americans.

Sincerely,

Thinking About It

1. Do you think that educational administrators and mental health providers understood laws governing the use and disclosure of students' mental or physical health?

____

across state lines, sorting out differences in state privacy laws presents a significant challenge. In states with more-protective laws, state law takes precedence over HIPAA. In states with laws that are less stringent than HIPAA requirements, the HIPAA rule applies. If health data are shared by individuals and organizations in different states, which state's law applies?

The "Privacy and Security Solutions for Interoperable Health Information Exchange" report released in the fall of 2007 identified the challenges that states encounter when applying HIPAA regulations and state laws to protect the privacy of electronic health information. This report on the Health Information Security and Privacy Collaboration (HISPC) review of policies, practices, and laws pertaining to interoperable health information exchange in thirty-four state HIEs discovered significant variation in the way individual providers, hospitals, public

Scroll down the page until you come to the section with the heading "Critical Information Sharing Faces Substantial Obstacles," which appears below. Read that section of the report, and answer the questions that follow.

Critical Information Sharing Faces Substantial Obstacles

We repeatedly heard reports of "information silos" within educational institutions and among educational staff, mental health providers, and public safety officials that impede appropriate information sharing. These concerns are heightened by confusion about the laws that govern the sharing of information. Throughout our meetings and in every breakout session, we heard differing interpretations and confusion about legal restrictions on the ability to share information about a person who may be a threat to self or to others. In addition to federal laws that may affect information sharing practices, such as the Health Insurance Portability and Accountability Act (HIPAA) Privacy Rule and the Family Educational Rights and Privacy Act (FERPA), a broad patchwork of state laws and regulations also impact how information is shared on the state level. In some situations, these state laws and regulations are more restrictive than federal laws.

A consistent theme and broad perception in our meetings was that this confusion and differing interpretations about state and federal privacy laws and regulations impede appropriate information sharing. In some sessions, there were concerns and confusion about the potential liability of teachers, administrators, or institutions that could arise from sharing information, or from not sharing information, under privacy laws, as well as laws designed to protect individuals from discrimination on the basis of mental illness. It was almost universally observed that these fears and misunderstandings likely limit the transfer of information in more significant ways than is required by law. Particularly, although participants in each state meeting were aware of both HIPAA and FERPA, there was significant misunderstanding about the scope and application of these laws and their interrelation with state laws. In a number of discussions, participants reported circumstances in which they incorrectly believed that they were subject to liability or foreclosed from sharing information under federal law. Other participants were unsure whether and how HIPAA and FERPA actually limit or allow information to be shared and unaware of exceptions that could allow relevant information to be shared.

Of course, a predicate to sharing information is recognizing when individuals pose a threat to themselves or others, and when intervention to pre-empt the threat is appropriate. In this regard, participants flagged the need for effective, evidence-based, inter-disciplinary tools to conduct a reliable assessment of the degree, type, and immediacy of safety risk the individual poses.

State and Local Recommendations

- *Increase information sharing and collaboration among state and local communities, educators, mental health officials, and law enforcement to better provide care and detect, intervene, and respond to potential incidents of violence in schools and other venues.*
- *Provide accurate information to help ensure that family members, educational administrators, mental health providers, and other appropriate persons understand when and how they are legally entitled to share and receive information about mental illness, and appropriately do so, particularly where college and school-age children and youth are involved, for the protection and wellbeing of the student and the community.*
- *Along with reviewing federal laws that may apply, clarify and promote wider understanding about how state law limits or allows the sharing of information about individuals who may pose a danger to themselves or others, and examine state law to determine if legislative or regulatory changes are needed to achieve the appropriate balance of privacy and security.*

Recommended Federal Action

- *The U.S. Departments of Health and Human Services and Education should develop additional guidance that clarifies how information can be shared legally under HIPAA and FERPA and disseminate it widely to the mental health, education, and law enforcement communities. The U.S. Department of Education should ensure that parents and school officials understand how and when post-secondary institutions can share information on college students with parents. In addition, the U.S. Departments of Education and Health and Human Services should consider whether further actions are needed to balance more appropriately the interests of safety, privacy, and treatment implicated by FERPA and HIPAA.*
- *The U.S. Department of Education should ensure that its emergency management grantees and state and local communities receiving training through the program have clear guidance on the sharing of information as it relates to educational records and FERPA.*
- *Federal agencies should continue to work together, and with states and appropriate partners, to improve, expand, coordinate, and disseminate information and best practices in behavioral analysis, threat assessments, and emergency preparedness, for colleges and universities.* [2]
- *The U.S. Department of Education, in collaboration with the U.S. Secret Service and the Department of Justice, should explore research of targeted violence in institutions of higher education*[3] *and continue to share existing threat assessment methodology with interested institutions*[4].

2. Did conflicts between state and federal privacy laws contribute to the lack of information sharing?

____

3. What does the report suggest could be done to fix some of the problems?

____

When you are finished viewing the website and answering the questions, close your web browser.

health officials, and others implemented privacy and security laws. These variations are viewed as potential barriers to the widespread implementation of HIEs.

The Importance of Public Trust

As a practical matter, individuals sometimes need to share sensitive information with their doctors. People feel that they can trust their physicians to keep the information confidential. All physicians take an oath, known as the Hippocratic oath, that includes agreeing to protect the confidentiality of patients' information. They consent to disclose protected health information only when it is authorized by the patient unless not disclosing the information could cause harm to the public.

If there is any doubt or lack of trust on the part of patients, they may withhold potentially embarrassing information; they worry that if the information got in the wrong hands, they could lose their jobs, their health insurance, or their life insurance or otherwise be harmed. At the same time, a doctor who lacks a complete picture of the patient's condition is more likely to make an incorrect diagnosis, which can lead to prescribing inappropriate medications and other treatments. The trust between a patient and a physician plays a major role in ensuring that individuals receive appropriate medical care.

PUBLIC ATTITUDES TOWARD THE ELECTRONIC USE OF HEALTH INFORMATION

A number of surveys highlight the public's concern about electronic health records and health information networks:

- A Gallup Poll conducted in 2000 found that 78 percent of respondents believe that keeping their medical records confidential is very important (Gallup Organization, 2000).
- A 2005 survey of consumer attitudes toward health privacy conducted by Forrester Research confirms public fears about health privacy:
  - Two out of three people expressed concerns about the privacy of their personal health information.
  - Twelve percent admitted to engaging in behaviors intended to protect their privacy, such as not being honest with doctors about symptoms or behaviors, refusing to provide information, and paying their own money for care that is covered by insurance to avoid filing insurance claims.

When stories of data breaches make the news headlines almost daily, maintaining patient-physician trust is not easy. However, if individuals do not feel that the information disclosed to their physicians will be protected, there will be no EHRs and no nationwide health information network. Clearly, the development of a widespread computer network that contains large amounts of personal health information requires the trust of the public.

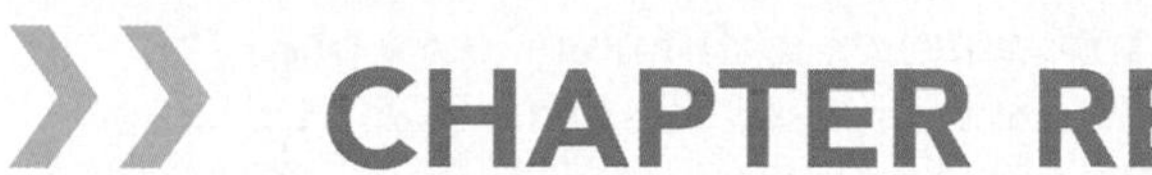

CHAPTER REVIEW

CHAPTER SUMMARY

1. The Health Insurance Portability and Accountability Act (HIPAA) of 1996 was the most significant legislation affecting the health care field since the Medicare and Medicaid programs were introduced in 1965. The Administrative Simplification provisions contained new requirements for the uniform transfer of electronic health care data such as for billing and payment; new patient rights regarding personal health information, including the right to access this information and to limit its disclosure; and broad new security rules that health care organizations must put in place to safeguard the confidentiality of patients' medical information.
2. The HIPAA Privacy Rule regulates the use and disclosure of protected health information (PHI). It requires covered entities (CEs) to have appropriate privacy policies and procedures and to notify patients about their privacy rights and about how their information can be used or disclosed. The CE must train employees so that they understand the privacy practices. The CE must appoint a staff member to be responsible for seeing that the privacy practices are adopted and followed. Finally, CEs must safeguard patients' health records.
3. Protected health information (PHI) can be released without patients' authorization when a covered entity uses it for health care treatment, payment, or operations. In addition, the rules for use and disclosure do not apply to the release of PHI in certain circumstances, such as public health, law enforcement, research, workers' compensation cases, and national security situations. There are no restrictions on the use or disclosure of de-identified health information.
4. Threats to the security of electronic information can come from a number of sources, including individuals; environmental hazards such as floods, wind, and lightning; and computer hardware, software, and networks.
5. The HIPAA Security Rule requires medical offices to establish safeguards to protect the confidentiality, integrity, and availability of health information that is stored on a computer system or transmitted across computer networks, including the Internet. The security standards are divided into three categories: administrative, physical, and technical safeguards. Administrative safeguards are policies and procedures designed to protect electronic health information. Physical safeguards are mechanisms to protect electronic systems, equipment, and data from environmental hazards and unauthorized intrusion. Technical safeguards are automated processes to protect data and to control access to data.

6. The rise in the use of information technology may place protected health information at increased security risk. A greater volume of confidential clinical patient information is available in electronic form, and there are many more points of access to that information. In addition, the use of portable computing and storage devices increases the possibility of lost data or stolen devices. Existing privacy laws may not cover some new types of companies that have entered the health care market.
7. Since HIPAA was enacted in 1996 and the HIPAA Privacy Rule (2003) and Security Rule (2005) went into effect, the field of health information technology has changed dramatically. Increasingly, an individual's personal health information is accessed, maintained, and exchanged by groups that may not be covered under current HIPAA privacy laws. Examples of groups that may not be covered are regional health information exchanges (RHIOs), providers of personal health records (PHRs), and overseas business associates. In addition, conflicts in state privacy laws must resolved to determine how state laws apply to transmission across state lines.
8. Patients must sometimes reveal sensitive information to their providers. They do this because they trust their providers to keep the information confidential. Individuals who lack trust may withhold important information, which could result in inappropriate diagnoses. Reports of computer security breaches appear in newspapers, on the Internet, and on television news on a regular basis. If individuals do not believe that their personal information will be secure in an electronic system, they may not share health information with their providers. This can undermine the public's willingness to participate in an electronic health record system.

CHECK YOUR UNDERSTANDING

Part 1. Write *T* or *F* in the blank to indicate whether you think the statement is true or false.

____ **1.** The HIPAA Privacy Rule does not apply to de-identified information.

____ **2.** Under the HIPAA Privacy Rule, patients' protected health information can be released to payers for payment purposes without patient authorization.

____ **3.** The HIPAA Security Rule allows organizations flexibility in determining what type of security mechanisms to implement.

____ **4.** The increased use of information technology places large amounts of protected health information at greater risk.

____ **5.** Companies that provide personal health records for their employees are considered business associates according to HIPAA.

_____ 6. The ability to access electronic health records from any location with an Internet connection presents a security challenge.

_____ 7. Laptops that contain personal health information are not allowed to be removed from the physician office.

_____ 8. All regional health information organizations (RHIOs) are covered by HIPAA privacy laws.

_____ 9. Laws that protect the privacy of personal health information vary from state to state.

_____ 10. If a state privacy law is more protective of patients' rights than the HIPAA Privacy Rule, the state law applies.

Part 2. Match each term below with its correct definition.

_____ 11. authorization

_____ 12. covered entities (CEs)

_____ 13. disclosure

_____ 14. HIPAA Security Rule

_____ 15. minimum necessary standard

_____ 16. administrative safeguards

_____ 17. encryption

_____ 18. physical safeguards

_____ 19. audit trails

_____ 20. protected health information (PHI)

_____ 21. HIPAA Privacy Rule

_____ 22. Administrative Simplification

_____ 23. role-based authorization

_____ 24. technical safeguards

_____ 25. de-identified health information

a. Permission to use and disclose information for uses other than treatment, payment, and operations.

b. Part of the Administrative Simplification provisions of HIPAA that provides protection for individually identifiable health information and grants certain rights to individuals in regard to their medical records.

c. Health care professionals and organizations that provide health care in the normal course of business and electronically transmit any information that is protected under HIPAA.

d. Part of the Administrative Simplification provisions of HIPAA that protects the confidentiality, integrity, and availability of electronic health information.

e. The mechanisms required to protect electronic systems, equipment, and data from threats, environmental hazards, and unauthorized intrusion.

f. Records that show who has accessed a computer or network and what operations were preformed.

g. The release of protected health information to an outside provider or organization.

h. Individually identifiable health information that is transmitted or maintained by electronic media or is transmitted or maintained in any other form or medium.

i. Safeguards to protect PHI from being accidentally released to those who do not need access to the information during an appropriate use or disclosure.

j. The name of Title II of HIPAA, which addresses the uniform transfer of electronic health care data as well as patient privacy protections.

k. The process of converting data into an unreadable format before it is distributed.

l. Limits access to patient information based on the user's role in an organization.

m. Information that neither identifies nor provides a reasonable basis to identify an individual.

n. Automated processes used to protect data and control access to data.

o. Policies and procedures designed to protect electronic health information.

THINKING ABOUT THE ISSUES

Part 3. In the space provided, write a brief paragraph describing your thoughts on the following issues.

26. With almost daily media coverage on breaches of computer security, how can a national health information system gain public trust?

____

____

27. With constant changes in computer technology and business practices, how can the HIPAA Privacy and Security Rules provide effective consumer protection?

____

____

7 Introduction to Practice Partner

CHAPTER OUTLINE

Practice Partner: An Ambulatory EHR
Passwords, Access Levels, and the Park Feature
Access Levels
The Park Feature
Exploring the Main Practice Partner Screen
The Dashboard
Schedule
Messages
Lab Review
To Do
Note Review
Patient Registration Information
The Lookup Function
The Patient Chart
Chart Summary
Progress Notes
Medical History
Hospital Reports
Order Entry
Problem List
Health Maintenance
Rx/Medications
Vital Signs
Laboratory Data
Patient Education
Images
HIPAA

LEARNING OUTCOMES

After completing this chapter, you will be able to define key terms and:

1. Explain how the use of access levels protects the privacy of information in a patient record.
2. Describe the purpose of the dashboard.
3. Explain where patient registration information is stored and accessed.
4. Explain the function of the Chart Summary.
5. Describe how progress notes can be entered.
6. Explain how Practice Partner assists with coding a patient encounter.
7. List two safety and cost-control features of electronic order entry.
8. Discuss the medication list in Practice Partner.
9. Explain how Practice Partner displays abnormal values in vital signs and lab results.
10. Describe how the HIPAA section of the patient chart can be used to document HIPAA compliance.

KEY TERMS

access levels
dashboard
evaluation and management codes (E/M codes)
Lookup
progress notes
SOAP
Web View

Why This Chapter Is Important to You

The information in this chapter will enable you to:

- ›› Understand how to enter information an EHR program through hands-on experience.
- ›› Understand how to locate information an EHR program through hands-on experience.
- ›› Understand how to review information an EHR program through hands-on experience.

Practice Partner: An Ambulatory EHR

Practice Partner is an electronic health record and practice management program for ambulatory practices. The electronic health record portion of the program, known as Patient Record, is widely used in medical practices throughout the United States. It has received certification from the Certification Commission for Healthcare Information Technology (CCHIT) as an ambulatory EHR product, having met the criteria for functionality, interoperability, and security.

The program includes many of the features and capabilities described throughout this book, including:

- › A choice of data entry methods for documentation including computer keyboard, voice recognition software, digital dictation, and traditional dictation

- Pre-defined templates for entering patient progress notes
- Electronic prescribing with built-in drug interaction and allergy checks
- Alerts for overdue health maintenance procedures
- Automated coding assistance for patient encounters
- Ability to import lab data electronically from outside facilities
- Alerts for lab results that are outside normal ranges
- Built-in access to patient education articles that can be printed and handed to patients
- Security features to protect the confidentiality of patient health information.

In this chapter, you will learn about the major features of Practice Partner. You will also have the opportunity to watch software demonstrations that are included on the CD inside the back cover of the book. After you watch a demonstration, you will gain hands-on experience as you practice entering information in Practice Partner.

Most of the concepts and techniques used in operating Practice Partner are similar to those in other EHR programs. Once you are familiar with Practice Partner, you should be able to transfer many skills taught in this book to other EHR programs.

Passwords, Access Levels, and the Park Feature

Before users can log in to Practice Partner, they must have a user name, password, and access level. The use of user names and passwords prevents unauthorized access to the program, safeguards critical patient information, and protects patient confidentiality. As passwords are entered, the characters are replaced with asterisks (*) on the screen so there is no chance of someone seeing the password. The system may be set up to limit the number of log on attempts. If the number of unsuccessful attempts exceeds the number permitted, the user will not be permitted to access the system until a system manager intervenes. In Practice Partner, passwords are encrypted for transmission between client workstations and the database located on the server. The Practice Partner sign in screen is illustrated in Figure 7-1.

ACCESS LEVELS

access levels a security feature that limits access to information based on the type of information each user will need to view or modify.

Access levels limit access to information based on the type of information each user will need to view or modify. Access levels play a major role in ensuring the security and confidentiality of patient records in a practice. In Figure 7-2, different access levels are created for different positions in the office—such as physician, nurse, billing, reception, etc. The access

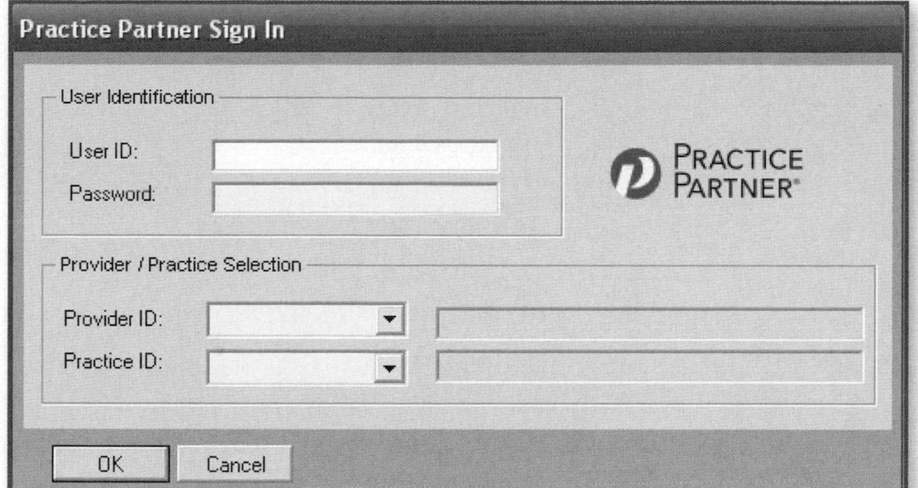

Figure 7-1

The Practice Partner Sign In screen.

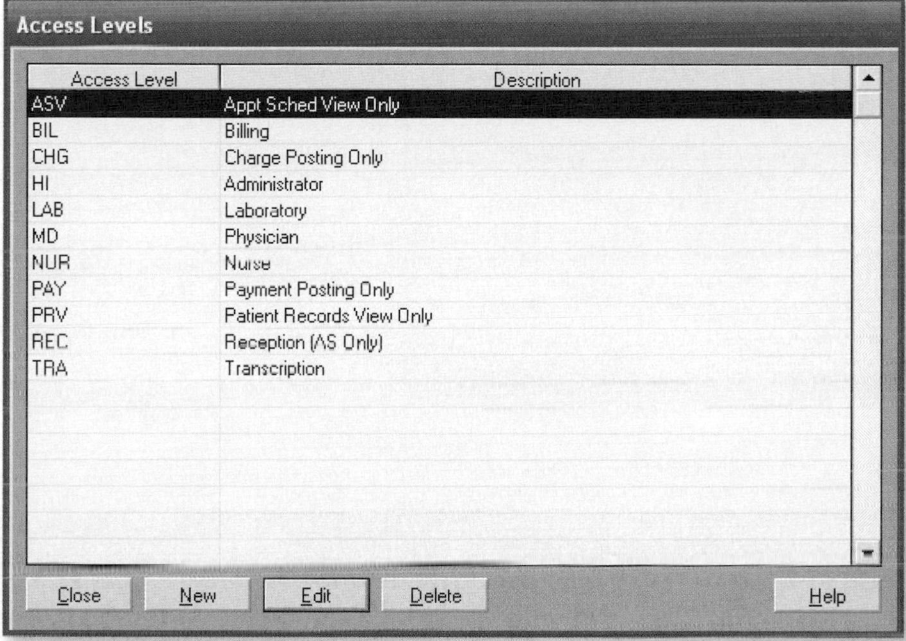

Figure 7-2

A list of access levels for office personnel.

levels define which areas of the program a user can view, and whether the user can add, edit, or delete information, or just view the information. The program can also specify whether a user has to enter a password to access certain areas of the program. Figure 7-3 on page 208 lists the access privileges for a staff member who can only view patient records.

THE PARK FEATURE

Another privacy and security feature in Practice Partner is known as "Park," which allows a user to leave a workstation for a brief time without having to exit the program. When a workstation is "parked" it cannot be accessed without re-entry of a valid operator's user name and password. If someone were to walk by and see the screen while the user was away from the computer, rather than seeing patient data, they would see the screen illustrated in Figure 7-4 on page 208.

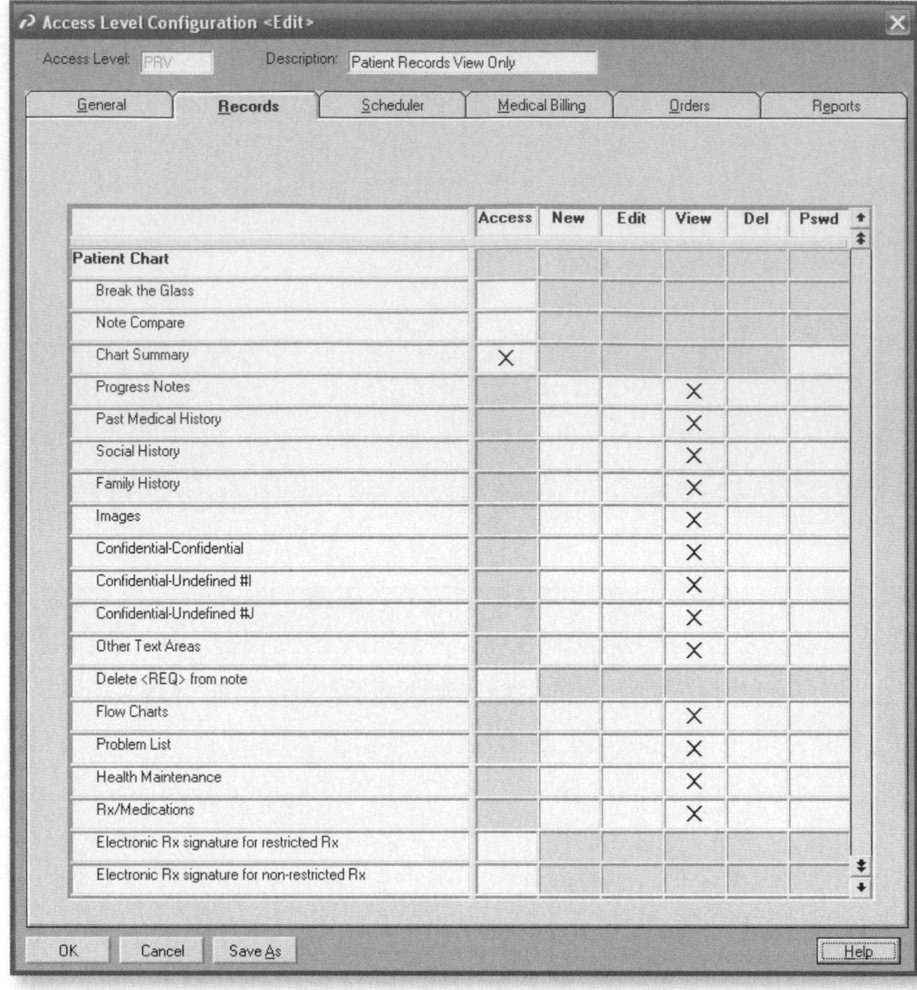

Figure 7-3

A screen showing the areas of the patient records program that a user of a particular access level can access, edit, or view.

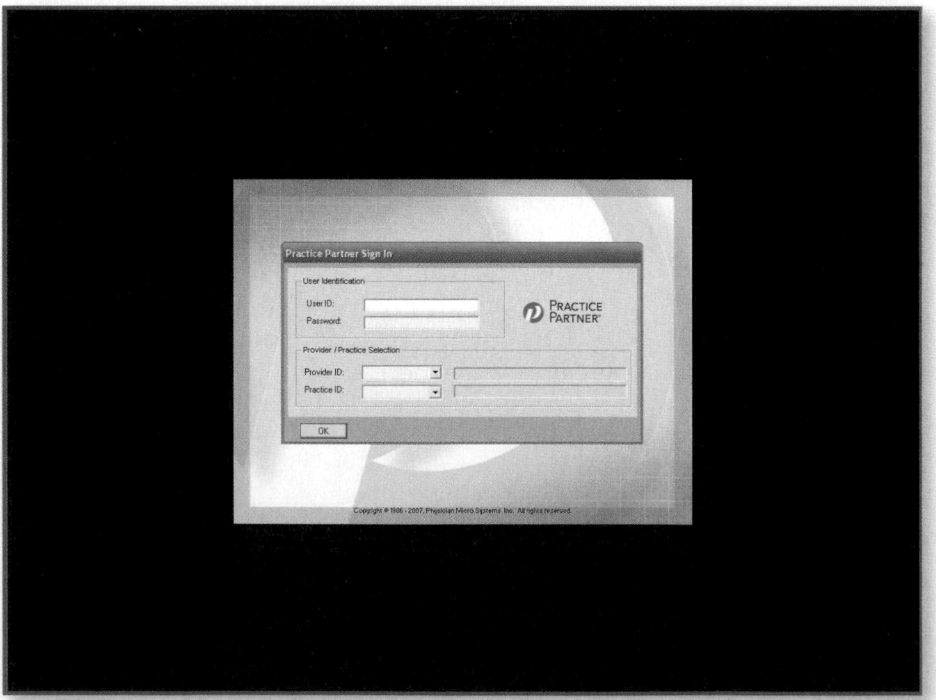

Figure 7-4

The Practice Partner screen in "Park" mode.

Exploring the Main Practice Partner Screen

Once a user has successfully logged in to the program, the main screen is displayed. To use Practice Partner effectively, it is important to understand the parts of the screen and the functions they perform. The main screen contains the following sections:

Title bar—The title bar states the title of the program. This is standard in all Windows packages, including Practice Partner.

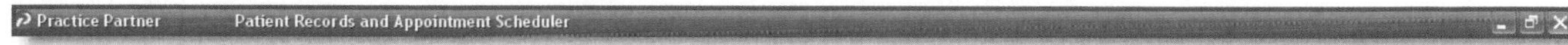

Menu bar—The menu bar contains the menus of Practice Partner commands. The menus and commands available may change depending on the task you are currently performing. For example, the Maintenance menu will not appear when you are in the patient chart, because you cannot perform maintenance tasks while you are working with patient information.

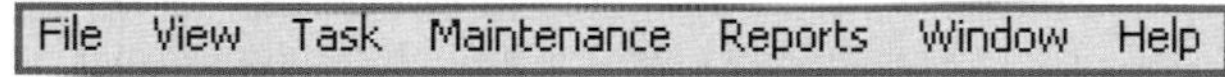

Toolbar—The toolbar provides instant access to important Practice Partner functions (Exit, Park, Chart, Schedule, and so on). You can click these buttons to activate the related function. The buttons on the toolbar vary depending on which function in the program is in use.

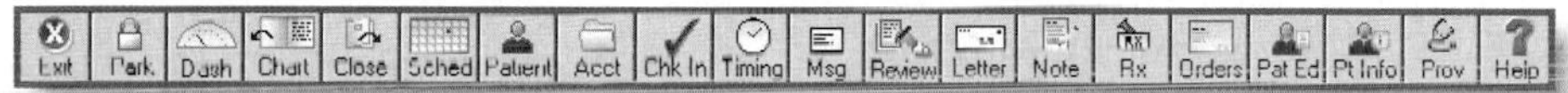

Status bar—The status bar (or message bar) at the bottom of the main Practice Partner screen, always displays the provider ID of the current provider. The status bar also displays additional information or messages about the task you are currently performing. For example, when a patient chart is open, the status bar displays the current patient's ID, sex, age, and whether Web View is enabled. **Web View** allows patients to view certain information from their chart via the Internet.

Web View a feature in Practice Partner that allows patients to view certain information from their chart via the Internet.

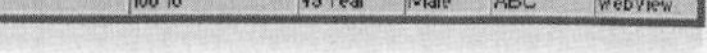

TABLE 7-1 **Icons in the Practice Partner Toolbar**

ICON	FUNCTION
Exit	Closes the chart(s) and exits out of the Practice Partner program.
Park	Protects your system from other viewers by locking the screen, requiring the next user to login with their user name and password.
Chart	Opens a chart. (More than one chart can be open at a time.)
Dash	Opens the Dashboard if it is not already open.
Close	Closes the chart you are viewing.
Sched	Opens the Appointment Scheduler program.
Patient	Opens a patient's registration screens for access to demographic information.
Acct	Only for Practice Partner Billing system.
Chk In	Checks in patients and tracks them through the visit.
Timing	This works with the Check In feature above.
Msg	Allows you to send messages (e-mail) to other staff members, regardless of which Practice Partner application they are using.
Review	Brings up the provider's review bin. All unsigned items go here automatically, including lab results, progress notes, and other incoming transmissions that await your sign off. This replaces the In basket on your desk.
Letter	Allows providers to write, store, and revise letters about specific patients and send them to consulting physicians.
Note	Starts a new progress note for a patient.
Rx	This is the Rx prescription writer.
Orders	This is the Order Entry module for ordering labs, x-rays, etc.
Pat Ed	This would launch the optional Patient Education modules.
Pt Info	Shows you all the demographic information for this patient.
Prov	Allows you to change to another provider or clinic registered to the system.
Help	Provides the user with on-line help for Patient Records.

The Dashboard

dashboard a feature in Practice Partner that offers providers a convenient view of important information at a glance.

The main screen also displays what is called the provider dashboard. The **dashboard** offers providers a convenient view of important information, including messages, to do list, unsigned lab orders, notes and more. Figure 7-5 shows a provider dashboard from Practice Partner.

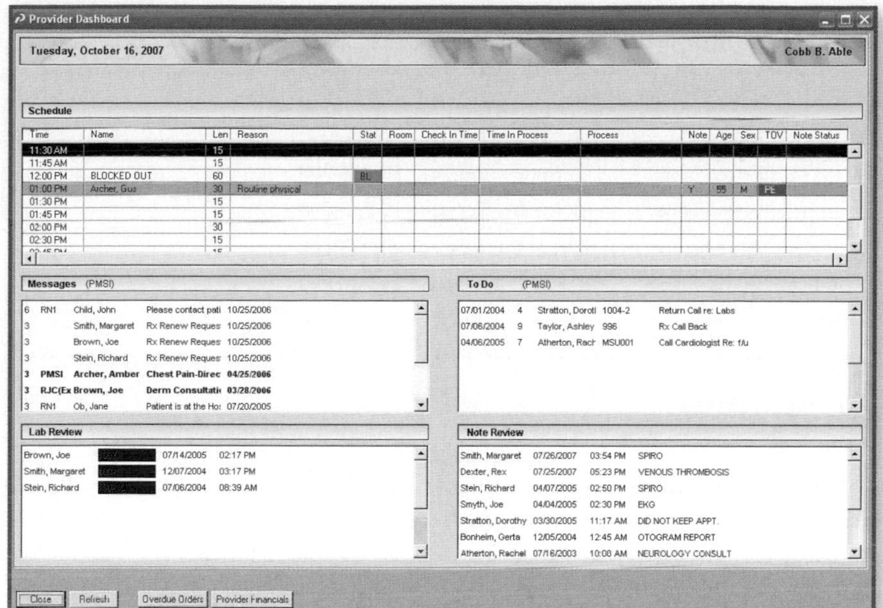

Figure 7-5

The provider dashboard in Practice Partner.

The main areas of the dashboard include:

- Schedule
- Messages
- Lab Review
- To Do
- Note Review

To access any of these features directly from the desktop, you would click on the title of that section, such as Messages or To Do.

SCHEDULE

The schedule area presents the daily schedule for the provider with appointment time, patient name, length of visit, reasons for visit, as well as whether the patient has checked in and if so, which room the patient is in (see Figure 7-6).

MESSAGES

The Messages section lists electronic messages for the provider. Unread messages appear in bold type. Information provided in this area includes the message priority (0-9), the sender of the message, the subject, and the date the message was received (see Figure 7-7 on page 212).

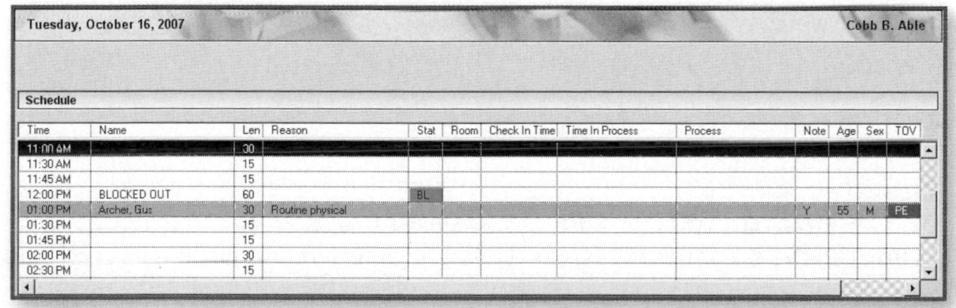

Figure 7-6

The Schedule section of the provider dashboard.

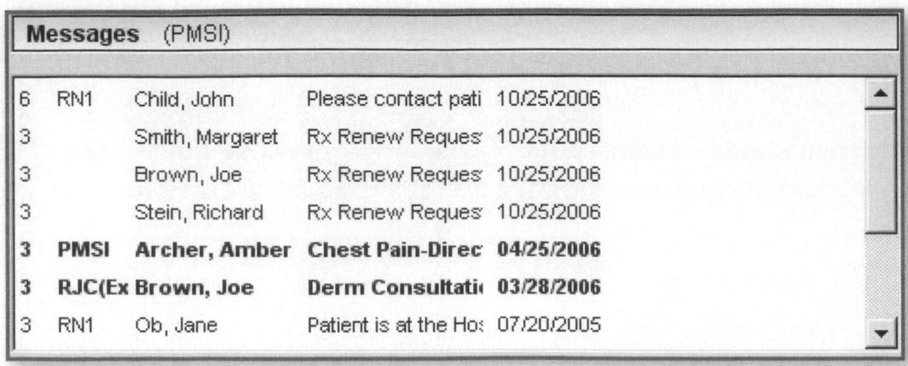

Messages (PMSI)
6 RN1 Child, John Please contact pati 10/25/2006
3 Smith, Margaret Rx Renew Reques 10/25/2006
3 Brown, Joe Rx Renew Reques 10/25/2006
3 Stein, Richard Rx Renew Reques 10/25/2006
3 PMSI Archer, Amber Chest Pain-Direc 04/25/2006
3 RJC(Ex Brown, Joe Derm Consultati 03/28/2006
3 RN1 Ob, Jane Patient is at the Ho: 07/20/2005

Figure 7-7
The Messages section of the provider dashboard.

LAB REVIEW

The Lab Review area presents lab results for the current provider that need to be reviewed. Information listed includes patient name, patient identification number, date of the lab work, and time the results were sent (see Figure 7-8).

TO DO

The To Do section of the Dashboard lists action items for the provider, including the date the item was added to the list, the priority assigned to the task (1-9), the patient's name, the patient's identification number, and the subject of the note (see Figure 7-9).

NOTE REVIEW

This area presents notes for the provider to review, and contains a patient name, date and time of the note, and the note's subject (see Figure 7-10).

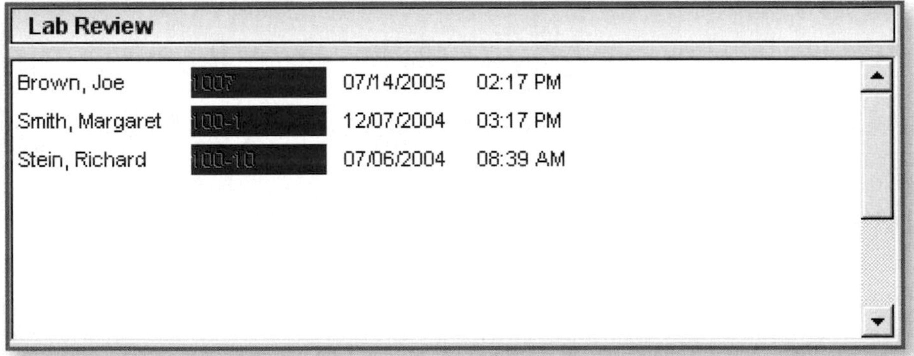

Lab Review
Brown, Joe 07/14/2005 02:17 PM
Smith, Margaret 12/07/2004 03:17 PM
Stein, Richard 07/06/2004 08:39 AM

Figure 7-8
The Lab Review section of the provider dashboard.

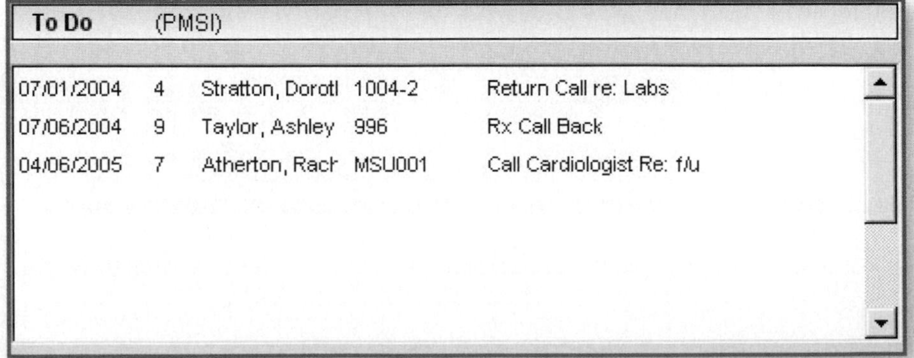

To Do (PMSI)
07/01/2004 4 Stratton, Dorotl 1004-2 Return Call re: Labs
07/06/2004 9 Taylor, Ashley 996 Rx Call Back
04/06/2005 7 Atherton, Racl MSU001 Call Cardiologist Re: f/u

Figure 7-9
The To Do section of the provider dashboard.

Note Review			
Smith, Margaret	07/26/2007	03:54 PM	SPIRO
Dexter, Rex	07/25/2007	05:23 PM	VENOUS THROMBOSIS
Stein, Richard	04/07/2005	02:50 PM	SPIRO
Smyth, Joe	04/04/2005	02:30 PM	EKG
Stratton, Dorothy	03/30/2005	11:17 AM	DID NOT KEEP APPT.
Bonheim, Gerta	12/05/2004	12:45 AM	OTOGRAM REPORT
Atherton, Rachel	07/16/2003	10:08 AM	NEUROLOGY CONSULT

Figure 7-10

The Note Review section of the provider dashboard.

Patient Registration Information

The Patient area contains demographic information about patients, such as name, address, date of birth, and so on. Clinical information, such as progress notes, lab results, and medications, is stored in the Chart section of the program.

Patients must be "registered" in Practice Partner before any clinical information can be added to their charts. This is accomplished using the Patient screen. Once a patient is registered, this screen is only used when patient information changes, such as when a patient moves or marries. Figure 7-11 displays one of the screens of the Patient function.

As with other functions in Practice Partner, the Patient screen can be accessed in two ways. The first option is to select Open Patient on the File menu. You can also click on the Patient button on the tool bar. Both methods lead to the same result: the display of the Lookup screen.

THE LOOKUP FUNCTION

Lookup a feature in Practice Partner that provides different search options for locating a patient's record.

The **Lookup** screen provides different search options, making it quick and easy to find the record you need. This screen appears in

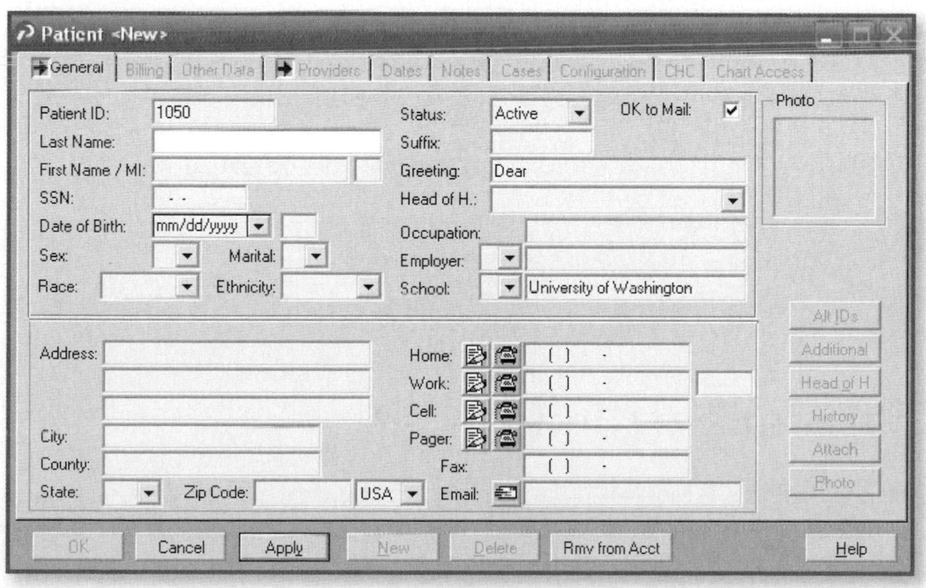

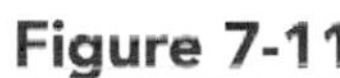

Figure 7-11

A screen from the Patient section of Practice Partner.

Figure 7-12

The Patient Lookup Screen.

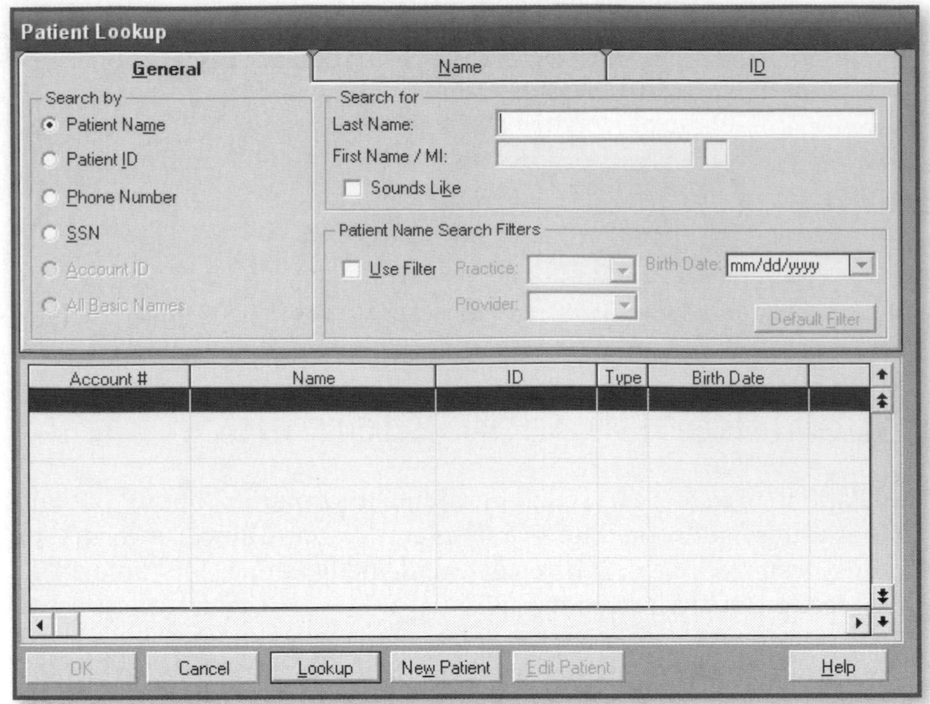

Practice Partner whenever you want to open and display more information about a patient. For example, using the three tabs on the Lookup screen, you can search for a patient by name, provider, telephone number, etc. The Patient Lookup screen is displayed in Figure 7-12.

Your Turn Exercise 1: Using the Lookup Feature

(Note: Make sure the CD is loaded in your drive before completing the exercise.)

Instructions: Double-click Tutorial 1 on the CD menu to launch the demonstration file. When the demonstration is finished, return to the CD menu.

Double-click Activity 1 on the CD menu and follow the on-screen instructions. Answer the question(s) listed below in the space provided.

1. Which patient's name appears at the top of the list of patients?

____

2. What is the patient's date of birth?

____

The Patient Chart

Most of the information in an electronic health record program such as Practice Partner is stored in the electronic version of the patient chart. In Practice Partner, the chart is organized in much the same

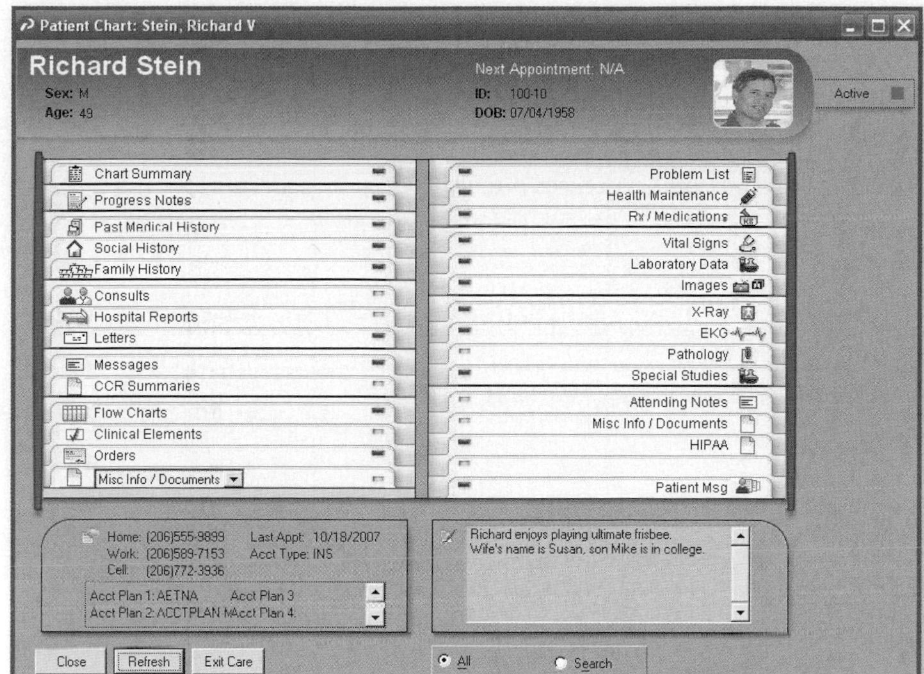

Figure 7-13

The Patient Chart screen in Practice Partner.

way as most paper-based medical records systems. As you can see in Figure 7-13, the chart contains a collection of folders designed to look like paper manila folders.

Charts can be opened by clicking the Chart icon on the toolbar, or by selecting Open Chart on the File menu.

Not all sections of the Patient Chart screen will be discussed in this chapter. The focus is providing an overall understanding of the features of an EHR system, and a closer look at some tasks often performed by allied health professionals.

Your Turn Exercise 2: Open a Patient Chart

(Note: Make sure the CD is loaded in your drive before completing the exercise.)

Instructions: Double-click Tutorial 2 on the CD menu to launch the demonstration file. When the demonstration is finished, return to the CD menu.

Double-click Activity 2 on the CD menu and follow the on-screen instructions. Answer the question(s) listed below in the space provided.

1. How many yellow folders does the patient chart contain?

____

2. What are the names of the three folders that contain information on the patient's history?

____

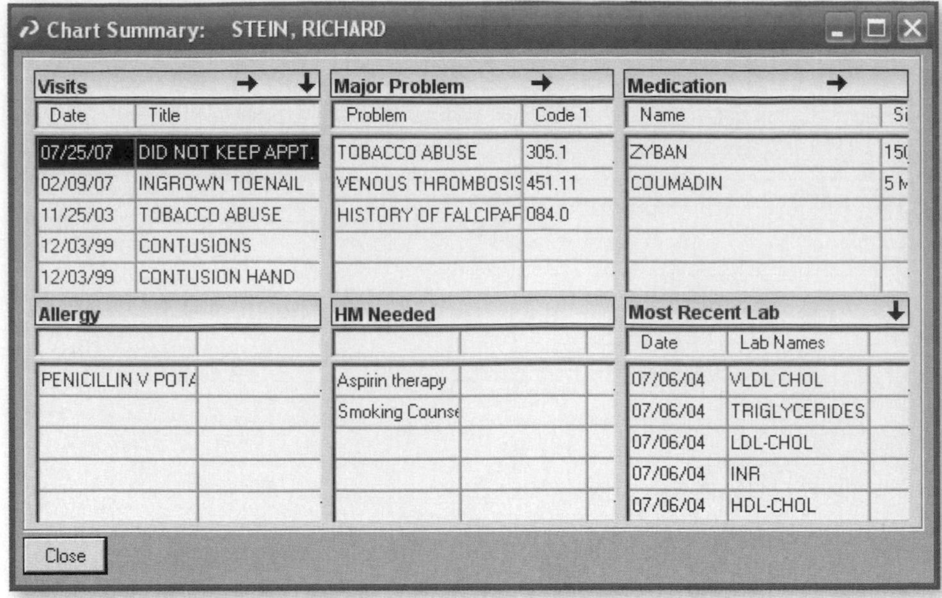

Figure 7-14
The Chart Summary screen.

CHART SUMMARY

The first folder listed is the patient chart is the Chart Summary folder, which provides an overview of a patient's most recent clinical information. The content of the Chart Summary can be changed to meet the needs of the provider. The Chart Summary that appears in Figure 7-14 shows the patient's most recent problems, along with the corresponding visit date. It also displays the patient's major problem list and current medications. Other information listed includes the patient's allergies, if any, and a summary of overdue health maintenance procedures. Clicking on any line of information takes you to that section of the patient's chart. For example, clicking on "Aspirin therapy" in the Health Maintenance section takes you to the Health Maintenance folder of the patient's chart.

The information displayed in the Chart Summary screen is for information only; it cannot be changed from this screen. For example, if you wanted to delete a medication, it would have to be done from the Rx/Medications folder, not from the Chart Summary folder. Whenever information is added or changed in any part of a patient chart, it is automatically updated in the Chart Summary screen.

PROGRESS NOTES

progress notes notes about a patient's medical condition that are made during or after a physician-patient encounter.

The Progress Notes folder stores records of a patient's visits. **Progress notes** are notes about a patient's medical condition that are made during or after a physician-patient encounter. In Practice Partner, notes can be entered in several ways. The program provides templates that can be inserted into a progress note. With a template, the user selects options such as "yes" or "no" to indicate whether the symptom or condition applies to the patient. This enables the program to easily code the information in the progress note. A user can also type information directly in to the progress note without using a template. In this approach, it is not easy for the program to code the information.

Progress notes can also be entered using by speaking. In digital dictation, the user speaks into a microphone that is connected to a computer. The program records the dictation and saves it as a digital.wav file. Then, the file is transmitted to the person responsible for transcribing the note, who can play back the dictation from any computer with Windows-based audio software, such as Windows Media Player. Finally, progress notes can be entered using voice recognition software, such as Dragon NaturallySpeaking. As a user speaks into a microphone that is attached to the computer, the software converts the spoken words into text in a word processing program. The file is then edited and saved as a progress note in Practice Partner. With voice recognition software, no transcription is required.

SOAP Format

The date and a title appear at the beginning of every progress note. Below that, the screen is set up for SOAP notes, but other formats can be used. **SOAP** is a widely used format for documenting patient encounters. SOAP stands for Subjective, Objective, Assessment, and Plan (see Table 7-2). A sample progress note is displayed in Figure 7-15.

SOAP a widely used format for documenting patient encounters, which stands for Subjective, Objective, Assessment, and Plan.

The Progress Notes section of Practice Partner provides many of the features available in word processing software. Text can be formatted by changing the font and size; bolding, italicizing, or underlining the text; centering or justifying the text; and indenting the text.

Evaluation and Management Coding

When billing for a patient visit, providers must submit a procedure code that represents the process performed to determine the best course for patient care. These CPT codes are known as **evaluation and management codes (E/M codes).** The process a physician uses to collect and analyze information about a patient's condition, and to make decisions about the best treatment, varies with each patient and illness.

evaluation and management codes (E/M codes) procedure codes that are used to represent the processes a physician performed in determining the best course of treatment for a patient.

Some conditions require little in the way of information gathering and analysis, such as a teenager with a case of poison ivy. Other cases, such as an adult with shortness of breath that seems unrelated to physical activity, are more complex, and require more time and evaluation. The

TABLE 7-2 **The SOAP Format for Progress Notes**

Subjective	Patient's complaints, presenting problems, etc.
Objective	Visible or observable findings
Assessment	Diagnostic process, impression based on subjective and objective observations
Plan	Treatment plan including tests, medications, follow-up care, etc.

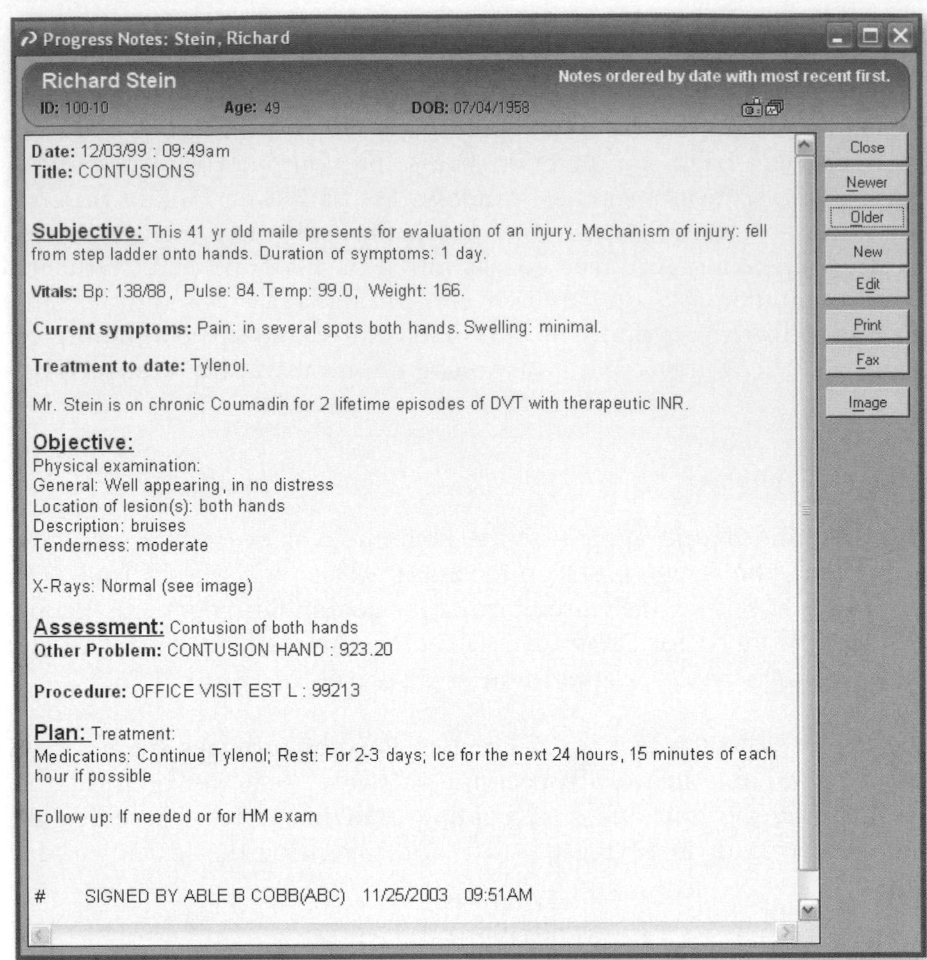
Progress Notes: Stein, Richard
Richard Stein
Notes ordered by date with most recent first.
ID: 100-10
Age: 49
DOB: 07/04/1958
Date: 12/03/99 : 09:49am
Title: CONTUSIONS
Subjective: This 41 yr old maile presents for evaluation of an injury. Mechanism of injury: fell from step ladder onto hands. Duration of symptoms: 1 day.
Vitals: Bp: 138/88, Pulse: 84. Temp: 99.0, Weight: 166.
Current symptoms: Pain: in several spots both hands. Swelling: minimal.
Treatment to date: Tylenol.
Mr. Stein is on chronic Coumadin for 2 lifetime episodes of DVT with therapeutic INR.
Objective:
Physical examination:
General: Well appearing, in no distress
Location of lesion(s): both hands
Description: bruises
Tenderness: moderate
X-Rays: Normal (see image)
Assessment: Contusion of both hands
Other Problem: CONTUSION HAND : 923.20
Procedure: OFFICE VISIT EST L : 99213
Plan: Treatment:
Medications: Continue Tylenol; Rest: For 2-3 days; Ice for the next 24 hours, 15 minutes of each hour if possible
Follow up: If needed or for HM exam
SIGNED BY ABLE B COBB(ABC) 11/25/2003 09:51AM
Close
Newer
Older
New
Edit
Print
Fax
Image

Figure 7-15

A progress note in Practice Partner.

following major elements are considered in the calculation of the E/M code for a patient's visit:

Extent of the History That Is Documented—how much information the provider collects from the patient about the chief complaint and other signs or symptoms, about all or selected body systems, and about pertinent past history, family background, and other personal factors.

Extent of the Examination That Is Documented—whether a particular body area or organ system is the focus of the examination or whether the provider conducts a multisystem examination.

Complexity of Medical Decision Making—how many possible diagnoses or treatment options were considered; how much information was considered in analyzing the patient's problem; and how serious the illness is, meaning how much risk there is for significant complications, advanced illness, or death.

Additional Factors Two additional factors are also considered: (1) how severe the patient's condition is, and (2) how much time the physician spends directly treating the patient. While not key components, these factors help in selecting the correct E/M level.

There are five different levels (level 1=simplest, level 5=most complex) of E/M codes to account for the different levels of information

TABLE 7-3 **List of E/M Codes**

CODE	DESCRIPTION
99201	Office visit level 1, new patient
99202	Office visit level 2, new patient
99203	Office visit level 3, new patient
99204	Office visit level 4, new patient
99205	Office visit level 5, new patient
99211	Office visit level 1, established patient
99212	Office visit level 2, established patient
99213	Office visit level 3, established patient
99214	Office visit level 4, established patient
99215	Office visit level 5, established patient
99241	Consultation visit level 1
99242	Consultation visit level 2
99243	Consultation visit level 3
99244	Consultation visit level 4
99245	Consultation visit level 5

gathering, analysis, and decision making by providers. Table 7-3 shows a list of the E/M codes for new patients, established patients, and consultations.

The correct code is determined by examining the provider's documentation of the patient encounter. The documentation must contain enough detail about the provider's work to support the selected E/M code.

In Practice Partner, the program analyzes information in the progress note and suggests the appropriate E/M code for the visit. Practice Partner automatically determines whether the patient is new or established, based on whether there are existing progress notes in the patient's chart. A patient is considered new if there are no existing progress notes for the patient or if the last progress note is more than 3 years old. Otherwise the patient is considered an existing patient. The codes can be modified if coding personnel determine that the program-generated entry is not accurate.

The Evaluation and Management Coding Results screen displays the E/M code that will be inserted in the progress note. Figure 7-16 on page 220

Figure 7-16

Evaluation and Management Coding Results screen.

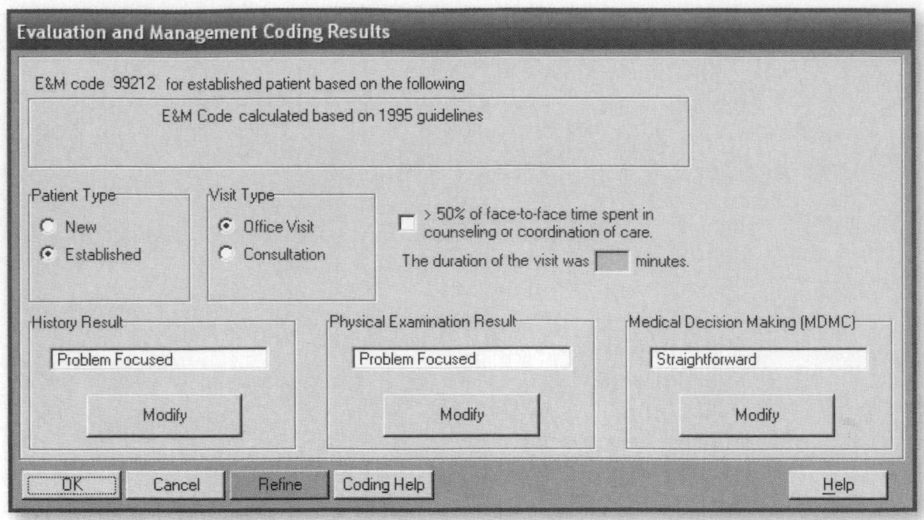

shows an Evaluation and Management Coding Results screen. If not enough information is available to calculate the code, the message "E/M code cannot be determined for new/established patient based on the following" is displayed, and additional information must be provided.

Your Turn Exercise 3: Review a Progress Note

(Note: Make sure the CD is loaded in your drive before completing the exercise.)

Instructions: Double-click Tutorial 3 on the CD menu to launch the demonstration file. When the demonstration is finished, return to the CD menu.

Double-click Activity 3 on the CD menu and follow the on-screen instructions. Answer the question(s) listed below in the space provided.

1. What is the patient's primary symptom?

   ____

2. What body systems are listed under the Review of Systems heading?

   ____

MEDICAL HISTORY

The medical history section of the patient chart includes three folders:

- **Past Medical History**—Chronic illnesses, hospitalizations, and other health information.
- **Social History**—Medically relevant information about the patient's life, such as marital status, tobacco and alcohol use, habits, work, etc.
- **Family History**—Medically relevant information about the patient's family, including major diseases and chronic conditions.

A sample of a Social History folder is illustrated in Figure 7-17.

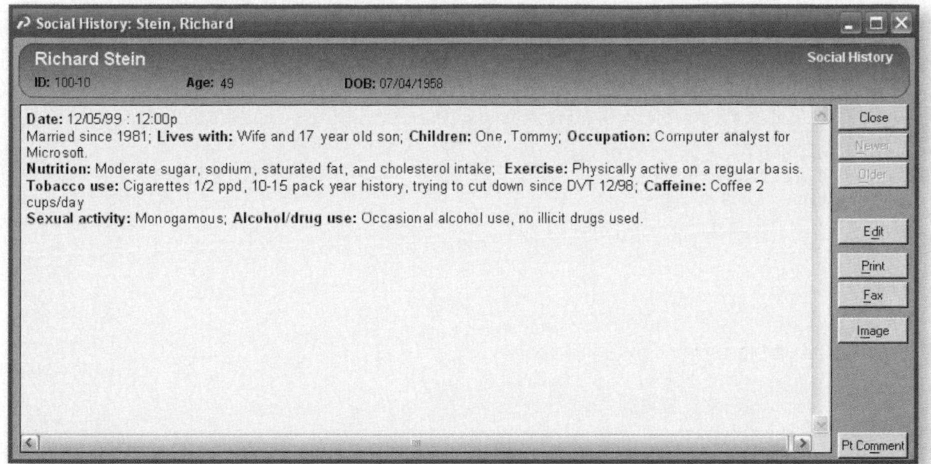

Figure 7-17

Content of a Social History folder.

Your Turn Exercise 4: Review a Patient's Family History

(Note: Make sure the CD is loaded in your drive before completing the exercise.)

Instructions: Double-click Tutorial 4 on the CD menu to launch the demonstration file. When the demonstration is finished, return to the CD menu.

Double-click Activity 4 on the CD menu and follow the on-screen instructions. Answer the question(s) listed below in the space provided.

1. What did the patient's father die of, and at what age?

____

2. Does the patient have any siblings, and if so, how many?

____

HOSPITAL REPORTS

The Hospital Reports section of the patient chart contains the physician's summaries of patient hospitalizations, and other relevant information about a patient's hospitalizations. Figure 7-18 shows a hospital report note entered by a provider.

ORDER ENTRY

The Orders folder is a computerized physician order entry (CPOE) module for Patient Records. It is used to electronically enter, review, and report on laboratory, radiology, pathology, and other diagnostic tests. Figure 7-19 shows the screen that is used to select orders for a patient.

Figure 7-18

A hospital report in a patient chart.

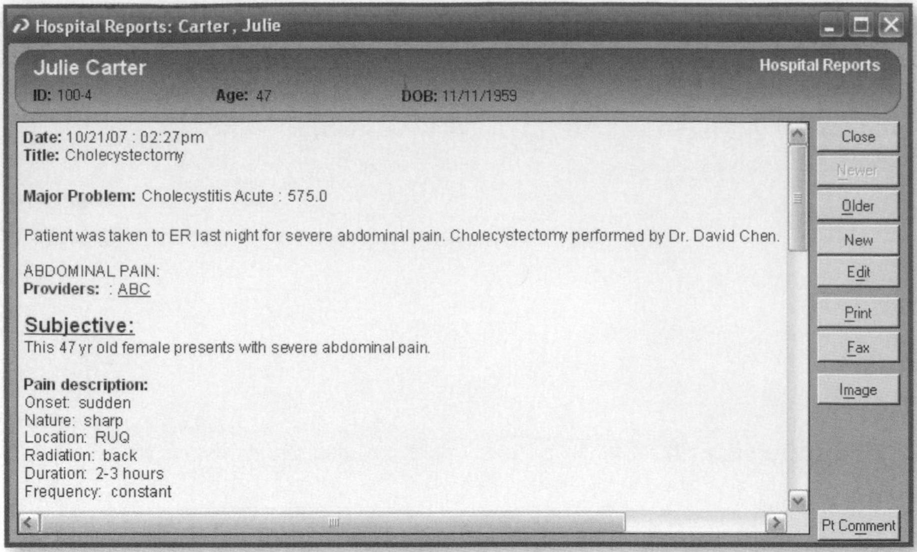

Figure 7-19

An order entry screen for a complete blood count (CBC) and a lipid panel.

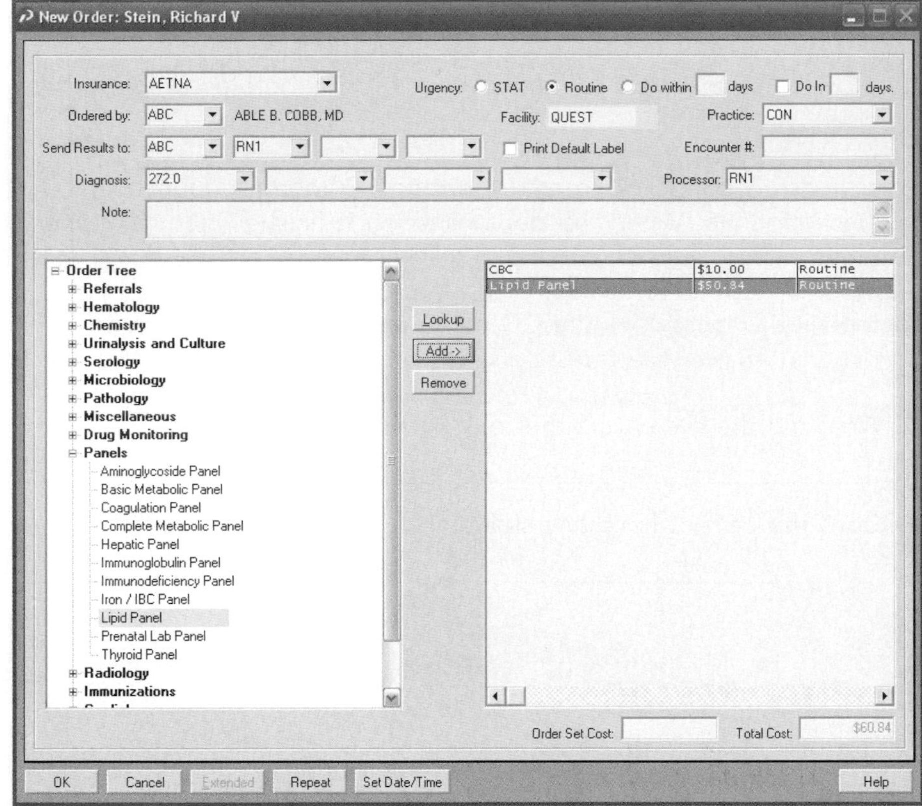

Electronic order entry is much more than a replacement for a paper order system; it provides numerous safety and cost-control benefits. For example, the software can incorporate the rules of different insurance carriers, making it easy to determine whether a test requires preauthorization and whether it is limited to specified diagnoses. The software can delay sending out these orders until approval is received. In addition, Practice Partner is capable of checking orders against information specific to the patient, such as whether the order would be inappropriate based on a patient's medications, lab tests, diagnoses, allergies etc.

Your Turn Exercise 5: Enter an Order for Blood Work

(Note: Make sure the CD is loaded in your drive before completing the exercise.)

Instructions: Double-click Tutorial 5 on the CD menu to launch the demonstration file. When the demonstration is finished, return to the CD menu.

Double-click Activity 5 on the CD menu and follow the on-screen instructions. Answer the question(s) listed below in the space provided.

1. What is the first entry under the heading Hematology?

___

2. List the individual tests that make up the order set you entered.

___

PROBLEM LIST

The Problem List section of the chart provides a longitudinal record of the problems for which the patient has sought treatment (see Figure 7-20). Problems are organized into the following six categories, each displayed on a separate tab:

- Major Problems—the patient's major medical problems
- Other Problems—problems of secondary importance, and/or chief complaints for individual patient visits
- Procedures—Significant procedures which the patient has undergone.
- Diagnoses—the diagnoses from specific patient visits.
- Risks—the conditions that put patients at risk for diseased states and other adverse health events.
- Hospitalizations—the problems for which the patient has been hospitalized.

The list screens contain a list of problems, the status of the problem, the date on which the patient first sought treatment for the problem, the date the problem last occurred, the provider, free-text notes about the problem, the problem's status, and two fields which can be used

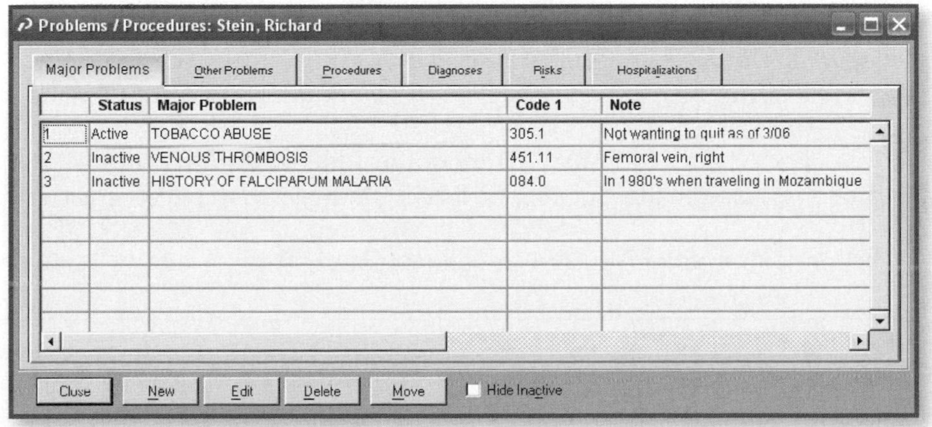

Figure 7-20

A patient's major medical problems displayed in the Problem List area of the patient chart.

Figure 7-21

A Health Maintenance Summary for a patient.

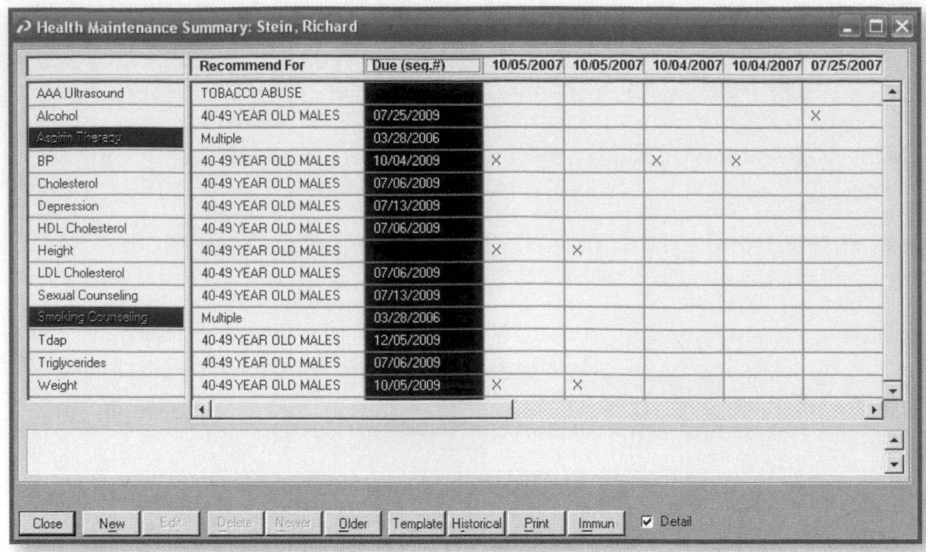

for codes from standardized terminology systems (such as ICD-9-CM or SNOMED-CT).

Health Maintenance Summary: Stein, Richard
Recommend For
Due (seq,#)
10/05/2007
10/05/2007
10/04/2007
10/04/2007
07/25/2007
AAA Ultrasound
TOBACCO ABUSE
Alcohol
40-49 YEAR OLD MALES
07/25/2009
Aspirin Therapy
Multiple
03/28/2006
BP
40-49 YEAR OLD MALES
10/04/2009
Cholesterol
40-49 YEAR OLD MALES
07/06/2009
Depression
40-49 YEAR OLD MALES
07/13/2009
HDL Cholesterol
40-49 YEAR OLD MALES
07/06/2009
Height
40-49 YEAR OLD MALES
LDL Cholesterol
40-49 YEAR OLD MALES
07/06/2009
Sexual Counseling
40-49 YEAR OLD MALES
07/13/2009
Smoking Counseling
Multiple
03/28/2006
Tdap
40-49 YEAR OLD MALES
12/05/2009
Triglycerides
40-49 YEAR OLD MALES
07/06/2009
Weight
40-49 YEAR OLD MALES
10/05/2009
Close
New
Edit
Delete
Newer
Older
Template
Historical
Print
Immun
Detail

HEALTH MAINTENANCE

The health maintenance feature is used to track a patient's periodic preventive tests and examinations. Practice Partner comes with built-in health maintenance templates, including the United States Public Health Service health guidelines. The program uses the templates to determine when patients are due for preventive exams, based on their age, gender, medications, problems, diagnoses, etc. Figure 7-21 shows the preventive health examinations and tests for a patient.

Practice Partner tracks patients' health maintenance visits and highlights exams and tests that are overdue on the Health Maintenance screen and in the Chart Summary screen. In addition, when a patient who is overdue schedules an appointment for any reason, the system alerts the scheduler to the health maintenance items.

Your Turn Exercise 6: Checking a Patient's Health Maintenance

(Note: Make sure the CD is loaded in your drive before completing the exercise.)

Instructions: Double-click Tutorial 6 on the CD menu to launch the demonstration file. When the demonstration is finished, return to the CD menu.

Double-click Activity 6 on the CD menu and follow the on-screen instructions. Answer the question(s) listed below in the space provided.

1. When is the patient due for a colonoscopy?

____

2. Is the patient overdue for any preventive screenings?

____

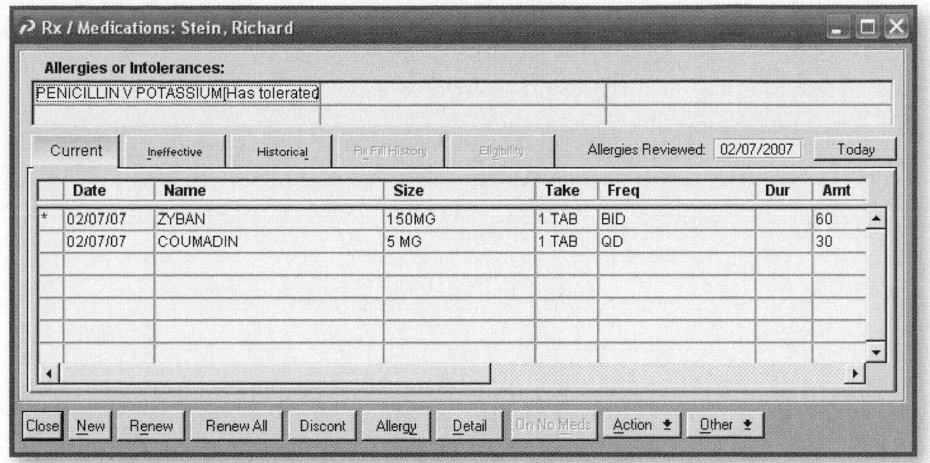

Figure 7-22

The Rx/Medication screen for a patient.

RX/MEDICATIONS

The Rx/Medications folder in a patient's chart is used to organize and maintain patients' medications. Figure 7-22 shows Rx/Medication screen for a patient, with the current medications listed. Notice that to the right of the Current tab there are tabs for tracking historical and ineffective medications. The Rx/Medications screen also stores information about patient allergies.

In some offices, a medical assistant or nurse is responsible for reviewing medication lists with patients when they come in for an office visit. The patient or a family member is asked to look at the list of current medications and indicate if anything has changed. Medications that have been added, discontinued, or changed are noted in the patient chart. A provider or licensed staff member updates the medication list after confirming the changes.

New prescriptions can be entered from the Rx/Medications folder in a chart, or by clicking the Rx/medication button on the toolbar. The screen for ordering new medications is displayed in Figure 7-23 on page 226.

To prevent unauthorized personnel from writing prescriptions, a special electronic signature (PIN) is required when writing prescriptions. The PIN serves as an electronic signature on the prescription. When a signature is required, the prescription cannot be transmitted until the PIN is provided.

Practice Partner contains a number of features to improve medication safety, including checking the new medications for interactions with current medications, patient allergies, diagnoses, and checking that the prescribed dose is appropriate.

Drug Interaction and Allergy Checking. New prescriptions are checked for interactions with the patient's current medications and allergies using an up-to-date drug database.

Drug Dosage Checking. The program checks the dosage in the prescription against standard dosages to ensure that the prescribed dose

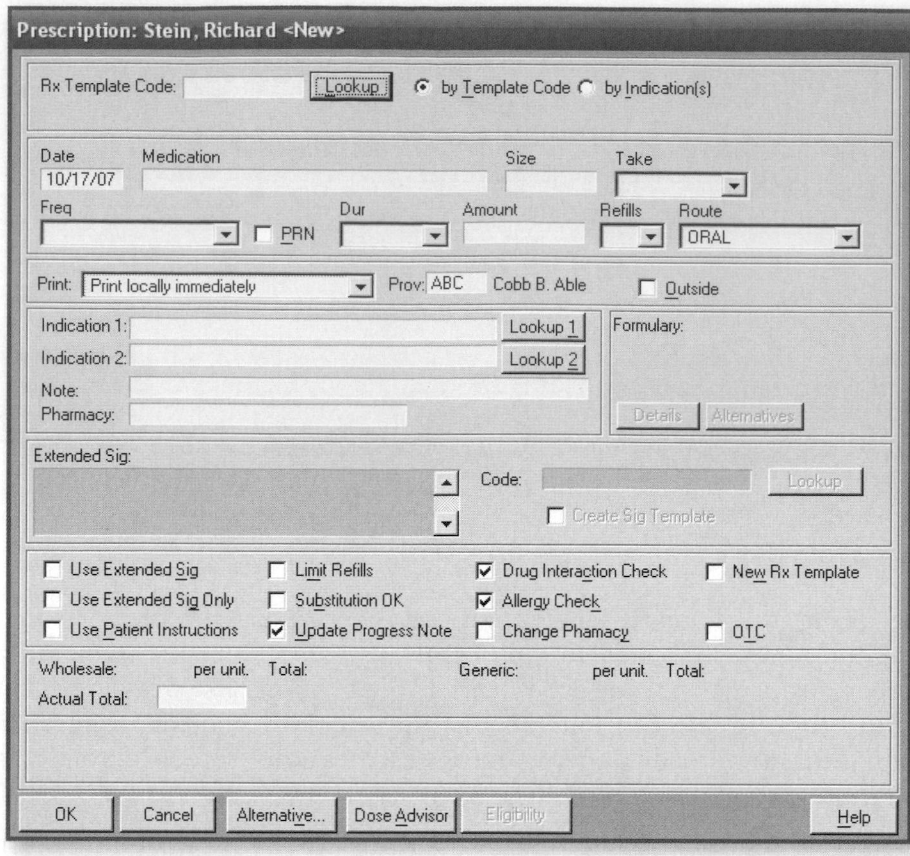

Figure 7-23

The screen used to enter a medication order.

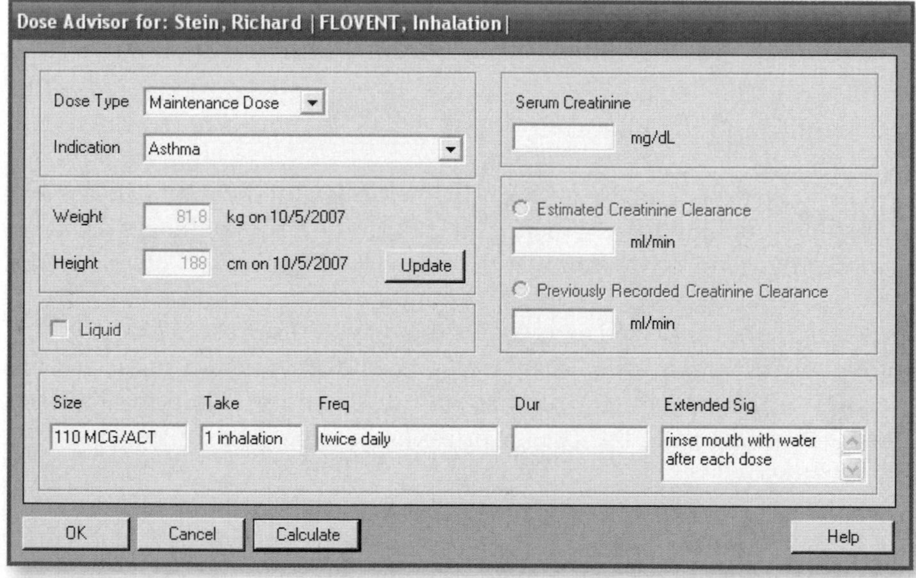

Figure 7-24

Practice Partner's built-in Dose Advisor.

is appropriate for the patient. Checks can be performed on the amount of the dose and whether it is age appropriate. If the dosage conflicts with standard dosages, a warning message is displayed. Practice Partner's built-in drug dosage advisor is shown in Figure 7-24.

Diagnosis Checking. New prescriptions are checked to make sure they are appropriate for the patient's diagnosis.

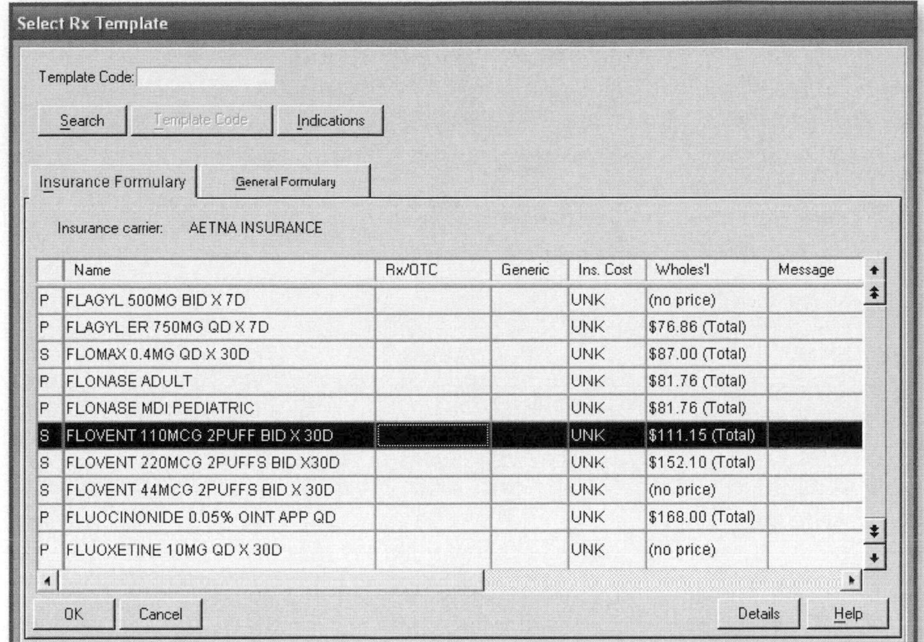

Figure 7-25

An insurance formulary list of medications.

Formulary Checking. This feature is used to look up whether a medication is covered by a patient's insurance plan, and the amount the patient is required to pay. It can also notify a provider if a medication requires pre-authorization. Figure 7-25 illustrates a formulary list for a patient's insurance plan.

Your Turn Exercise 7: Order a Medication

(Note: Make sure the CD is loaded in your drive before completing the exercise.)

Instructions: Double-click Tutorial 7 on the CD menu to launch the demonstration file. When the demonstration is finished, return to the CD menu.

Double-click Activity 7 on the CD menu and follow the on-screen instructions. Answer the question(s) listed below in the space provided.

1. What is the estimated wholesale cost of the medication?

 ____

2. Does the new medication interact with any of the patient's current medications? If so, which one?

 ____

VITAL SIGNS

Patients' vital sign measurements are entered in the Vital Signs folder in the patient chart. The screen displayed in Figure 7-26 is used to

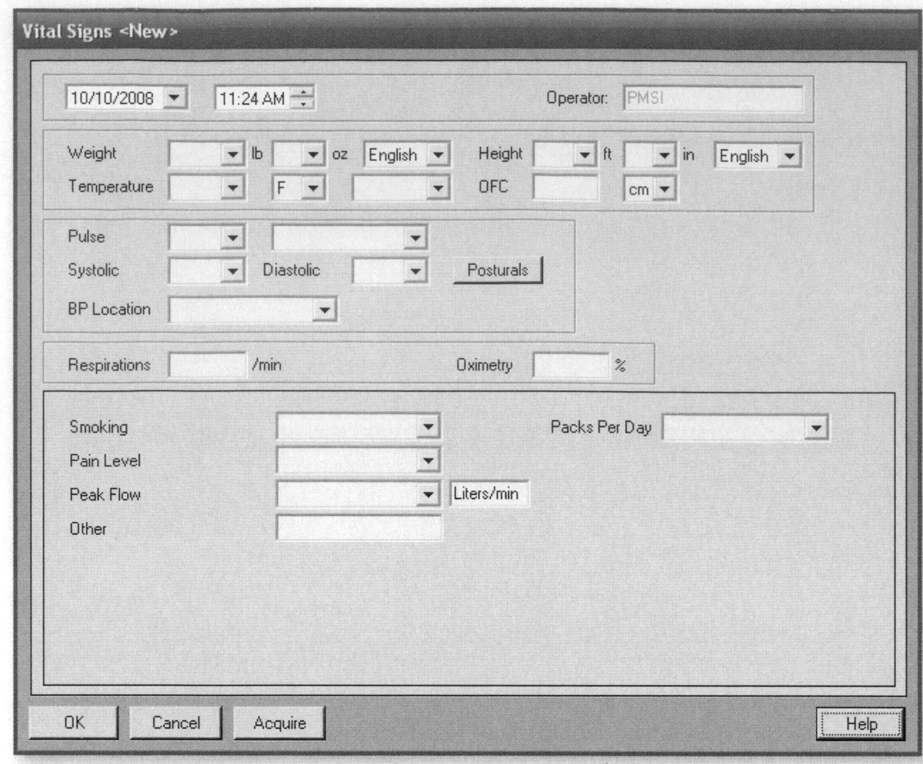

Figure 7-26

The screen for entering a patient's vital signs.

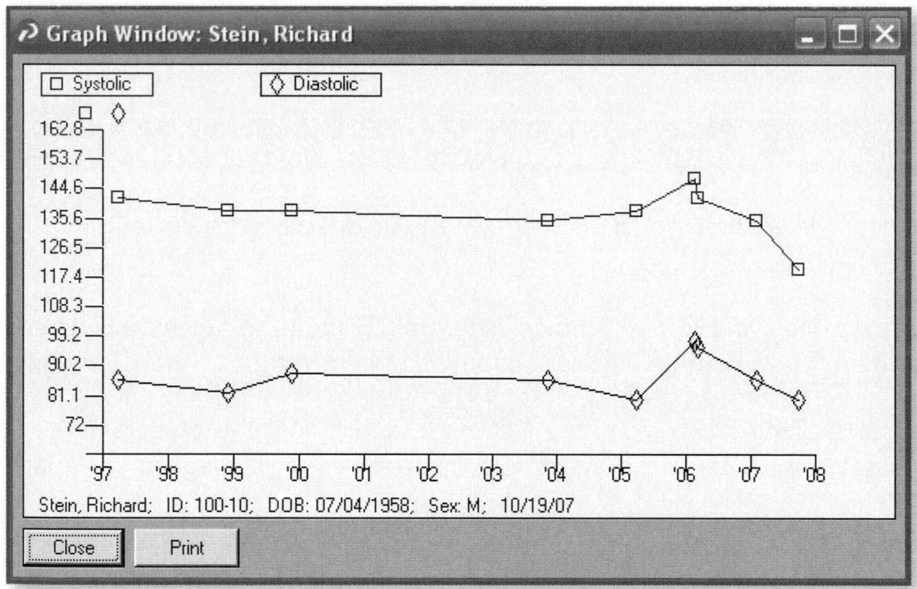

Figure 7-27

A patient's blood pressure readings viewed in a graph.

record vital signs, including: height, weight, temperature, pulse, systolic blood pressure, diastolic blood pressure, and others. Patient vital signs taken over a period of time can be viewed in a table or a graph (see Figure 7-27 for a sample graph). Abnormal values are highlighted on the Vital Sign screen. Blood pressure readings can be entered manually or imported from a digital vital sign monitor.

Your Turn Exercise 8: Enter a Patient's Blood Pressure Reading

(Note: Make sure the CD is loaded in your drive before completing the exercise.)

Instructions: Double-click Tutorial 8 on the CD menu to launch the demonstration file. When the demonstration is finished, return to the CD menu.

Double-click Activity 8 on the CD menu and follow the on-screen instructions. Answer the question(s) listed below in the space provided.

1. What was the patient's blood pressure the last time it was taken?

   ____

2. Are any of today's vital signs outside the standard range?

   ____

LABORATORY DATA

There are several ways to enter laboratory data. Information can also be entered manually, through a progress note. A special program within Practice Partners can be used to import laboratory test results provided electronically by outside laboratory facilities. An interface exists that can handle file formats provided by most outside labs.

The Laboratory Data screen can display four different types of information:

- **Most Recent Lab Data**—Provides a convenient display of the most recent information for each category of laboratory data. Figure 7-28 illustrates a sample screen with a patient's most recent lab data.

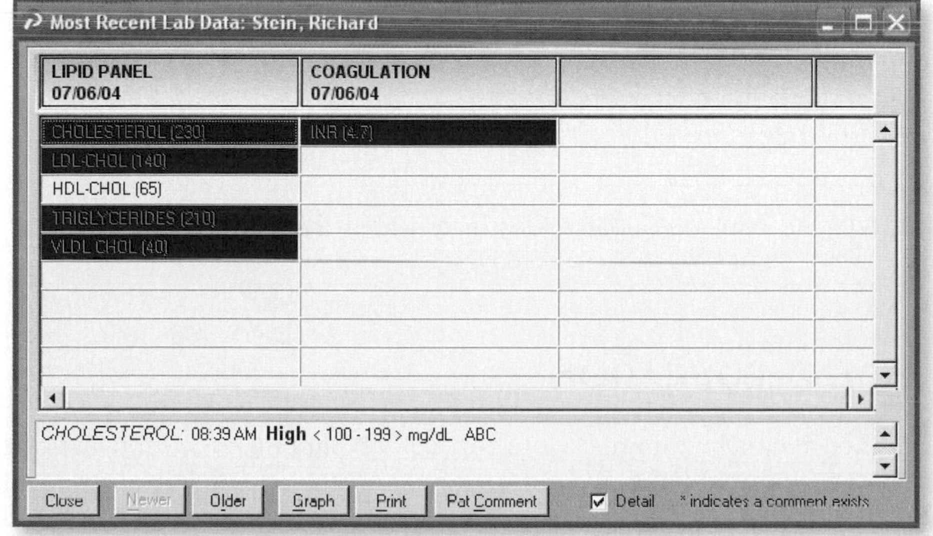

Figure 7-28
A screen showing a patient's lab data, with abnormally high readings shaded in red.

- **Lab Data Tables**—Users can add, view, edit, or graph numeric laboratory data for any laboratory data category.
- **Microbiology**—Users can view and edit text information about microbiology data.
- **Miscellaneous**—Users can view and edit text information about miscellaneous laboratory data.

Abnormal lab values are highlighted in color:

- Red indicates a result above normal range.
- Bright Green indicates a result below normal range.
- Dull Green indicates abnormal.

If test results are in the critical range, an alert is automatically sent to the patient's provider and other staff members, if appropriate. The message contains the critical value for the test performed, the date and time of the test, and the normal and critical ranges for the test.

The Laboratory Data folder also allows providers to add comments that can be viewed by the patient via the Internet. Once a comment has been created, the patient can log in to Practice Partner's Web View site and view the note.

Your Turn Exercise 9: Review a Patient's Test Results

(Note: Make sure the CD is loaded in your drive before completing the exercise.)

Instructions: Double-click Tutorial 9 on the CD menu to launch the demonstration file. When the demonstration is finished, return to the CD menu.

Double-click Activity 9 on the CD menu and follow the on-screen instructions. Answer the question(s) listed below in the space provided.

1. What was the date of the patient's last lipid panel?

   ____

2. Was the patient's Triglycerides level within the normal range?

   ____

PATIENT EDUCATION

Practice Partner contains a built-in set of patient education articles that can be printed and given to patients. A sample article is illustrated in Figure 7-29. Many of the articles are available in Spanish as well as English.

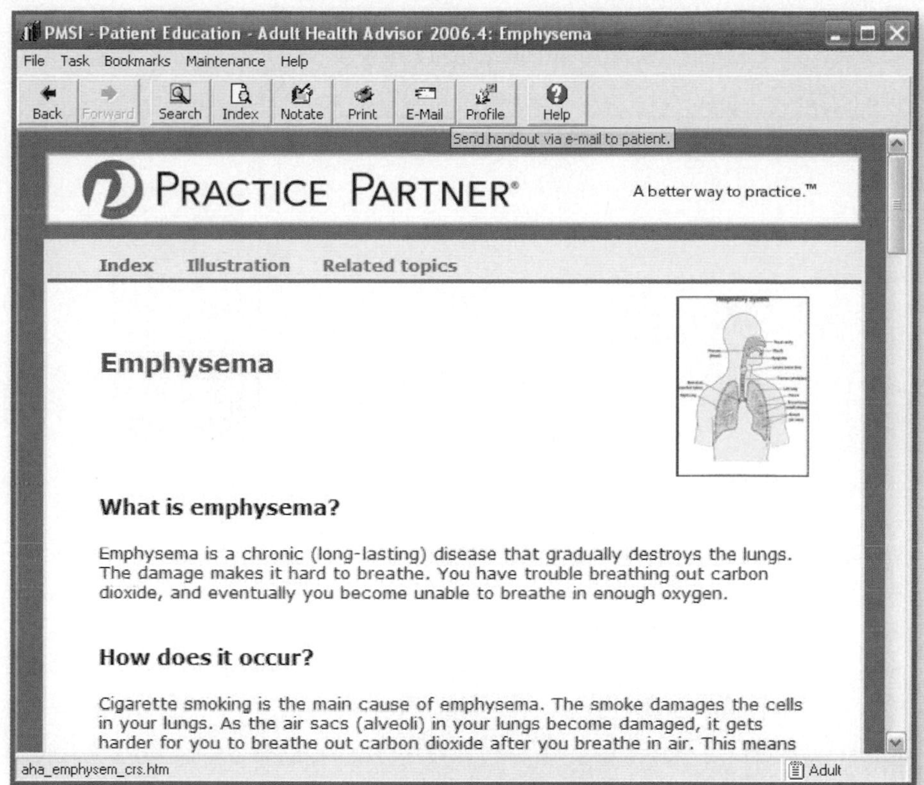

Figure 7-29
A screen from Practice Partner's built-in patient education module.

Your Turn Exercise 10: Locate a Patient Education Article

(Note: Make sure the CD is loaded in your drive before completing the exercise.)

Instructions: Double-click Tutorial 10 on the CD menu to launch the demonstration file. When the demonstration is finished, return to the CD menu.

Double-click Activity 10 on the CD menu and follow the on-screen instructions. Answer the question(s) listed below in the space provided.

1. What is the title of the article you found?

____

2. Is a Spanish version of the article available?

____

IMAGES

Images can be added to progress notes and other areas of the patient chart. Images come from several sources:

- an image may be created by the user using Practice Partner's built-in drawing capabilities

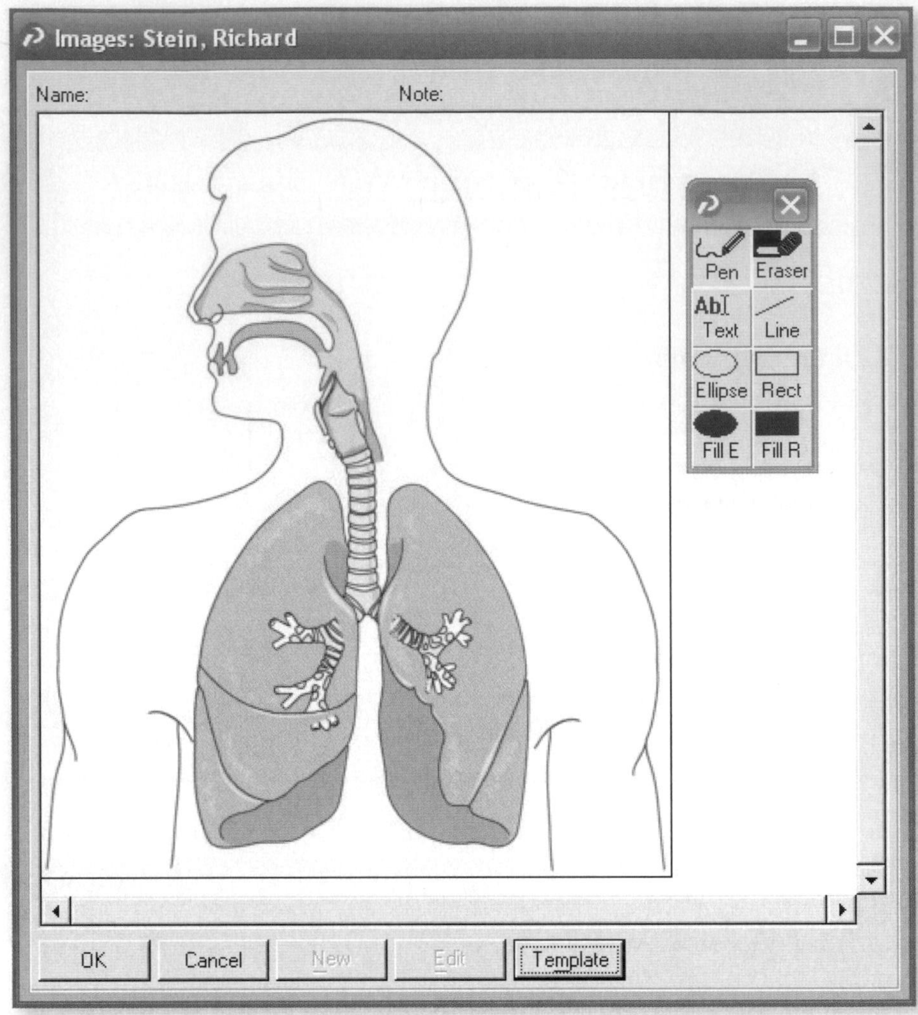

Figure 7-30
A built-in image template with a palette of tools for annotating the image.

- An image template provided by the program can be used
- An image may be scanned in using a scanner

Images can be black and white or color. Figure 7-30 shows an image from a template that can be edited using the drawing tools on right side of the screen.

HIPAA

A section of the patient chart can be used to store HIPAA-related notes and documents. For example, a practice may use this section to document when a patient was given a Notice of Privacy Practices, and whether or not the patient signed to Acknowledgment of Receipt of Privacy Practices. In addition, paper documents can be scanned and saved in this part of the patient chart. Figure 7-31 shows a signed patient consent form for a patient.

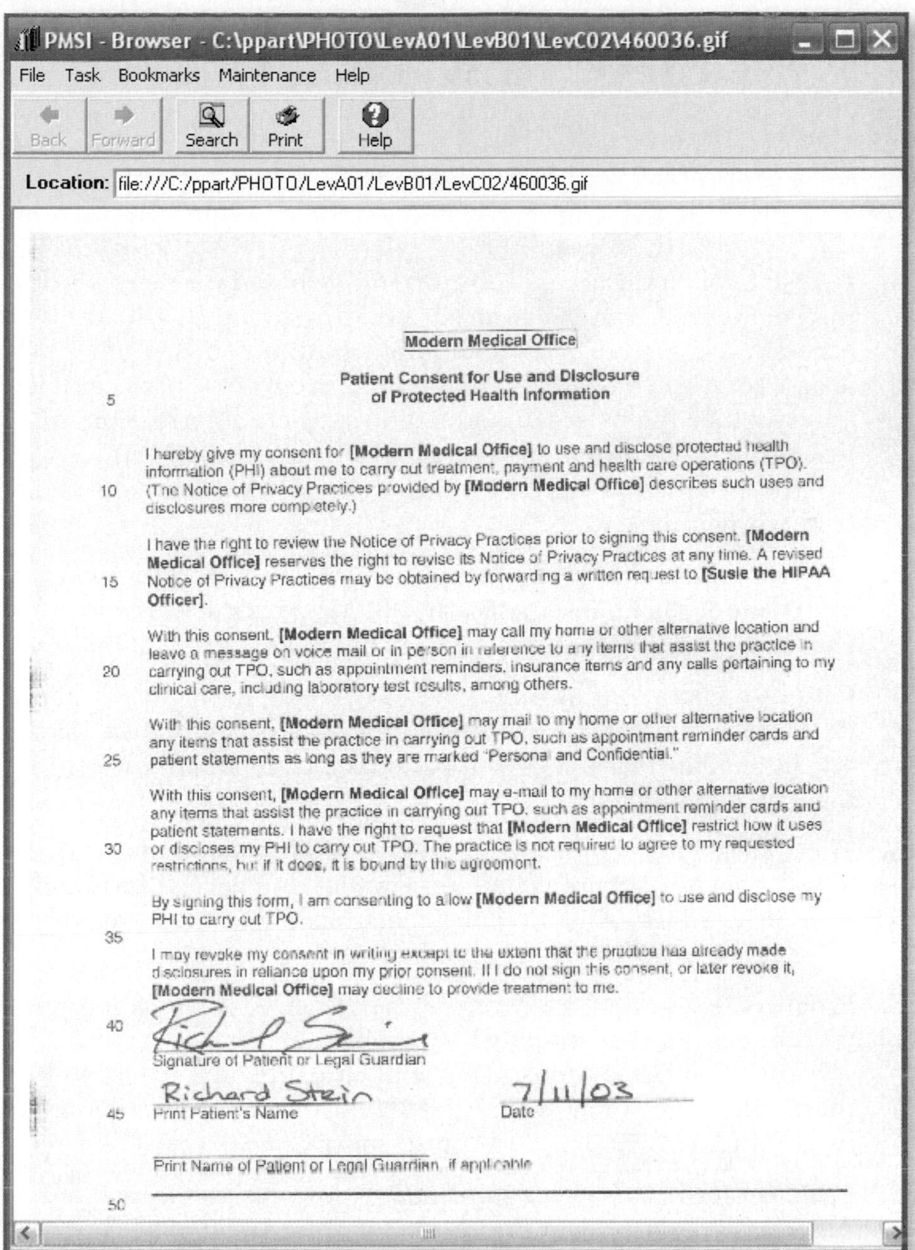

Modern Medical Office

Patient Consent for Use and Disclosure of Protected Health Information

I hereby give my consent for **[Modern Medical Office]** to use and disclose protected health information (PHI) about me to carry out treatment, payment and health care operations (TPO). (The Notice of Privacy Practices provided by **[Modern Medical Office]** describes such uses and disclosures more completely.)

I have the right to review the Notice of Privacy Practices prior to signing this consent. **[Modern Medical Office]** reserves the right to revise its Notice of Privacy Practices at any time. A revised Notice of Privacy Practices may be obtained by forwarding a written request to **[Susie the HIPAA Officer]**.

With this consent, **[Modern Medical Office]** may call my home or other alternative location and leave a message on voice mail or in person in reference to any items that assist the practice in carrying out TPO, such as appointment reminders, insurance items and any calls pertaining to my clinical care, including laboratory test results, among others.

With this consent, **[Modern Medical Office]** may mail to my home or other alternative location any items that assist the practice in carrying out TPO, such as appointment reminder cards and patient statements as long as they are marked "Personal and Confidential."

With this consent, **[Modern Medical Office]** may e-mail to my home or other alternative location any items that assist the practice in carrying out TPO, such as appointment reminder cards and patient statements. I have the right to request that **[Modern Medical Office]** restrict how it uses or discloses my PHI to carry out TPO. The practice is not required to agree to my requested restrictions, but if it does, it is bound by this agreement.

By signing this form, I am consenting to allow **[Modern Medical Office]** to use and disclose my PHI to carry out TPO.

I may revoke my consent in writing except to the extent that the practice has already made disclosures in reliance upon my prior consent. If I do not sign this consent, or later revoke it, **[Modern Medical Office]** may decline to provide treatment to me.

Signature of Patient or Legal Guardian

Richard Stein
Print Patient's Name

7/11/03
Date

Print Name of Patient or Legal Guardian, if applicable

Figure 7-31

A patient consent form that has been scanned and saved in a patient chart.

CHAPTER REVIEW

CHAPTER SUMMARY

1. Access levels limit access to information based on the type of information each user will need to view or modify. Different access levels are created for different positions in the office. The access levels define which areas of the program a user can view, and whether the user can add, edit, or delete information, or just view the information. The program can also specify whether a user has to enter a password to access certain areas of the program.
2. The dashboard offers providers a convenient view of important information, including the Schedule, Messages, Lab Review, To Do, and Note Review.
3. Patient registration information is stored in the Patient section of the program, which is accessed by clicking the Patient icon on the toolbar or by selecting New Patient or Open Patient on the File menu.
4. The Chart Summary is a section of a patient chart that provides an overview of key information in a patient chart. Information cannot be added, edited, or deleted from the Chart Summary screen; it is used for viewing only.
5. Progress notes can be entered by typing directly in the progress note screen on the computer, by the use of voice recognition software that takes a provider's spoken words and transfers them into a word processing document; by digital dictation, and by traditional dictation and transcription.
6. Practice Partner analyzes information in a progress note and suggests an appropriate E/M code for the patient visit. The coding/billing staff can override the automated entry if necessary.
7. Electronic order entry checks whether an insurance plan requires preauthorization before a test or procedure can be performed. It also checks that the order is appropriate for the patient in light of a patient's age, diagnoses, allergies, medications, etc.
8. The medication list in a patient's chart organizes the medications into three groups: current, ineffective, and historical.
9. Abnormal results in vital signs or lab tests are displayed in different colors, making it easy to notice an abnormal result. Providers are immediately sent an electronic message if results are in a critical range.
10. The HIPAA section of the patient chart can be used to document when a patient was given required forms, such as the Notice of Privacy Practices. Signed consent forms can be scanned and saved in the patient chart.

CHECK YOUR UNDERSTANDING

Part 1. Write *T* or *F* in the blank to indicate whether you think the statement is true or false.

_____ **1.** The toolbar provides quick access to commonly used features of Practice Partner.

_____ **2.** The Orders folder in the patient chart is used to order a new medication for a patient.

_____ **3.** In addition to a sign-on password, an additional password may be required for a user to access certain areas of the program.

_____ **4.** Patient registration information is located in a patient's chart in Practice Partner.

_____ **5.** The patient chart in Practice Partner contains folders that resemble paper folders in a paper-based recordkeeping system.

_____ **6.** A speech recognition program creates a word processing file out of a provider's spoken words.

_____ **7.** Evaluation and management coding (E/M) is used to indicate the patient's diagnosis to a patient's insurance plan.

_____ **8.** Physician's notes in regard to a patient's hospitalization are stored in the patient chart.

_____ **9.** Orders entered electronically can be assigned a priority status including STAT, routine, or do within a specified number of days.

_____ **10.** Practice Partner takes into account a patient's age and gender when determining health maintenance schedules for patients.

Part 2. Match each term below with its correct definition.

_____ **11.** access levels

_____ **12.** Dashboard

_____ **13.** evaluation and management codes (E/M codes)

_____ **14.** Lookup

_____ **15.** progress notes

_____ **16.** SOAP

_____ **17.** Web View

a. A feature in Practice Partner that provides different search options for locating a patient's record.

b. A security feature that limits access to information based on the type of information each user will need to view or modify.

c. A widely used format for documenting patient encounters.

d. A feature in Practice Partner that allows patients to view certain information from their chart via the Internet.

e. A feature in Practice Partner that offers providers a convenient view of important information at a glance.

f. Procedure codes that are used to represent the processes a physician performed in determining the best course of treatment for a patient.

g. Notes about a patient's medical condition that are made during or after a physician-patient encounter.

THINKING ABOUT THE ISSUES

Part 3. In the space provided, write a brief paragraph describing your thoughts on the following issues.

18. Based on your experience with Practice Partner, what do you see as the major advantages of electronic health records?

____

____

19. Would you be more interested in working for a physician's office that used an EHR, or would you prefer an office still using paper records? Explain the reasons behind your choice.

____

____

Glossary

A

access levels In electronic health records software, a security feature that limits access to information based on the type of information each user will need to view or modify.

acute care Inpatient treatment for urgent problems.

administrative safeguards Policies and procedures designed to protect electronic health information.

Administrative Simplification HIPAA Title II rules on the uniform transfer of electronic health care data and privacy protection.

adverse drug event (ADE) Side effect or complication from a medication.

adverse event Patient harm resulting from health care treatment.

ambulatory care Treatment provided without admission to a hospital, on an outpatient basis.

antivirus software Software that scans for viruses and attempts to remove them.

application service provider (ASP) An electronic health record model in which software and data are housed on an external company's servers or off-site from a medical practice, as opposed to a locally hosted model.

audit trails Records of who has accessed a computer or network and the operations performed.

authentication Confirmation of the identity of a computer user.

authorization Permission to use and disclose information for uses other than TPO.

availability Accessibility of systems for delivering, storing, and processing electronic protected health information.

B

business associates Entity that works under a contract for a covered entity and is therefore subject to the CE's HIPAA policies and procedures.

C

chronic diseases Prolonged conditions that rarely improve and often cannot be cured.

classification systems Software systems that organize related terms into categories.

clearinghouses Companies that process health information and execute electronic transactions.

clients Computers that access a server through a network.

clinical guidelines Recommended patient care based on the best available scientific evidence.

clinical templates Structured progress notes that document patient encounters in an EHR.

clinical vocabularies Common definitions of medical terms that minimize ambiguity.

computer-assisted coding Software that automates part of the coding process.

computerized physician order entry (CPOE) Application for health care providers to enter patient care orders.

confidentiality Sharing of electronic PHI among authorized individuals or organizations only.

consumer-driven health plans (CDHPs) Health plans with high deductibles, low premiums, and tax-free savings accounts.

content standards Standards that specify the functional content of an information system.

continuity of care Delivery of appropriate and consistent care over time.

covered entities (CEs) Professionals and organizations that normally provide health care and electronically transmit PHI.

Current Procedural Terminology (CPT) A coding classification system maintained by the American Medical Association for reporting medical services and procedures performed by physicians.

D

dashboard A feature in Practice Partner that offers providers a convenient view of important information at a glance.

decision-support tool Computer-based program that make the latest clinical information available.

de-identified health information Information that neither identifies nor provides a basis to identify an individual.

designated record set (DRS) Information that includes PHI and is maintained by a covered entity.

desktop computer Fixed, hardwired computer.

Digital Imaging and Communications in Medicine (DICOM) Standards that enable electronic information exchange between imaging systems.

disclosure Release of PHI to an outside provider or organization.

disease management (DM) Systematic approach to improving health care for people with chronic diseases.

E

electronic health record (EHR) A computerized lifeloqng health care record with data from all sources.

electronic medication administration records (e-MARs) Electronic log with information about a medication order that enables electronic tracking of medication administration at the bedside.

electronic medical record (EMR) A computerized record of one physician's encounters with a patient over time.

electronic prescribing A computer-based communication system that transmits prescriptions electronically.

electronic protected health information (ePHI) PHI created, received, maintained, or transmitted in electronic form.

encryption Process of converting data into an unreadable format.

evidence-based medicine Medical care based on the latest and most accurate clinical research.

evaluation and management codes (E/M codes) Procedure codes that are used to represent the processes a physician performs in determining the best course of treatment for a patient.

F

firewall A software tool that examines traffic entering and leaving a computer network.

five rights Five safety rules followed during the administration of medication—1. right patient; 2. right medication; 3. right dose; 4. right time; 5. right route of administration.

formulary Pharmaceutical products and dosages deemed the best, most economical treatments.

H

Healthcare Common Procedure Coding System (HCPCS), Level II Classification codes for products, supplies, and certain services not included in Current Procedural Terminology (CPT).

health information exchange An electronic network that securely moves clinical information among a variety of health information systems.

health information technology (HIT) Technology that is used to record, store, and manage patient health care information.

Health Insurance Portability and Accountability Act of 1996 (HIPAA) Federal legislation the main purpose of which is to protect patient's private health information, ensure continuation of health care coverage, and uncover fraud and abuse.

Health Level Seven (HL7) An electronic messaging standard used to send data from one application to another.

health plan Insurance plan that provides or pays for medical care.

HIPAA Privacy Rule HIPAA rule that provides protection for individually identifiable health information.

HIPAA Security Rule HIPAA rule that protects the confidentiality, integrity, and availability of electronic health information.

hybrid conversions Paper to electronic document conversion process that combines approaches.

I

incremental conversion Gradual paper to electronic document conversion process.

Institute of Electrical and Electronics Engineers 1073 (IEEE1073) A standard developed to provide communication among medical devices at a patient's bedside.

integrity Authenticity, completeness, and reliability of electronic PHI.

International Classification of Diseases, Ninth Revision, Clinical Modification Internationally accepted rules for selecting and sequencing diagnosis codes in both the inpatient and the outpatient environments; standard that categorize diseases.

interoperable Able to exchange electronic information and use the information in a meaningful way.

intrusion detection system (IDS) A software tool that provides surveillance of a computer network.

L

laptop computer Fully functioning portable computer.

locally hosted EHR model in which hardware and software are housed onsite in a medical practice.

Logical Observation Identifiers Names and Codes (LOINC) Universal terms and codes for electronic exchange of laboratory results and clinical observations.

Lookup A feature in Practice Partner that provides different search options for locating a patient's record.

M

medical error Adverse medical event that could have been prevented, such as an incorrectly filled prescription, a surgical mistake, and so on.

medical record Chronological record generated during a patient's treatment.

Medicare Part D Voluntary prescription drug benefit plan under Medicare.

Medicare Prescription Drug, Improvement, and Modernization Act of 2003 (MMA) Federal legislation creating a prescription drug benefit plan that encourages electronic prescribing.

medication administration record (MAR) Log with information about a medication order.

medication reconciliation Process of obtaining and updating an accurate list of all of a patient's medications.

messaging standards Electronic standards that allows data transfer to an electronic health record system.

minimum necessary standard Required safeguards to protect PHI from being accidentally released.

N

National Council for Prescription Drug Program (NCPDP) Code sets or standards for exchanging prescription information in the retail pharmacy environment.

Nationwide Health Information Network (NHIN) Nationwide computer network facilitating the exchange of health care information.

network Equipment that enables computers to exchange information electronically.

networked personal health record PHR that transfers information to and from multiple health information systems.

Notice of Privacy Practices (NPP) Document describing practices regarding use and disclosure of PHI.

O

order sets Predefined groupings of standard orders for a condition, disease, or procedure.

Office of the National Coordinator for Health Information Technology (ONC) The organization that serves as the recognized certification authority for electronic health records (EHR) and their networks.

outsourcing The process of an organization contracting with an outside company for completion of all or part of a job.

P

passwords Codes for gaining access to information on a computer or network.

patient portal Website that allows patients to interact with provider or facility.

pay for performance (P4P) The use of financial incentives to improve health care quality and efficiency.

personal digital assistants (PDA) Handheld computer devices used to search for information, write prescriptions, and handle e-mail.

personal health record (PHR) An individual's comprehensive record of health information.

physical safeguards Mechanisms to protect electronic systems, equipment, and data.

picture archiving and communication system (PACS) Electronic image management system.

point-of-care Setting in which a physician makes decisions about a patient's illness and treatment.

progress notes Notes about a patient's medical condition that are made during or after a physician-patient encounter.

protected health information (PHI) Individually identifiable health information transmitted or maintained by electronic media.

providers People or organizations that furnish, bill, or are paid for health care in the normal course of business.

R

regional health information organization (RHIO) A group of health care organizations that share information.

role-based authorization A tool that limits access to patient information based on the user's organizational role.

S

scanning Method for electronically capturing text and images from paper documents.

server Powerful computer that houses software applications and data.

smart phones handheld devices similar to personal digital assistants (PDAs) that are also cell phones.

SOAP A widely used format for documenting patient encounters. It stands for Subjective, Objective, Assessment, and Plan.

standards A set of commonly agreed-on specifications.

Systematized Nomenclature of Medicine Clinical Terms (SNOMED-CT) Internationally recognized comprehensive clinical vocabulary of all terms used in medicine.

T

tablet computer Portable computer with built-in handwriting and voice recognition software.

technical safeguards Automated processes to protect and control access to data.

tethered Information system attached to another information system.

total conversion Paper to electronic document conversion method by an external company.

transition points Times when patients move from one setting to another.

treatment, payment, and operations (TPO) Conditions under which PHI can be released without patient consent.

U

Unified Medical Language System (UMLS) Major thesaurus database of medical terms.

untethered Information system not connected to another information system.

V

voice recognition Method of entering information via a microphone connected to a computer.

W

Web View A feature in Practice Partner that allows patients to view certain information from their chart via the Internet.

wired network Network in which computers are connected via Ethernet cable.

wireless network Network in which computers access servers without cables.

workstations Hardware devices used to access the electronic health record and other software.

Index

A

B

C

D

I

J

L

M

N

O

P

Q

R

S

T

U

V

W